Praise for
Eat To Beat Disease

"Molecular medicine has finally been joined by molecular nutrition! Human health care can now be truly transformed by integration of the two most powerful determinants of health and disease: the medicine we take and the food we eat. As a physician-scientist, Dr. Li has a distinguished career of contributing to stunning progress in our elucidation of the genetic, molecular, and cellular mechanisms determining our health and disease. This knowledge has enabled researchers and clinicians to unleash powerful, targeted medicines to prevent, eliminate, or control disease and ushered in the modern era of 'precision medicine.' Medical science has long recognized that in addition to pharmaceuticals, diet also played a significant part in modulating our heath but we did not understand how and why. In EAT TO BEAT DISEASE, Dr. Li presents a scientifically rigorous and comprehensive exposition of the molecular nutrients contained in our diets and their relationship to prevention of disease and restoration of health, thereby providing for 'precision molecular nutrition.' It's a truly historic compendium.

"This book is extraordinary in the depth of its providing an elucidation of the unique micronutrient of an extensive variety of food and its specific interaction with cells and tissues of the body. For decades, we captured a primitive understanding of 'healthy foods' and applied maxims like 'An apple a day keeps the doctor away.' In this book, Dr. Li not only tells us why an apple has health benefits but even more importantly tells us which variety of apple is best!

"This book is brilliantly written in a style that first explains the key mechanisms the body employs to maintain the health and integrity of our bodies when confronted by invading infections, a breakdown in genetic controls that can lead to cancer or the simple process of aging. Those principal mechanisms are angiogenesis, regeneration, the microbiome, DNA protection and immunity. Dr. Li then offers us detailed exposition of the molecular nutrients most effective in support of these mechanisms and the specific foods in which they are found in sufficient abundance. In effect this creates a precision dietary prescription, and the great pleasure and perhaps surprise is that the formulary is filled with things we like to eat!

"Throughout the extensive exposition of the interaction between the micronutrients of various foods on the functions of the body, Dr. Li provides ample documentation with data derived from scientific experiments and well-conducted clinical research trials, but beyond sound nutritional prescriptions the latter portion of the book becomes quite practical with his presentation of his 5 x 5 x 5 plan that matches the condition to be addressed with the foods you like the best and the practical way to incorporate this kind of healthy eating into your life style.

"In summary, EAT TO BEAT DISEASE is the best guide to using food to enhance heath that I am aware of for both professionals and the public. It is scientific, it is comprehensive, it links logic with prescription, and most important it is practical! It will not only transform the way you eat—it will transform health care."

—*Andrew C. von Eschenbach, MD, president, Samaritan Health Initiatives, former director of the National Cancer Institute, former commissioner of the Food and Drug Administration*

"A groundbreaking physician shares how we can use food to hack our natural defense systems and hard-wire ourselves for health."

—*Mehmet Oz, MD, host,* The Dr. Oz Show

"EAT TO BEAT DISEASE is a trailblazing book. Author, world-renowned physician, and medical scientist Dr. William Li explains how we have the power to help control our own health destiny by making decisions that help the body heal itself. Dr. Li describes how more than two hundred foods amplify our body's defenses, which can result in beneficial health outcomes. EAT TO BEAT DISEASE is a must read—I strongly endorse it."

—*Dean Ornish, MD, founder and president, Preventive Medicine Research Institute, clinical professor of medicine, University of California, San Francisco, author,* UnDo It!

"With EAT TO BEAT DISEASE, Dr. William Li tells us why your fork is your most powerful tool for health. This book reveals powerful new discoveries about how the body naturally resists disease through specific health defense systems. Dr. Li takes us on an epic journey, accompanied by scientific evidence, that shows us what we eat can activate these defenses. Unlike so many books that turn people away from the foods they enjoy, EAT TO BEAT DISEASE shows us how the foods we love actually support our well-being and vitality. I recommend that every health seeker should read this new classic and tell their friends and family all about it."

—*Mark Hyman, MD, director, Cleveland Clinic Center for Functional Medicine, and #1* New York Times *bestselling author,* Food: What the Heck Should I Eat?

"An ode to one of life's greatest pleasures and a convincing case for a healthy appetite. This book will entertain, educate, devour, and then empower you. Dr. William Li, pioneer of angiogenesis-based therapy, teaches us that we have radically underestimated our own power to transform and restore our health. And we can do so by making choices and applying our creativity to something we do every day: eat! Dr. Li reminds us that we are not passive actors in the play of diseases attacking our health, or reliant on elitist treatment or expensive medical innovations, but that we as individuals have agency to strengthen all of our five defense systems through our diet. This is a fascinating story of the power of food, a reflection on what we mean by health, and practical tool with the 5 x 5 x 5 framework to make sure we are around to enjoy life's pleasures for as long as possible."

—*Bono*

"Finally! A book that tells us the truth about what we can eat to be healthy, based on real science, from a true expert. EAT TO BEAT DISEASE will completely change the way you think about your body and the choices you make when you grocery shop, cook for your family, or dine out. Read this book from cover to cover if you want to be on top of your game for health, beauty, and fitness, from the inside out. When it comes to food and health, I'm so happy to have Dr. Li in my camp!"

—*Cindy Crawford*

"As the former secretary of agriculture, one of my tasks was to promote good health and nutrition by giving the public modern, scientifically based information on the foods they eat. Dr. Li's transformational book is one of the best narratives I have read on the scientific relationship between healthy food, nutrition, and the fight against disease. I recommend it highly."

—Dan Glickman, former US secretary of agriculture, vice president, Aspen Institute, former chairman, Motion Picture Association of America

"The time has come for 'health' to be properly defined and for us to understand clearly how food impacts health. EAT TO BEAT DISEASE delivers on this vision in a big way—and with real science to back it up. Dr. Li's highly enjoyable and informative book spreads the word that achieving great health is within reach for all of us, using the very foods that we love. EAT TO BEAT DISEASE will excite, amaze, and inspire us all to eat healthy and defeat disease. And remember—you are in control of your own destiny."

—Louis J. Ignarro, 1998 Nobel laureate in medicine

"Among the many diet and health books of recent years, this book should top the list. Dr. William Li, an experienced internal medicine physician, also has an outstanding professional reputation in medical research. He knows science and how to present it to the public. His facts can only lead to a more fulfilling way to think about health for all of us."

—T. Colin Campbell, PhD, Cornell University, author, The China Study and Whole

" 'We are what we eat' goes the old cliché, but it would be more accurate to say that 'we are what we extract from our food.' What if food is more than energy and more than nutrition, but a form of medicine? In his groundbreaking book EAT TO BEAT DISEASE, Dr. William Li brings the discipline of clinical medical research to bear on a new analysis of the relationship between food and health. Piecing together the puzzle of the how the food we consume impacts on how the human body functions and how it protects itself from disease, Dr. Li puts forward a new paradigm to explain this relationship: 'Food as Medicine.' EAT TO BEAT DISEASE heralds a revolution in thinking about how the food we eat dictates our health."

—*The Edge, U2, director, the Angiogenesis Foundation*

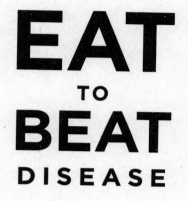

EAT
TO
BEAT
DISEASE

EAT

TO

BEAT

DISEASE

THE NEW SCIENCE OF HOW YOUR BODY CAN HEAL ITSELF

WILLIAM W. LI, MD

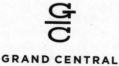

GRAND CENTRAL
PUBLISHING

New York   Boston

Grand Central Publishing
Hachette Book Group
1290 Avenue of the Americas, New York, NY 10104
grandcentralpublishing.com
twitter.com/grandcentralpub

First edition: March 2019

Grand Central Publishing is a division of Hachette Book Group, Inc. The Grand Central Publishing name and logo is a trademark of Hachette Book Group, Inc.

The publisher is not responsible for websites (or their content) that are not owned by the publisher.

The Hachette Speakers Bureau provides a wide range of authors for speaking events. To find out more, go to www.hachettespeakersbureau.com or call (866) 376-6591.

Library of Congress Cataloging-in-Publication Data

Names: Li, William W., author.
Title: Eat to beat disease : the new science of how the body can heal itself / William W. Li, MD.
Description: First edition. | New York : Grand Central Publishing, 2019. | Includes bibliographical references and index.
Identifiers: LCCN 2018041407| ISBN 9781538714621 (hardcover) | ISBN 9781538715499 (large print) | ISBN 9781549117183 (audio download) | ISBN 9781549117190 (audio book) | ISBN 9781538714638 (ebook)
Subjects: LCSH: Nutritionally induced diseases—Prevention. | Nutrition.
Classification: LCC RC622 .L5 2019 | DDC 616.3/9—dc23
LC record available at https://lccn.loc.gov/2018041407

ISBNs: 978-1-5387-1462-1 (hardcover), 978-1-5387-1463-8 (ebook), 978-1-5387-1549-9 (large print)

Printed in the United States of America

LSC-C

10 9 8 7 6 5 4 3 2 1

This book is dedicated to my family, my mentors, and the patients who have inspired me to pull the future of health closer to those who need help today.

Contents

Contents

PART III
PLAN, CHOOSE, AND ACT:
Putting Food to Work

Introduction

We are truly at a turning point in the fight against disease. Each of us has an enormous opportunity to take charge of our lives using food to transform our health. You can make decisions about what to eat and drink based on scientific evidence gleaned from testing foods with the same systems and methods that have been used to discover and develop drugs. The data generated when we study food like medicine clearly show that food can influence our health in specific and beneficial ways.

First, a bit about myself. I'm a medical doctor, an internal medicine specialist, and a research scientist. In college, I studied biochemistry (now called molecular and cellular biology), and I spent the first half of my career immersed in the world of biotechnology. For the past twenty-five years, I've led the Angiogenesis Foundation, a nonprofit organization that I cofounded in 1994 with a unique mission: to improve global health by focusing on a "common denominator" shared by many diseases: angiogenesis, the process our bodies use to grow new blood vessels.

As a scientist, finding common denominators of disease has long been my interest and passion. Most medical research is dedicated to exploring the individuality of disease, searching for what makes each disease distinct from every other as the path toward finding cures. My approach has been the complete opposite. By looking for common threads shared by many diseases and asking if those threads might lead to new treatments, I've found it is possible to achieve breakthroughs for not only one disease, but many diseases at the same time.

Early in my career, I chose to study angiogenesis. Blood vessels are essential for health because they bring oxygen and nutrients to every cell in our body. My mentor, Judah Folkman, was a brilliant surgeon-scientist at Harvard who first came up with the idea that targeting abnormal blood vessels feeding cancer could be an entirely new way to treat the disease. Angiogenesis gone awry is not just a problem in cancer, but also a common denominator in more than seventy different diseases, including the world's other top killers: heart disease, stroke, diabetes, Alzheimer's disease, obesity, and more. In 1993, I had an inspiration: what if controlling blood vessel development could be a singular approach to address all of these serious diseases?

Over the past twenty-five years, along with a long roster of amazing colleagues and supporters, this work is precisely what the Angiogenesis Foundation has been doing. We have coordinated research and advocated for new treatments taking this common-denominator approach. We've worked with more than three hundred of the brightest scientists and clinicians from North America, Europe, Asia, Australia, and Latin America; more than one hundred innovative companies in biotechnology, medical devices, and diagnostic and imaging technologies; and visionary leaders from the National Institutes of Health, the Food and Drug Administration, and major medical societies from around the world.

We have been very successful. By coordinating collective efforts, a new field of medicine called angiogenesis-based therapy has been created. Some of the innovative treatments stop blood vessels from growing in diseased tissues, such as in cancer or in blinding diseases like neovascular age-related macular degeneration and diabetic retinopathy. Other treatments that have changed medical practice spark new blood vessels to heal vital tissues, such as in diabetic and venous leg ulcers. Today, there are more than thirty-two FDA-approved drugs, medical devices, and tissue products based on angiogenesis.

These treatments, once just glimmers of ideas, have become

important new standards of care in oncology, ophthalmology, and wound care, helping patients live longer and better lives. We've even worked with veterinarians and developed new treatments that have helped save the lives of pet dogs, dolphins, reef fish, raptors, a rhinoceros, and even a polar bear. I'm proud to have been part of these advances, and given the more than 1,500 ongoing clinical trials in angiogenesis, there are certainly more to come.

*   *   *

But, despite all of the success, the sobering fact is that the rates of new disease are skyrocketing. The biggest health threats for people worldwide are the noncommunicable diseases, which include cancer, heart disease, stroke, diabetes, obesity, and neurodegenerative conditions. We each know someone in our lives who has suffered from or succumbed to one of these diseases. According to the World Health Organization, cardiovascular disease killed 17.7 million people in 2015; cancer, 8.8 million; and diabetes, 1.8 million.

Even with remarkable treatment breakthroughs and FDA approvals, treatment of disease alone is not a sustainable solution for noncommunicable diseases, in part because of the stratospheric cost of new drugs. It can cost more than $2 billion to develop a single new biotechnology drug. The expense of using some of the latest drugs after they've received FDA approval is staggering, ranging in some cases from $200,000 per year to more than $900,000 per year. Since few can afford these price tags, the most advanced treatments don't get to everyone who needs them, while the growing and aging population keeps getting sicker.

Drug treatments alone cannot keep us healthy. The question then becomes, how can we do a better job at preventing disease, before we have to cure it? One modern answer: food. Every doctor knows that poor diet is linked to preventable disease, and food is becoming a topic of ever greater importance in the medical community. Some avant-garde medical schools have even added culinary classes to their curriculum. Food is easily accessible and dietary interventions do not rely on expensive pharmaceutical treatments.

Not many doctors know how to discuss a healthy diet with their patients. This is through no fault of the individual doctors, but rather a side effect of how little nutrition education they receive. According to David Eisenberg, a professor at the Harvard T.H. Chan School of Public Health, only one in five medical schools in the United States requires medical students to take a nutrition course. On average, medical schools offer a mere nineteen hours of coursework in nutrition, and there are few postgraduate continuing education classes on nutrition for doctors already in practice.

Compounding this problem is that the different branches of science that study food and health have traditionally worked independently, as separate fields. Food technologists study chemical and physical properties of edible substances. Life science researchers study living organisms, including humans. Epidemiologists study real-world populations. Each field contributes important perspectives and ideas, but they rarely converge to answer practical questions about which foods and beverages might be responsible for a health benefit in the human body, in what amounts, and what is within a specific food that causes the effect.

What this all means for you is that your doctor, while armed with deep skills and invaluable knowledge about medicine, may not be fluent in advising you on what to eat for your health to beat disease.

I experienced the ramifications of this firsthand in my own practice of medicine. When I was taking care of older patients at a hospital for veterans, I often wondered what had happened to their bodies. These patients, mostly men, were once specimens of perfect fitness, trained as warriors to fight for their country. By the time I saw them decades later, they were often overweight, if not downright obese, diabetic, ravaged by terrible heart and lung diseases and, often, cancer.

As their doctor, I would give them the news of a terrible diagnosis. They would ask me: *How bad is it? What is the treatment? How long do I have to live?* I would give them my best estimate. Then, as they were leaving my office, they would almost invariably turn and ask me: "Hey doc, what can I eat so that I can help myself?"

I didn't have an answer to that question—because I hadn't been educated or trained to deal with it. That struck me as wrong, and thus I began the journey to seek the answers that led me to write this book.

*   *   *

In order to understand the benefits of food for health, we need to first understand the definition of *health*. To most people, health is the absence of disease. But it is much more than that. In fact, the definition of health needs a major upgrade.

What is clear is that our health is an active state, protected by a series of remarkable defense systems in the body that are firing on all cylinders, from birth to our last day alive, keeping our cells and organs functioning smoothly. These health defense systems are hardwired in our body to protect us. Some are so powerful they can even reverse diseases like cancer. And while they function as separate systems of defense, they also support and interact with one another. These defense systems are the common denominators of health. By recalibrating our approach to disease prevention and focusing on these common denominators, we can take a unified approach to intercepting diseases before they set in. This can be as powerful as finding common denominators to treat disease, as we did two decades ago.

Five defense systems form key pillars to your health. Each of the systems is influenced by diet. When you know what to eat to support each health defense, you know how to use your diet to maintain health and beat disease.

When I teach other doctors and students about diet and health, I use the analogy that the body is like a medieval fortress, protected not only by its stone walls, but by a host of other clever built-in defenses. Indeed, in castles, some of these defenses, such as the talus, the trou de loup, and murder hole, were not even apparent until the enemy tried to invade. Think of your health defense systems as the hidden defenses of the body fortress. These defenses heal the body from within, so it is now possible to systematically examine how to shore up your health.

The five defense systems are angiogenesis, regeneration, microbiome, DNA protection, and immunity.

Angiogenesis

Sixty thousand miles of blood vessels course throughout our bodies and bring oxygen and nutrients to all of our cells and organs. Angiogenesis is the process by which these blood vessels are formed. Foods like soy, green tea, coffee, tomatoes, red wine, beer, and even hard cheese can influence the angiogenesis defense system.

Regeneration

Powered by more than 750,000 stem cells distributed throughout our bone marrow, lungs, liver, and almost all of our organs, our body regenerates itself every day. These stem cells maintain, repair, and regenerate our bodies throughout our lives. Some foods like dark chocolate, black tea, and beer can mobilize them and help us regenerate. Other foods, like purple potatoes, can kill deadly stem cells that spark cancer growth.

Microbiome

Almost 40 trillion bacteria inhabit our bodies, most of which act to defend our health. Not only do these bacteria produce health supporting metabolites from the foods that we swallow and deliver to our gut, but they also control our immune system, influence angiogenesis, and even help produce hormones that influence our brain and social function. We can boost our microbiome by eating foods like kimchi, sauerkraut, cheddar cheese, and sourdough bread.

DNA Protection

Our DNA is our genetic blueprint, but it is also designed to be a defense system. It has surprising repair mechanisms that protect us against damage caused by solar radiation, household chemicals, stress, compromised sleep, and poor diet, among other insults. Not only can certain foods prompt DNA to fix itself, but some foods turn on helpful genes and turn off harmful ones, while other foods lengthen our telomeres, which protect DNA and slow aging.

Immunity

Our immune system defends our health in sophisticated ways that are much more complicated than we previously thought. It is influenced by our gut, and it can be manipulated to successfully attack and wipe out cancer, even in the elderly. Recent discoveries have completely changed our understanding of the immune system. Foods like blackberries, walnuts, and pomegranate can activate the immune system, while other foods can dampen its activities and help reduce the symptoms of autoimmune diseases.

* * *

This book was written to give you the knowledge and tools to make better decisions when you choose what to eat every day. It is intended to help you live longer by eating foods that you actually like. If you are fit and in good health and want to stay that way, this book is for you. If you are starting to feel your age, and you want to prevent decline and stave off chronic diseases, this book is for you. If you're one of the millions of people living with heart disease, diabetes, autoimmune disease, or another chronic condition, this book is for you. And if you are actively battling a feared disease like cancer, or your family history makes it very likely that you someday will, this book is for you.

I want to make it clear that this book is not presenting a "total diet." If you are using a diet plan to lose weight, deal with gluten intolerance, manage your blood sugar, slow Alzheimer's disease, or reverse heart disease, you need to know that my goal is not to replace these specialized diets, but rather to provide you with the scientific evidence and recommendations about foods you may want to incorporate into your plan, choices that will make the plan even better. I've also included some tasty recipes to help you do just that.

Everyone is afraid of disease. If your goal is to stay healthy, and especially if you are battling a disease, you want reliable information based on science and fact, and actionable steps that you can take right away to improve your situation. The advice on foods I've included in this book is not intended to take the place of good medical care. I am not one of those doctors who rejects Western biomedicine and suggests that food is the magic solution. Quite the opposite: my training and experience in internal medicine guides my judicious use of evidence-based medicine, including surgery and cutting-edge medications, when it comes to diagnosis and treatment.

What's missing in the toolkit of most doctors is the ability to guide an individual, whether they are healthy or sick, on how they can use food as a way to resist disease. How many people do you know who have asked their doctor about what they should eat to help themselves and gotten back either a blank stare or the flip answer: "Eat whatever you want"? This book provides a very different and empowering set of answers.

Eat to Beat Disease has three parts. In part 1, I share the fascinating story behind the power of the health defense systems, how they were discovered, how they work, and how we can harness their healing powers. Even more exciting, scientists are now studying food with the same tools and methods used to study pharmaceutical therapies. In part 2, I will reveal the foods that activate the health defense systems, including some surprises. I will tell you about astonishing research into more than two hundred health-boosting foods, with some results that will make your jaw drop. In part 3, I will give you easy and practical ways to incorporate these foods into your life. I have designed a flexible tool called the 5 × 5 × 5 framework that makes it easy for you to boost your health by choosing foods you love every day.

To get the most out of this book, I recommend that you first read it once, cover to cover, to get a total picture of how to eat to beat disease. You'll learn about health defenses, foods, and why and how to eat them.

Next, return to the many tables and charts I've included that summarize the different foods (and beverages) and how they positively affect your health. Keep an eye out for the foods you know you like, and foods you don't yet know but might be willing to try. You should *always* be eating foods you enjoy and that interest you.

When you are ready, go back to part 3, but now pull out a pen and paper. Make your personalized preferred foods list and complete the 5 × 5 × 5 Daily Worksheet in appendix A, as described in chapter 11. Then, go for it: use your worksheet to make choices about what you will eat each day to beat disease.

* * *

There is no "silver bullet" for any one disease or for overall health and longevity. No single factor in our life is going to prevent sickness. But my research shows we have something even better. There is a way to boost our own defense systems, so the body will heal itself. These revelations tell us that we have radically underestimated our power to transform and restore our own health.

If your goal is to extend the number of healthy years you have ahead, your food choices can tip the odds in your favor. By boosting your defense systems and keeping them in good shape, you'll have a better shot at beating back disease and extending not just the length but also the quality of your life.

The decisions you make on food every day throughout your lifetime offer perfect opportunities for you to stay healthy while enjoying life. Just like taking the extra step of locking the doors before we go to bed at night or checking to be sure the stove is off before we leave the house, taking deliberate preventive measures using our diet is just plain common sense. Combined with regular exercise, good quality sleep, stress management, and strong social bonds, your diet can help you realize your full health potential.

We live in a time of enormous and exciting scientific progress, so good health should be within reach of most everyone. And yet millions suffer and die from avoidable chronic illnesses, even as more high-tech treatments are invented. Between the rising costs of health care and an increasingly toxic and imbalanced environment, better health is an issue of equality that affects us all. The crushing cost of medical care continues to rise, creating a precarious situation where the entire system of modern medicine is on the brink of collapse. The only way to comprehensively bring down the cost of health care is to decrease the number of people who are sick.

We each need to do our part, and the best way to make the world a healthier place is to start with the choices you make for yourself and the people you care about. Let go of the idea that health is the absence of disease and start eating to beat disease every day. *Bonne santé,* and *bon appétit.*

PART I

HARDWIRED FOR HEALTH

Our Body's Natural Defense Systems

Natural forces within us are the true healers of disease.
—*Hippocrates*

Health is not simply the absence of disease. Health is an active state. Your body has within it five health defense systems: angiogenesis, regeneration, the microbiome, DNA protection, and immunity. These systems are responsible for maintaining our health and resisting the regular hazards we all face every day as part of ordinary life—and they heal us when incursions from disease inflict damage in our body. By knowing about how these systems defend your body like a fortress, you can tap into their healing powers to live a longer, healthier life.

Each of your health defense systems has a fascinating story of research and discovery. Each is supported by a well-orchestrated symphony of players: organs, cells, proteins, and more. Each is a common denominator for preventing not one, but many diseases. And all five systems work together to keep you in great health, from the time you are in your mother's womb until your last breath. Join me in the next five chapters to get to know these systems and the benefits they can offer.

CHAPTER I

Angiogenesis

We all have cancer growing in our body. Every single one of us, even you.

In autopsy studies on individuals who never received a diagnosis of cancer during their lifetimes, almost 40 percent of women between the ages of forty and fifty had microscopic tumors in their breasts, about 50 percent of men between fifty and sixty had microscopic cancer in their prostate, and almost 100 percent of people over the age of seventy had microscopic cancers in their thyroid gland.[1] Tumors such as these develop when healthy cells make natural errors during cell division or when a cell's DNA is mutated by environmental exposures. Up to ten thousand mistakes occur in the DNA of dividing cells in your body every day, making the formation of cancers not only common but inevitable.[2] And yet, these microscopic cancers are completely harmless. Most of them never become dangerous. They start out tiny, smaller than the tip of a ballpoint pen, and as long as they cannot enlarge and invade organs, they cannot spread and kill.

Your body has a remarkable defense system that keeps microscopic cancers small by starving them of the blood supply and nutrients they would need to grow—and you can optimize this defense system through the foods you eat. More than one hundred foods can enhance your body's ability to starve cancer and keep those tumors small and harmless, among them soy, tomatoes, black raspberries, pomegranate, and even some surprising ones, like licorice, beer, and cheese. Your defense weapons to keep these tumors at bay can be found at the grocery store, the farmers market, and in your garden.

The defense system that allows our bodies to intercept cancer this way is called angiogenesis. Angiogenesis is the process our bodies use to grow and maintain blood vessels. In ordinary circumstances, blood vessels are supporters of life, delivering oxygen and vital nutrients to all of our organs. But when abnormal blood vessels grow, they can nourish microscopic cancers. A healthy angiogenesis system regulates when and where blood vessels should grow and can prevent tumors from recruiting a private blood supply for the oxygen they need to expand. When the body loses this ability to control blood vessels, a wide range of diseases can occur, including cancer.

As long as the angiogenesis system operates properly, blood vessels grow in the right place at the right time—not too many, not too few, but just the right amount. Keeping this perfect balance in the circulatory system is at the heart of how angiogenesis defends health by keeping us in a state called homeostasis. Homeostasis is defined as maintaining stability in the body for normal function while adjusting to constantly changing conditions. Angiogenesis plays a vital role by creating and maintaining your entire circulatory system and adapting it to various situations over the course of our lives to protect our health.

Because of this powerful health defense system that naturally cuts off the blood supply to tumors, cancer doesn't have to be a disease.[3] In part 2, I will share how the latest science of angiogenesis is shaping our understanding of which foods can help your angiogenesis system maintain homeostasis and how you can eat to starve cancer, grow vessels to feed your heart, and stave off deadly diseases to live a longer, healthier life. But in order to fully appreciate how food influences angiogenesis and your health, let's first take a look at how blood vessels go to work for you every day.

Angiogenesis at Work

Inside you, there are sixty thousand miles of blood vessels whose job it is to deliver oxygen and nutrients to keep cells alive. These are the vessels of life that nourish our healthy organs and protect us against disease. If all your blood vessels were lined up end to end, they would encircle the earth twice. Remarkably, it takes only sixty seconds from the time your heart pumps out a drop of blood for it to circulate throughout the body and back again.

The smallest blood vessels are called capillaries. They are finer than a hair, and your body has 19 billion of them. Capillaries have a unique relationship with all other cells because they are the final link in the chain of the blood vessel delivery system to your cells. Because they are at the end of the line, virtually every cell in the body is located within two hundred micrometers from a capillary.[4] That's really close proximity, just a little more than the width of a human hair. Each organ has its own unique density and pattern of capillaries, depending on what the organ does and how much blood flow it needs. Your muscles, for example, have a huge oxygen demand, so they need four times more blood supply than your bones, which act as structural support. Other high-demand organs for blood flow are your brain, heart, kidneys, and liver. All of these have a capillary density of an amazing three thousand vessels per cubic millimeter, which is thirty times that of bone.

Under the microscope, capillaries look like works of art, sculpted to fit the organ in which they are growing. The ones feeding your skin look like rows of Velcro hooks, with loop after loop of vessels providing the blood that gives warmth and color to your body's surface. Along your nerves, from spinal cord to fingertips, capillaries course along like telephone lines feeding neurons and keep your senses sharp. In the colon, capillaries are formed in a beautiful geometric honeycomb pattern, so that they can stretch with the colon as it fills with digested matter, while providing maximum surface area to absorb fluid back into your bloodstream.

The importance of angiogenesis to support life is so fundamental that it begins in the reproductive system, even before conception. By the time a sperm meets an egg, the womb has already been prepared with the endometrium, a lining of new blood vessels ready to receive and nurture the fertilized egg. If no pregnancy occurs, this lining is sloughed off every month during menstruation. If the fertilized egg is implanted, the blood vessels act as the first supply lines for the developing fetus. About eight days after implantation, a new vascular organ, the placenta, is created to bring blood from the mother to the fetus.[5] Over the next nine months, a symphony of angiogenesis takes place within the fetus, forming an entire circulatory system from scratch, and then filling up each organ in the developing body. Toward the end of pregnancy, as the body prepares for birth, the placenta releases a natural antiangiogenic factor, called soluble Flt-1, which slows down the building of blood vessels. This ability to turn on, turn down, and turn off is a hallmark of the angiogenesis health defense system, not only for building life during pregnancy, but for protecting our health for life's duration.

Angiogenesis defense is a method to protect all animals with a circulatory system, including humans. Whenever you've suffered a deep cut, whether from surgery or trauma, you've no doubt noticed the wounded area starts to undergo changes within seconds, launching a process that continues until the wound is healed. If you've ever scraped your knee badly enough to bleed and later form a scab, and if that scab pulled off too early, you have seen this process unfolding before your eyes. Underneath the scab, the tissue was bright red and glistening. In that red patch, thousands of new blood vessels were growing in the wound to restore the injured tissue back to health.

When you see this process, you are witnessing angiogenesis, which is jump-started in wounded tissue as soon as bleeding begins. The trigger is hypoxia, or lowered oxygen levels, caused by the interruption of normal blood flow in the injury. Lack of oxygen is the signal for more blood vessels to grow to bring in more oxygen. Hypoxia causes wounded cells to start releasing protein signals called growth factors, whose job is to stimulate angiogenesis. Inflammation is very important at the beginning of healing. Inflammatory cells called macrophages and neutrophils crawl into a wound to clean up any bacteria and debris from the injury, and they themselves release their own angiogenic growth factors, amplifying the blood vessel generating response.

From here, several events unfold on the cellular level to grow blood vessels. Thanks to special cells lining your veins called endothelial cells, a rescue team is waiting to receive the growth factor signals that instruct the endothelial cells to deploy. Roughly a trillion endothelial cells line your circulatory system, making them one of the most abundant cell types in your body. Think of each of these endothelial cells as a car engine, connected to an ignition switch. Now, imagine the growth factors that were released from the site of the injury as car keys. The growth factors fit into specific receptors studding the surface of endothelial cells, just as car keys fit into ignition switches. When the right key goes in the right switch, the engine turns on, and the endothelial cells are ready to start migrating toward the source of the protein growth factors and start dividing and forming tubes that will turn into new blood vessels. But first, the endothelial cells need to get out of the vein. They release enzymes that digest the sleeve-like wall of the vein outside the cell, creating holes in the vein wall. From this point on, the activated endothelial cells begin sprouting out of these holes, following the gradient of growth factors being sent from the injured area, and building new blood vessels in that direction. As blood vessel sprouts elongate, they roll up lengthwise to create tubes. Tubes eventually connect at their tips to form capillary loops. As more and more capillary loops form in the healing zone, a new circulation for healing is born.

Freshly formed blood vessels are way too fragile to support blood flow on their own, so they are assisted by another type of cell, the pericyte, which helps them mature. Pericytes help out in a couple of ways. First, they wrap themselves around the endothelial tubes like a tube sock over an ankle to provide architectural stability. Simultaneously, the pericytes slow down angiogenesis, so there isn't a super overage of blood vessels.[6] The pericyte cells are shape-shifters. Once anchored to a new blood vessel, they extend tentacle-like arms to embrace the endothelial cells around them. A single pericyte can touch as many as twenty cells at a time and release a chemical signal that turns off the frenzied activity surrounding angiogenesis.[7]

Once the new vessels have sprouted and been stabilized, blood flow begins. The flood of new oxygen turns down the switch for growth factor signals, slowing the engines of angiogenesis until they finally grind to a halt. At the same time, natural angiogenesis inhibitors are released in the area, further suppressing new blood vessel growth. When the new blood vessels are solidly in place, the endothelial cells lining them churn out proteins, called survival factors, that help heal cells in the neighborhood where angiogenesis took place. When properly constructed, these defensive new blood vessels can last for a lifetime, keeping the skin and other organs alive.

The angiogenesis system constantly senses where and when more vessels are needed to keep organs healthy and functioning. Like a master builder, blood vessels detect the need from your muscles after a workout: more blood flow is needed to build the muscles. On the other hand, the system is also constantly on the lookout for situations where blood vessels should be pruned back. Not too few or too many but just the right balance and mix of blood vessels is what a healthy angiogenesis system is designed to accomplish, twenty-four hours a day.

It's like a dimmer switch. The intensity can be upped to grow more blood vessels when there's a need. When it needs to be dimmed, your body has endogenous (naturally occurring in the body) inhibitors of angiogenesis that squelch the process. These stimulators and countermeasures are everywhere, including our muscles, blood, heart, brain, breast milk, and even semen.

Your body's control of angiogenesis needs to be perfect to optimize your health. Over the course of a lifetime, however, many factors can derail this defense system, leading to either excessive angiogenesis, which can feed diseased tissues, or, on the other hand, insufficient angiogenesis, which can lead to tissue loss and death. You are going to learn about the foods that help shore up your angiogenesis defenses to help your body resist diseases in part 2. But first, let's return to the microscopic cancers growing in your body to see how breakdown of the defenses happens and its dire consequences—so you can learn why it is so important to eat the right foods for health. The main reason microscopic cancers don't grow is your body's natural angiogenesis inhibitors. These countermeasures keep tumors in check by depriving them of a blood supply. As researchers at Harvard Medical School discovered as early as 1974, so long as no blood vessels grow to feed tumors, the cancer cells will remain dormant and harmless. Your immune system, which I'll tell you about later in chapter 5, eventually spots them and destroys them. Over time, however, some tiny nests of cancer can overwhelm the defense system and overcome antiangiogenic countermeasures by releasing huge amounts of the same growth factor signals involved in wound healing. In lab experiments, once new blood vessels sprout into the small cluster of cancer cells, a tumor can grow exponentially, expanding up to sixteen thousand times in size in only two weeks after angiogenesis starts.[8] When tumors hijack the angiogenesis defense system to grow their own circulation, a harmless cancer quickly becomes a potentially deadly one. Worse yet, the same blood vessels that feed cancer tumors also serve as exit channels for malignant cells to escape into the bloodstream. This is known as metastasis, and is the most dangerous aspect of cancer. Patients with cancer rarely die from their initial tumor, which can often be removed by surgery—it's the metastases that pepper the body like buckshot that kill.

Helping the body prevent unwanted angiogenesis can have the

powerful effect of suppressing cancer. The goal is to boost your angio-genesis defenses, helping your body's natural countermeasures keep blood vessels in the normal zone of balance, which means cancer cells do not have the advantage of being fed so they can't grow. The first patient to benefit from an antiangiogenic treatment was a 12-year-old boy named Tom Briggs, who lived in Denver, Colorado. He was diagnosed with a condition called pulmonary capillary hemangiomatosis, in which tumors grew in his lungs. As the tumors expanded, his breathing became dif-ficult and it interfered with his ability to play his favorite sports like baseball, and sometimes, even to get a good night's sleep. As a last-ditch measure, he received a medicine called interferon alfa, which his doctors knew could stop angiogenesis. Over the course of a year, his lung tumors shrank away, and Tom returned to living life as a normal kid. Tom's case was so remarkable that it was published as a "first human case" in the *New England Journal of Medicine* as a glimpse into the future of treating tumors.[9]

Biotech companies began developing targeted drugs to treat tumor angiogenesis starting in the 1990s. The first cancer to show the benefit of antiangiogenic therapy was colorectal cancer, where targeting tumor blood vessels improved patient survival using a treatment called Avastin. Many other cancers have become treatable by boosting the body's own angiogenesis countermeasures, using Avastin and more than a dozen other designer medicines that inhibit angiogenesis. These include kidney, lung, brain, thyroid, liver, cervical, ovarian, and breast cancers, as well as multiple myeloma. In 2004, the U.S. Food and Drug commissioner Mark McClellan declared, "Angiogenesis inhibitors can now be considered as the fourth modality of cancer therapy (after surgery, chemotherapy, and radiation)."[10]

Excessive angiogenesis drives disease in many other conditions beyond cancer, such as vision loss. In the healthy eye, vision is possi-ble because light can pass through crystal clear fluid to the retina and be registered by the brain, without interference from blood vessels.

Angiogenesis in the eye is so tightly controlled that the endothelial cells lining the blood vessels in the retina normally divide only twice in a person's lifetime. But in both age-related macular degeneration (AMD), the leading cause of blindness worldwide in people age sixty-five and older, and diabetes-related vision loss, angiogenesis leads to abnormal tangles of blood vessels being formed, which leak fluid and bleed. This disastrous consequence of unwanted angiogenesis destroys vision. Fortunately, these conditions can now be treated using FDA-approved biological medicines that are injected by ophthalmologists into the eye to halt the destructive angiogenesis, stop the leaking, and protect vision. Some patients can even regain lost vision. I had one patient who became legally blind from macular degeneration and could not drive or play golf, her favorite pastime. After treatment, she could safely drive again and got back to working on her backswing on the golf course.

In both rheumatoid arthritis and osteoarthritis, inflammation in the joints leads to new blood vessels that release destructive enzymes. These enzymes destroy your cartilage which causes crippling joint pain. In psoriasis, a disfiguring skin condition, abnormal angiogenesis under the skin helps grow the patches of raised red skin plaques that are accompanied by swelling, irritating itchiness, and pain.

Alzheimer's disease has been discovered to involve excessive and abnormal angiogenesis. In 2003, along with psychiatrist Dr. Anthony Vagnucci, I proposed that abnormalities in brain blood vessels contributed to Alzheimer's disease in a paper that was published in *The Lancet*.[11] Today, we know that blood vessels in Alzheimer's-affected brains are abnormal and do not actually improve blood flow but instead they release neurotoxins that kill brain cells.

Even obesity has a powerful angiogenesis connection. Although obesity is a multifactorial disease, overeating and eating the wrong foods generate high levels of angiogenesis-stimulating growth factors circulating in the blood.[12] Just like tumors, a mass of fat requires new blood vessels to grow and feed fat cells.[13] For all of these health concerns, and many others, exciting new angiogenesis-targeting drug treatments are showing promising results in the laboratory and in clinical trials.

Pruning away excessive blood vessels is important, but just as important is maintaining the body's capacity to grow an adequate circulatory system to protect organs that need to increase or restore their blood supply. As we age, our circulation often naturally wanes, and this ability needs to be coaxed and boosted to feed and maintain healthy tissues and organs. When compromised, the inability to mount a defensive angiogenic response has dire consequences.

One such consequence is neuropathy. Neuropathies occur when the function of your nerves is compromised. This can lead to numbness or pain that range from mild to crippling. Your peripheral nerves are your electrical wiring running throughout your body, relaying directions from your brain to your muscles telling them to contract and relax. The nerves also send sensations from your skin and muscles back to your brain. These electrical cables have their own mini circulatory system called the vasa nervorum, which keeps blood flowing to nerves. When the vasa nervorum goes down, nerves begin to die. The symptoms can range from tingling to unbearable pain to complete numbness of the hands, legs, and feet.

People with diabetes can develop a compromised nerve blood supply, especially if their blood sugar is not well managed. Diabetes also slows down angiogenesis, which damages nerves. Researchers have been working on new ways to improve nerve blood flow using therapeutic angiogenesis. In the lab, researchers inject the muscles of diabetic animals with the gene for the angiogenic protein VEGF (vascular endothelial growth factor) and find they can increase blood flow to the nerves and restore their function close to normal levels.[14] Another common cause for peripheral neuropathy is cancer chemotherapy, which not only kills cancer cells, but can be highly toxic to nerves and destroy their mini circulatory system. In the lab, gene therapy using VEGF completely protects the nerves and their blood supply against loss of function.[15]

When your angiogenesis defenses are crippled, many other diseases can intrude on your life. Chronic wounds are another example. While normal wounds heal in under a week's time, chronic wounds are slow to heal or don't heal at all. These open sores become infected, gangrenous, and often lead to the need to amputate an effected limb. This affects more than 8 million people in the United States alone, specifically striking people with diabetes, atherosclerosis, or malfunctioning valves in their leg veins, or those who are confined to bed or use a wheelchair. It's a silent and deadly epidemic with a mortality rate greater than breast and colon cancer.[16] If you have a chronic wound, one of the primary goals of your doctor should be to jumpstart angiogenesis to improve blood flow and speed up healing. This can be done with a variety of medical devices and other techniques, including diet. We'll talk about angiogenesis-stimulating foods in chapter 6.

Your heart and brain also rely on the angiogenesis defense system to respond whenever there is any threat to their own circulation. Restoring blood flow quickly to these organs is literally a matter of life and death. When there are blockages to their blood vessels, which happens with atherosclerosis, your defense system will kick into gear and grow new blood vessels to help form a natural bypass around the blocked channels. Natural bypasses, called collateral vessels, form when the blockages occur slowly with gradual narrowing of the coronary vessels or carotid arteries. People can live for years or decades with their coronary heart disease or carotid disease if their angiogenesis defense system does its job. Even in the case of sudden blockages, such as happens with a heart attack or an ischemic stroke, if the patient survives, the angiogenesis defense will kick in to form natural bypasses.

This defense happens slowly if a patient has a condition that stymies angiogenesis, such as diabetes or hypercholesterolemia, or is a smoker or is elderly. Clinical trials for therapies that stimulate angiogenesis in the heart or brain have shown it is possible to deliver new therapies to speed this process, but these are still in experimental stages and years away from being used to treat patients. In part 2, I'm going to tell you about foods that you can use at home to aid cardiovascular angiogenesis and healing.

Foods and Angiogenesis

Clearly, a fully functioning angiogenesis defense system protects us against many diseases. Your health depends on a normal balance of the circulatory system, without excessive or insufficient blood vessels in your organs. When this balance is upset, your body needs help. Researchers at biopharmaceutical and medical device companies are racing to develop new life-, limb-, and vision-saving treatments, but creating a new therapy can take a decade or more, cost more than $1 billion, and even if successful may not be accessible to everyone who needs it due to the cost and availability. Even more, these drugs and devices are intended for disease treatment, not prevention.

Your diet can be used for disease prevention as well as to help aid treatment. Research being conducted from all corners of the world is revealing that specific foods and beverages, including many that we recognize and enjoy, can boost your angiogenesis defenses on both sides of the equation. Even the way you prepare and combine food ingredients can influence angiogenesis. This brings an entirely new perspective to how to think about which foods you eat and how to eat them. And it opens new doors if you want to increase your odds for preventing diseases influenced by angiogenesis. If you are currently battling an angiogenesis-dependent condition, choosing the right foods may help you control or even beat that disease.

There's mounting evidence for the power of this approach. People in Asia who consume lots of soy, vegetables, and tea in their diet have a significantly lower risk for developing breast and other cancers. In Japan, there are more than sixty-nine thousand people who are older than one hundred years of age.[17] China also has a rising population of centenarians. My great-uncle, who lived to a healthy 104, resided in the town of

Changshu, outside of Shanghai, at the base of the Yushan mountain, where green tea is grown. The vibrant centenarians of Ikaria, Greece, and in central Sardinia eat the Mediterranean diet, which is chock-full of angiogenesis-defense-boosting ingredients and not strictly vegan. Understanding that angiogenesis is one of your key health defense systems is key to unlocking new secrets for long-lasting health inside your body and outside of the health-care system.

CONDITIONS WHERE ANGIOGENESIS DEFENSES ARE BREACHED

Excessive Angiogenesis	Insufficient Angiogenesis
Age-related macular degeneration	Alopecia
Alzheimer's disease	Diabetic foot ulcers
Brain cancer	Erectile dysfunction
Breast cancer	Ischemic heart disease
Cervical cancer	Heart failure
Colorectal cancer	Neuropathy
Diabetes-related vision loss	Peripheral arterial disease
Endometriosis	Peripheral neuropathy
Kidney cancer	Pressure ulcers
Leukemia	Venous leg ulcers
Liver cancer	
Lung cancer	
Lymphoma	
Multiple myeloma	
Obesity	
Ovarian cancer	
Prostate cancer	
Psoriasis	
Rheumatoid arthritis	
Thyroid cancer	

CHAPTER 2

Regeneration

If angiogenesis grows new blood vessels to feed your organs as health defense, what grows and maintains the organs? The answer: stem cells. Stem cells are so vital to your health that if they suddenly stopped working, you'd be dead in a week. From the time you were conceived, stem cells have played a key role in generating and maintaining your body and health. We are literally made from stem cells. Around five days after your father's sperm met your mother's egg, you started life as a small ball of roughly fifty to one hundred embryonic stem cells (ESC) in the womb. The remarkable thing about these stem cells is they are pluripotent, meaning they can form any cell or tissue in the body, from muscle to nerve to skin to brain to eyeball. As you "the embryo" matured over twelve weeks into you "the fetus," all your basic organs were created from stem cells that morphed into more specialized cells to perform the functions of each organ. Soon, your specialized organ cells began to outnumber the unspecialized stem cells as your body was built.

Stem cells in the fetus not only build the organism but also provide health defense—even for the mother. Scientists at the Mount Sinai School of Medicine in New York performed a landmark lab experiment in which they studied heart attacks in pregnant mice. The heart attacks were serious enough to damage 50 percent of the heart's main pumping chamber. In a human, this degree of damage would be enough to cause heart failure, if not swift death.[1] In the surviving mice, as the weeks passed after the heart attack, the research discovered that stem cells from the fetus had migrated from the womb into the mother's bloodstream. From there, remarkably, the fetal stem cells homed in on the damaged area of their mother's heart and began regenerating and repairing it. By a month after the heart attack, 50 percent of the migrating fetal stem cells in the mother's heart had become her adult heart cells, capable of spontaneous beating. This study was one of the first to show that stem cells from the fetus can help defend the health of the mother.

By the time of birth, most cells in the developing human have transformed into their final organ form, leaving only a tiny fraction of stem cells remaining. After childbirth, some stem cells are left stranded in the umbilical cord and in the placenta. The ones in the umbilical cord can be collected as cord blood, which can be sent to a stem cell bank, where the cells are frozen and reserved for future medical use. These may be someday useful for your child or even to you and your family members to help regenerate or heal damaged organs in the future. It's a one-time deal, and I definitely recommend collecting and banking cord blood.

Despite their low numbers, stem cells continue to play a critical role in adult life. They quietly regenerate most of our organs "behind the scenes" as we age. The process happens at its own pace, different for each organ[2]:

- Your small intestine regenerates every two to four days.
- Your lungs and stomach, every eight days.
- Your skin, every two weeks.
- Your red blood cells, every four months.
- Your fat cells, every eight years.
- Your skeleton, every ten years.

The pace of regeneration also changes with age. When you are twenty-five years old, about 1 percent of cells in your heart are renewed annually, but things slow down as you age. By the time you are seventy-five, only 0.45 percent of heart cells are renewed each year.[3]

Your immune cells are regenerated every seven days, so if your stem cells disappeared, you'd likely die of an infection soon after. If you somehow survived infection, then you'd die of hemorrhage, because blood elements called platelets, responsible for clotting, are replaced every ten days. If you made it past that, your skin would slough off in six weeks. Then your lungs would collapse, and you would suffocate. Our stem cells defend our health, and are one of our lifelines.

The Healing Power of Stem Cells

What we know about our body's stem cells goes back to the atomic bomb. The nuclear annihilation of Hiroshima and Nagasaki killed an estimated two hundred thousand people in 1945, ending World War II. Doctors observed that some people who survived the initial blast later succumbed in a second wave of death because radiation exposure destroyed their body's ability to renew its own cells in the bone marrow. As governments made preparations for future nuclear wars, scientists went on the hunt for stem cells that could be used to treat and protect survivors from deadly radiation fallout. Two Canadian researchers, James Till and Ernest McCullough, showed in 1961 that stem cells were present in the bone marrow and spleen, and they could regenerate blood cells. Till and McCullough discovered that, if injected in time, these stem cells could rescue lab animals exposed to lethal amounts of radiation.[4]

Till and McCullough's work led to the development of bone marrow transplantation, a lifesaving procedure now performed around the world to rescue cancer patients who are being treated with the harshest chemotherapies and highest doses of radiation. Although the chemo and radiation do kill cancer cells, they also demolish the healthy stem cells in the bone marrow. Without stem cells, the cancer patient's immune system crashes, and they can die of overwhelming infection. By transplanting stem cells taken from the bone marrow of a donor into the cancer patient, however, doctors can rescue patients from this certain death. The donor stem cells circulate into the patient's bone marrow and engraft themselves. They then reconstitute the immune system. This bone marrow transplantation technique using donor stem cells was deemed a medical breakthrough. Its pioneer, E. Donnall Thomas, won the 1990 Nobel Prize in Medicine or Physiology, along with kidney transplant pioneer Joseph Murray. But even without being damaged by chemotherapy or radiation exposure, your body needs its stem cells because they continuously rebuild your body from the inside out.

Among the 37.2 trillion cells in your body, stem cells make up a tiny but powerful subset, only 0.002 percent, which are capable of regenerating your health.[5] Stem cells repair, replace, and regenerate dead and worn out cells on demand. Like special forces soldiers in your body, they gather intelligence, conduct reconnaissance, and execute missions to keep organs in optimal shape. Whenever you suffer an injury or develop a disease, your stem cells swing into action: to create new tissues that heal or help your body overcome the condition. This is your regenerative health defense system. And just like the angiogenesis system, the latest research is showing that your stem cells are powerfully influenced by diet.

Whether you are an athlete building your muscles, or a pregnant mother building a fetus, or someone who is fighting the ravages of aging, the right foods can help boost the number and performance of your stem cells and their ability to regenerate your body. You can eat to protect your heart, keep your mind sharp (brain regeneration), heal your wounds, and keep your body in a youthful shape. I'm going to tell you about the foods that can help your stem cell health defenses in part 2, but first I'm going to give you a primer on regeneration, so you can see why eating the right foods might save your life.

Stem Cells and Injury

The regeneration defense system is hardwired to be at the ready at any time to respond to injury or trauma. Adult stem cells remain unspecialized, lying in wait until they are needed and called into action. They can renew and replicate by cell division and still maintain their pluripotency. When they're in mission mode, they sense their environment and use the cues around them as the instructions for turning into the exact type of cell that needs to be regenerated. If they find themselves in a lung, they become lung. If they find themselves in the liver, they become liver.

The story of how stem cells accomplish these protective functions begins with where they live in their inactive, undifferentiated, and renewable state. They reside in special hideouts called niches. Niches are found in skin, along the walls of intestines, at the base of hair follicles, in testes and ovaries, in fat, in the heart and brain, and especially in bone marrow, the spongy material inside the hollow of our bones.

The bone marrow is a storage unit for at least three different types of stem cells. The hematopoietic stem cells (HSC) turn into blood-forming cells. Mesenchymal stromal cell (MSC) precursors form muscle, fat, cartilage, bone, and other non-blood elements. Endothelial progenitor cells (EPC) contribute to building new blood vessels in regenerating organs. Collectively, they are labeled bone-marrow-derived mononuclear cells (BM-MNC) because they all reside in the bone marrow.

When stem cells are called into action by a body part that needs to be regenerated, a series of events takes place to bring the stem cell from their niches into your circulatory system. The stem cells in bone marrow are alerted by growth factor signals released by the organ in distress. One particular growth factor, vascular endothelial growth factor (VEGF), is a powerful stem cell activator. This distress signal reaches the bone marrow through blood vessels that penetrate bone. Once inside, these signals travel along a system of capillaries called sinusoidal channels within the marrow that floats the signal to stem cells attached to the channel walls. These stem cells interpret the signal as a chemical alert and respond accordingly. What starts as a distress call ends with swarms of stem cells flying like bees out of a hive from the bone marrow into the body's circulatory system.[6] This important step in regenerating an injured part of your body is called stem cell mobilization.

What happens next is a powerful illustration of the cleverness of how stem cells are designed to act. Stem cells get to the front lines of injury quickly whenever there is an emergency. Carried in the swift current of the bloodstream and propelled by the heart's pumping action, stem cells use a biological homing device to locate the exact place in the organ that sent the distress call. Like a guided missile zeroing in on its target, the stem cell finds its landing spot. Proteins on the stem cell called receptors attach to proteins in the landing zone. They hook together like cellular Velcro, ensuring that stem cells attach only to the site of injury.[7] All this happens very quickly after the distress signal is sent. Research has shown, for example, that forty-eight hours after a surgeon has made an incision, there is a fourteenfold increase in the number of endothelial progenitor cells in the circulatory system compared to before surgery, because of the need for healing.[8]

Once they've attached to the landing zone, stem cells take stock of the organ environment in which they've landed, and they execute their mission based on instructions given by their environment. If they are in skin, they become skin cells and respond in the ways that meet the needs of skin. If in the heart, they become heart muscle cells (cardiomyocytes) and respond to the heart's needs. The stem cells do their job as part of a larger set of players after an injury. An entire disaster response team, including inflammatory and other immune cells, blood vessel cells, and blood clotting cells, all show up with their own specific tasks to perform.

What stem cells do exactly once they are embedded in the injured tissue is still somewhat of a mystery. We know they differentiate into and regenerate the local tissue. But, stem cells don't stick around for long. They last for only a few days, at most. Scientists are working to document what actually happens to them. A couple of theories: the stem cells morph their appearance and disappear into the background becoming indistinguishable from the normal tissue they are repairing. Or, it is possible they play a vital but short-lived role, then die after their mission is complete.

What we do know is that stem cells are factories for proteins called growth factors, cytokines, and survival factors that are needed in organs that are growing or being repaired. They also can release special molecular containers called exosomes and microvesicles filled with a cargo of proteins and genetic information. When these are released in an organ, they instruct other cells on what to do next to fix the damage.[9] Stem cells release this cargo to encourage other cells to help build a healthier neighborhood around the landing zone. This is called the paracrine effect. One study examining bone regeneration showed that at least forty-three growth factors can be released by stem cells that help improve the neighborhood of injured bone.[10]

Some of the same growth factors involved in the stem cell response are the exact same ones that trigger angiogenesis, linking these two health defense systems. When vascular endothelial growth factor is released by cells due to lack of oxygen (hypoxia) or by injury, for example, it triggers angiogenesis locally, while farther away, in the bone marrow niche, stem cells become alerted by this factor. If a new mass of tissue is regenerated, it will need a fresh blood supply. Angiogenesis kicks in at this point and supplies the nourishment needed to support the regenerated tissue by forming new blood vessels. Conversely, stem cells also contribute to building new angiogenic blood vessels, too, so it's a win-win relationship. Anywhere from 2 to 25 percent of cells in new blood vessels come from stem cells.

Causes of Stem Cell Damage

As vital as our regenerative defense system is for good health and healing, our stem cells are highly vulnerable to common factors that assault our bodies throughout our life span. One of the most damaging is tobacco smoke. The oxygen deficit that occurs when a smoker inhales cigarette smoke starts the recruitment of stem cells into the bloodstream. But habitual smoking eventually depletes the number of stem cells stored in the bone marrow, leaving fewer cells overall available for regeneration and repair over time.[11] Even worse, the remaining stem cells in smokers do not function properly—their ability to multiply themselves is reduced by as much as 80 percent, and their participation in regeneration is reduced by almost 40 percent.[12] These compromises in the number and function of stem cells help explain, beyond the direct damage smoking does to blood vessels, the increased risk of cardiovascular and lung disease in smokers.

Even if you don't smoke yourself, you are not safe if you are nearby those who do. Secondhand smoke can be almost as bad. Even as little as thirty minutes of exposure to tobacco smoke exhaled by someone else is enough to stun your stem cells.[13] Not surprisingly, air pollution is similarly damaging. Researchers have found that in people living in communities with major air pollution problems, exposure to fine particulate matter during pollution flares lowers the number of endothelial progenitor cells in their blood.[14]

Heavy drinking kills stem cells. Alcohol affects stem cells in a number of ways. Researchers studied monkeys who were given small daily amounts of alcohol to drink, and remarkably, they had *more* stem cells in their circulatory system than nondrinking monkeys. The stem cells of drinking monkeys, however, were impaired and less effective in their ability to take part in regeneration.[15] Think of these as inebriated stem cells that have difficulty walking a straight line. Fetal alcohol syndrome is a disastrous consequence when pregnant women consume lots of alcohol. The developing fetus suffers permanent brain damage and growth abnormalities. Alcohol is toxic to fetal stem cells, so the devastation of fetal alcohol syndrome may be due, in part, to damaged stem cells, which indeed was found by researchers from Louisiana State University studying mouse models of fetal development.[16] Binge drinking delivers another blow to stem cell health. Researchers at the University of Kentucky found that binge drinking lowers the activity of brain stem cells called oligodendrocyte progenitors that are needed to make new neurons. The effect was especially pronounced in the brain's hippocampus region. This is the part of the brain responsible for building short- and long-term memory.[17] The good news here is that the damage was able to be reversed when binge drinking stopped.

We can avoid some risk to our stem cells by reducing our exposure to air pollution, tobacco, and alcohol, but some other risks are harder to avoid. Aging, for example, relentlessly wears down our ability to regenerate. As we get older, we naturally have fewer stem cells in our bone marrow. Not only do our reserves become depleted over time, but also the remaining stem cells are less active than they were during our younger years.[18] High blood cholesterol also impairs stem cell function, although not all cholesterol is equal.[19] High-density lipoprotein (HDL), the "good" cholesterol, slows down the programmed cell death of endothelial progenitor cells. Dietary strategies that increase HDL are protective for these cells.[20] This pays dividends for our health, because endothelial progenitor cells can help prevent atherosclerosis, protect against the buildup of fatty plaque on the walls of blood vessels that reduces blood flow, and repair the lining of blood vessels. This kind of vascular protection by stem cells is yet another reason why HDL is considered "good" cholesterol.

Chronic diseases also can have a deleterious effect on stem cells. Diabetes is a stem cell killer. People with diabetes have fewer stem cells, and the ones that exist are unable to do their job properly. High blood sugar is the problem. Stem cells exposed to a high-sugar environment are less capable of regenerating tissue. They can't multiply normally to make more of themselves, and they can't move around in the body very well. They are thus unable to properly participate in building new tissue. On top of that, they secrete fewer survival factors than normal stem cells.[21] Researchers have found that high blood sugar affects stem cells even in normal healthy adults who do not have diabetes.[22] This is another reason to watch your sugar intake.

Stem cell damage is seen in both type 1 and type 2 diabetes. Type 1 diabetes is a disease in which the body's own immune system destroys the insulin-producing cells needed to properly control the metabolism of sugar. Type 2 diabetes similarly is a problem of blood sugar metabolism, but it is not caused by an autoimmune attack. Instead, due to genetics, an inactive lifestyle, and/or obesity, the body either stops responding properly to insulin or doesn't make enough insulin. A study from New York University showed that endothelial progenitor cells are compromised in their ability to grow by almost 50 percent in type 2 diabetes, with worse impairment if the individual's blood sugar levels were not under control.[23] When researchers tested the performance of endothelial progenitor cells, taken from people with diabetes, in helping to form blood vessels, they were 2.5 times less likely to participate in the process than nondiabetic stem cells. A similar defect was found by researchers in the Netherlands studying stem cell impairment in type 1 diabetes.[24]

Stem cell crippling is a problem of gigantic proportions when you realize that diabetes is a pandemic that affects more than 422 million people worldwide, and leads to 1.6 million deaths each year. Diabetes is a major underlying cause of heart attack, stroke, blindness, kidney failure, chronic wounds, and disability caused by lower extremity amputations. These are all medical complications that are tied in one way or another to the dysfunctional stem cells. Any methods to protect or improve the performance of stem cells in diabetes, hyperlipidemia, and aging could be a lifesaver.[25]

Peripheral vascular disease is a severe condition accompanying atherosclerosis and often occurs after long-standing diabetes. In this condition, the severe atherosclerotic narrowing of the arteries chokes off the oxygen supply to the legs. This is a condition that gets worse over time, and blood flow to muscles, nerves, and skin of the leg becomes increasingly poor. The cells in the leg become oxygen starved and eventually die, leading to skin breakdown and gaping wounds called ischemic leg ulcers. Because wound healing itself is already slowed in diabetes, when ischemic leg ulcers occur in people with diabetes, infection can easily set in, leading to gangrene. Often, amputating the leg is needed to save the patient's life. Researchers at the University of Padova in Italy have studied circulating stem cells in patients with type 2 diabetes and peripheral vascular disease, and compared them with healthy subjects without diabetes.[26] Patients with diabetic vascular disease had 47 percent fewer stem cells, and those with the fewest stem cells also had ischemic foot ulcers, reflecting just how important stem cells are for wound regeneration and repair.

The lesson here is that good diabetes management is absolutely critical for protecting your regenerative defense system. Better blood sugar control leads to better stem cell health. By contrast, poor control of diabetes seriously impairs the function of your stem cells. Improving your blood sugar control can increase the number and improve the function of endothelial progenitor cells. So if you have diabetes, make sure you are on top of your game with blood sugar management—it could literally save your life.[27]

Benefits of Boosting Stem Cells

When our stem cell system goes down, so goes our health. But when we take measures to boost our stem cells, the effect on our health can be positive. Consider cardiovascular disease. Researchers from Homburg,

Germany, published a study of 519 individuals in the *New England Journal of Medicine* that showed that measuring baseline levels of circulating endothelial progenitor cells could predict whether an individual would have a heart attack or a stroke during the next twelve months, and the levels could even forecast whether the individual would live or die from their event.[28] In this particular study, people who had higher baseline levels of endothelial progenitor cells had a 26 percent lower risk of experiencing a first major event. People with higher baseline stem cell levels also had a 70 percent lower risk of dying from a cardiovascular cause.

Another landmark study, the Malmo Diet and Cancer Study from Sweden, also examined the connection between stem cell levels and cardiovascular disease.[29] The study began in 1991 with a group of middle-aged participants. For nineteen years, the researchers followed the participants' health by regularly sampling their blood and giving them nutrition questionnaires to explore correlations with disease. Of this group, the researchers measured a blood marker called stem cell factor in 4,742 people. Stem cell factor is a protein made in the bone marrow that nurtures the hive of stem cells waiting in reserve. The protein is also found in the bloodstream, where it guides stem cells in their actions, such as multiplying, migrating, and eventually transforming on demand into specific tissue, a process called differentiation. Stem cell factor is essential for healthy stem cell function. Among the Malmo participants, researchers found that those with the highest levels of stem cell factor had a lower risk of heart failure by 50 percent, a lower risk of stroke by 34 percent, and a lower risk of death from any cause by 32 percent compared to those participants with the lowest levels of stem cell factor. Not surprisingly, the study also found that people with the lowest level of stem cell factor in their blood also tended to be those who were smokers, have high alcohol intake, or diabetes, clearly showing the close connection between lifestyle, stem cell function, and risk of chronic disease.

Within your cardiovascular system, stem cells have unique protective functions. Endothelial progenitor cells not only contribute to forming new blood vessels in regenerating organs, but they also play an important role in repairing damage within existing blood vessels. Atherosclerosis, a process that hardens and narrows your arteries, increases your risk for heart attack, stroke, peripheral vascular disease, and even erectile dysfunction. The plaques that tend to form in the walls of the arteries grow wherever the inner lining of the blood vessels are damaged, like rust growing on a scraped up drainpipe.

If the damage on the lining is not repaired, more and more plaque will accumulate, eventually piling up to narrow the diameter of the blood vessel and close off blood flow. Like a cellular seamstress, endothelial progenitor cells can repair the lining. Damage to your stem cells, therefore, reduces your regenerative defenses against atherosclerosis. Keeping your stem cells healthy reduces the risk of atherosclerotic buildup and protects you from developing cardiovascular disease.

Loss of brain stem cells is implicated in the development of dementia.[30] These stem cells, called oligodendrocyte progenitors, regenerate and replace neurons in your brain and are critical for maintaining sharp mental function as you age. These are the same stem cells affected by binge drinking. Researchers are now working on finding ways to support and boost brain stem cells to treat Alzheimer's disease. Another type of specialized brain cells called microglia develop from hematopoietic stem cells. These microglia are responsible for cleaning up the brain and removing the brain-killing beta amyloid plaques that form in Alzheimer's. In the lab, scientists from Huazhong University of Science and Technology in China injected a protein called stem cell recruitment factor (SDF-1) into the brains of mice with Alzheimer's disease. They found that this protein could recruit the hematopoietic stem cells from the bone marrow into the brain, which then morphed into microglia and improved the cleanup of amyloid debris that accumulates in the disease.[31]

Stem Cells in Medicine

The importance of stem cells in health is undeniable, and clinical trials are underway around the world to develop stem cell therapies. While there are many ways to create regenerative therapy, one common way is to inject stem cells into the body to enhance organ regeneration for diseases of heart, brain, eyes, kidney, pancreas, and liver. If you are searching for a clinical trial of regenerative therapy, go to clinicaltrials.gov, the world's most comprehensive database of human research studies. Maintained by the U.S. National Library of Medicine, this site is an extremely valuable resource for patients or caregivers seeking the latest treatments in development. To find clinical trials in regenerative medicine, enter the search term "BM-MNC" (shorthand for bone marrow derived mononuclear cells) or "progenitor" or "regenerative," along with the name of the disease you are interested in treating.

The results will show you specific trials, what they are testing, where the trial is being conducted, whether the study is enrolling patients, and often, if the study has been completed, the results. There are presently more than six thousand trials listed for regeneration, making this one of the most intense areas of clinical research in medicine. Among the most provocative and intriguing trials using stem cells are those aimed at reversing multiple sclerosis, Parkinson's disease, and even autism.[32]

The stem cells being used in regenerative therapy come from a variety of sources, and it's important for you to know how stem cell therapies are performed in medical centers. Common sources for the stem cells used in these treatments are bone marrow, blood, fat, and even skin. The stem cells from bone marrow, for instance, are removed by placing a large needle into the hip bone and suctioning out some liquid marrow. Alternatively, stem cells can be removed from the blood through a process called apheresis and then concentrated before being injected into the patient.

Often, harvested stem cells undergo a few processing steps to ensure they are in top form and safe before doctors put them back into the body.

Imagine this: a plastic surgeon performs liposuction to remove adipose tissue (fat) from the belly of a patient with heart disease. The removed tissue is then processed in the clinic to separate the adipose stem cells from the fat, and then the stem cells are handed to a waiting cardiologist, who injects them into the patient's heart. This is being done in clinical trials right now. The early results in patients showed that the injection of 20 million fat-derived stem cells led to a 50 percent decrease in the size of the damage caused by a heart attack.[33]

Another truly unique stem cell source is the skin, which contains a type of cell called inducible pluripotent stem cell (iPSC). These stem cells are not your garden-variety stem cell. They are a special kind of mature skin cell that can actually be reverse-morphed back into a stem cell, and from there, redirected to become a new specialized cell of an entirely different organ.

This discovery, made by medical researcher Shinya Yamanaka in 2006, caused entire textbooks on biology to be rewritten. Yamanaka shared the Nobel Prize in Physiology or Medicine for this work with Sir John B. Gurdon in 2012. The science is already being translated into practice. In 2014, a research group at the Riken Center for Developmental Biology in Kobe, Japan, was treating a seventy-seven-year-old woman with progressive vision loss caused by neovascular age-related macular degeneration, a condition sometimes called wet AMD.

For her treatment, the researchers surgically removed a BB-size piece of her skin, then collected iPSCs from this tissue. The researchers then reprogrammed her iPSCs to form a sheet of special retinal cells that are found naturally in the eye, called retinal pigment epithelium (RPE). They then transplanted the regenerated RPE cells into her retina and found not only that the transplant was safe and well-tolerated even after two years, but also that the cells prevented further vision loss and even partially restored her eyesight.[34]

While the widespread clinical use of stem cells for regenerative medicine is still many years away for most applications, patients in clinical trials and a few private centers are already benefiting. I witnessed this firsthand in 2016, when I participated in a conference convened by the Vatican called Cellular Horizons, bringing together world leaders in medicine, science, philanthropy, and faith to share progress on the potential of harnessing adult stem cells to defend health and cure disease. I was invited to present new concepts using a dietary approach to regenerate ailing tissues, and other researchers presented their own amazing work and results.

Among the most memorable cases were those of Richard Burt of Northwestern University, who treated patients so crippled by autoimmune diseases that they had been living on a ventilator. One woman, Grace Meihaus, was diagnosed with scleroderma at the age of seventeen, an extremely painful disease in which the immune system attacks the body and creates inflammation and the overproduction of collagen. Scleroderma eventually turns the skin and organs into stone-like hardness. Patients can literally become hard like sculptures. Grace felt her body became tight and constricted, and she had shortness of breath and became easily fatigued. Another young woman, Elizabeth Cougentakis, had been suffering from myasthenia gravis to the point where her muscles were so weakened that she was bedridden, supported by a ventilator, and fed by feeding tube. Her regular doctors had little else to offer. Burt felt regenerative therapy could be beneficial, and he injected each patient with their own stem cells.[35] After the treatments, the patients soon felt improvement and rapidly recovered their function. They both went on to live normal lives and were vibrant and able to travel to the Vatican, completely well, to tell us in person about their experience. In April 2018, the Vatican convened another medical event called Unite to Cure, in which other remarkable stem cell applications were described, including the treatment of cerebral palsy and autism, with exciting early signs of benefit.

Regenerative healing, however, doesn't rely only on injecting stem cells. Some techniques coax the patient's own stem cells to spring into action. Recall that the placenta is a reservoir for cells and proteins needed for tissue regeneration during pregnancy. The thin membrane of the placenta, called the amniotic membrane, has been used by surgeons to heal wounds. The amniotic membrane contains more than 256 growth and regenerative factors and cytokines that can attract stem cells. When a surgeon places the membrane on a slow-to-heal wound, the regenerative factors are released, stem cells are recruited from the patient's bone marrow, and they home in on the wound. Clinical trials using this membrane have shown vastly improved healing in patients with diabetic foot ulcers and in venous ulcers compared to conservative wound care techniques.[36] In 2012, I identified the mechanism involving recruiting a patient's own stem cells and coined the term *stem cell magnet* to describe any method in which a technology outside the body can be applied to attract a patient's own stem cells to a site that needs to be regenerated.[37]

Another approach to attract a patient's own stem cells for healing involves delivering ultrasound waves to the skin. A special device called MIST sprays a fine shower of water droplets in front of a beam of low-frequency ultrasound. When the spray is aimed at a wound, the water drops pick up the sound energy and land on the patient's wound, where it is released into the tissue. This sends a signal to stem cells in the bone marrow and recruits them into the circulatory system and then to the wound. Because this approach regenerates tissue from the inside out, MIST has even been used to prevent bedsores, also known as pressure ulcers. These are wounds that form when a person lies in one position for an extended period of time without moving, such as in a hospital or nursing home. Up to one-third of nursing home patients have these wounds.[38] They can swiftly become a medical catastrophe as infection sets in and the wound worsens until muscle and bone are exposed. Before a bedsore opens up, the entire area under the skin starts to die. This is known as deep tissue injury. If nothing is done, the skin will eventually break down and a wound cavity opens up, exposing flesh underneath. MIST has been used to prevent bedsores by treating deep tissue injury. The treatment is aimed at reversing the injury underneath dying but still intact skin. Sound-energized water droplets hit the skin, and the energy recruits stem cells that home to the deep tissue injury and improve its blood flow, thus preventing a wound from occurring.

Simply put, regenerative medicine is already changing the way medicine is practiced, and it will lead to future ways to conquer diseases that are now considered vexing and unbeatable.

Foods and Stem Cells

Regeneration doesn't rely only on advanced technologies in the medical clinic. Now you can jump-start your body's regenerative defense in your kitchen. Foods and beverages can activate a person's own stem cells, boosting the body's capacity to regenerate and heal itself from within. This is an entirely new approach to regeneration that doesn't require a doctor, hospital, or injections. Dietary regeneration taps into your own stem cell reservoir to restore health. Some foods enhance stem cell activity and foster regeneration, while other foods have been found to injure stem cells, rendering them impotent. Stunning your stem cells is obviously not a desirable goal—unless they are cancer stem cells, in which case, it could be life-saving. Some foods can do that as well. Whether you are healthy and want to optimize your strength or simply age gracefully, or you have a serious chronic condition, like heart disease, Alzheimer's disease, diabetes, or even cancer, there's a way to use diet to direct stem cells to help you heal from inside out. In part 2, I will tell you all about the foods that influence your stem cells and how they can be used to improve your health.

SOME CONDITIONS IN WHICH REGENERATION IS NEEDED

Acute brain injury	Heart failure
Age-related macular degeneration	Hypercholesterolemia
Alopecia	Kidney failure
Alzheimer's disease	Liver disease
Atherosclerosis	Multiple sclerosis
Autism	Myasthenia gravis
Blindness	Myocardial infarction
Cancer (all)	Osteoarthritis
Cerebral atrophy	Osteoporosis
Cerebral palsy	Parkinson's disease
Chronic wounds	Peripheral arterial disease
Deep tissue injury	Scleroderma
Dementia	Spinal cord injury
Depression	Stroke
Diabetes	Vascular dementia
Erectile dysfunction	

CHAPTER 3

Microbiome

In an age of ever-expanding identities, here's a new one. You are no longer simply human—you are a holobiont. The term *holobiont* describes an organism that functions as an assemblage of multiple species that are mutually beneficial. You are a holobiont because your body is not a singular entity, but rather a highly complex ecosystem including 39 trillion bacteria, mostly good, teeming inside and on your body's surface. These bacteria are plentiful: their quantity roughly matches that of your own cells (about 37 trillion), and combined, they weigh about three pounds, the equivalent heft of your brain.[1] They are amazingly hardy, resisting stomach acid and the chemical cauldron of your intestines.

While the medical community once thought of microorganisms as nasty disease vectors that should be scrubbed off, sterilized, and killed with antibiotics, we now know that the majority of bacteria within our body work in highly sophisticated ways to defend our health and even influence our behavior. Far from being passive squatters, healthy bacteria, collectively called the microbiome, form a complex biological system that interacts with your cells and organs in many ways. (This system also includes fungi, viruses, and microorganisms known as archea, but bacteria will be the focus of this chapter.)

We are learning more every day from researchers around the world about our microbiome and how it fosters health and even helps to conquer diseases like cancer. Some gut bacteria, like *Lactobacillus plantarum*, *Lactobacillus rhamnosus*, and *Bacillus mycoides*, have endocrine or hormonal functions and can even produce and release brain neurotransmitters such as oxytocin, serotonin, GABA (γ-aminobutyric acid), and dopamine. These chemicals activate brain signals that profoundly influence our mood.[2] Some bacteria release metabolites that can protect us against diabetes. Others control the growth of abdominal fat. One type of gut bacteria, *Bifidobacteria*, was shown to reduce stress and anxiety through a unique gut-brain interaction.[3] Our bacteria influence angiogenesis, stem cells, and immunity. They can even influence our hormones, sexual fitness, and social behavior. They can nurture our human cells, or they can irritate and inflame them. Our microbiota can make the difference between life and death, between developing a serious disease or resisting it.

Food has an astonishing ability to influence these powers of the microbiome. After all, our bacteria eat what we eat. They metabolize the food and drink we consume and create beneficial (or harmful) byproducts that influence our health. But before we delve into the specifics of how foods influence bacteria, I want to share with you what we are learning about these helpful colonists in our body. There is surprising new research about where they come from and what they do. This is an emerging medical revolution that is harnessing the untapped power of the microbiome defense system in our body to prevent and treat disease.

The Relationship between Humans and Bacteria— Good and Bad

Humans evolved together with bacteria on this planet. At the dawn of *Homo sapiens* three hundred thousand years ago, our hunter-gatherer ancestors ate what they could forage: ancient grains, nuts, legumes, and fruits, all of which contain the high amounts of fiber on which microbes thrive.[4] Food was handpicked from bacteria-laden soil and vegetation, so every bite our remote ancestors swallowed was loaded with microbes from the environment that entered their gut. Even after the first Agricultural Revolution of 10,000 BC, when humans moved away from hunting and gathering to rely on cultivated foods, the staple ingredients remained mostly plant-based. This dietary pattern, high in the fiber that microbes consume and full of bacteria from the environment, shaped our bodies for survival during evolution.[5]

As closely as our destinies were intertwined, for most of history, humans had no idea that bacteria even existed, let alone had knowledge of the role that healthy bacteria plays inside our bodies. But over the last few centuries, science has transformed our understanding of how bacteria contribute to both disease and health. It started with disease. In the early days of the field of microbiology, most of what we learned about bacteria focused on "bad" bacteria—but with good reason. After all, throughout history, devastating epidemics swept the world, indiscriminately killing most everyone in their path. During the Dark Ages, dreaded diseases such as typhoid fever, plague, dysentery, and leprosy were rampant, bringing suffering and death to untold millions. Doctors of the time only had theories about the causes of these diseases. They had even less idea that the unsanitary conditions around them allowed the bacteria to spread. During those times, in most communities around the world, feces, urine, rancid food, and pests all mixed together in homes and in the streets, creating ubiquitous cesspools that allowed bacterial swarms to flourish and spread.

One of medicine's eureka moments came in 1861 during an epidemic of high maternal mortality rates in Vienna. A shocking number of women were dying of infection after delivering babies in one particular obstetric clinic. Ignaz Semmelweis, a doctor at the clinic, noticed a pattern: doctors delivering babies whose mothers died were moving directly from the morgue, where they conducted autopsies on the dead women, back to the delivery suite, where they attended to the next mother in labor. Semmelweis wondered: could whatever had killed the deceased women be traveling back with their doctors to claim new victims? He developed a novel idea: doctors should scrub their hands with an "antiseptic" solution between autopsies and deliveries to clean off the threat. It worked. Maternal mortality rates from infection plummeted to the single digits.[6]

Semmelweis's discovery was a critical moment in the development of sanitary medical procedures. In a next major milestone, Joseph Lister (namesake of the mouthwash) cautioned that hand washing was not nearly enough: all surgical instruments also had to be sterilized in a chemical solution.[7] The result was a reduction of gangrene after surgery. Innovations such as these led to the high standards of sanitization and sterilization in hospitals, operating theaters, and doctors' offices that we take for granted today—and they continue to save millions of lives.

Yet there was an unintended consequence. The more that people learned how to control and eliminate bacteria that could lead to infection, the more pervasive became the idea that all bacteria were harmful. Thus launched the era of germaphobia that continues to this day. Most of us grew up scrubbing off, sterilizing, and avoiding bacteria everywhere we could. The familiar message of bacteria being bad and needing to be destroyed with antibiotics permeated public health and public consciousness. Disinfectants, hand sanitizers, and antimicrobial soaps became household items. In our food system, pesticides, pasteurization, and antibiotics for livestock became widespread, killing bacteria everywhere. In fact, the antibiotic revolution completely changed modern medicine—largely eliminating the destructive epidemics of the past by putting life-saving bacterial killing power in the hands of doctors, hospitals, and public health offices around the world.

Quietly, however, science has been making counterintuitive discoveries. Some bacteria actually confer life-saving health benefits. As early as 1907, one prominent Russian zoologist, Ilya Metchnikoff, began to question if the "all bacteria are bad" orthodoxy might be flawed. During the cholera epidemic of 1892 in France, Metchnikoff mixed bacteria together in a petri dish and found that some bacteria could stimulate cholera growth, but to his surprise found that other bacteria hindered it.[8] This led him to speculate whether swallowing some types of helpful bacteria might be useful for preventing deadly diseases. He was also struck by the fact that some people lived to a ripe old age despite harsh rural conditions and poor hygiene associated with poverty. In Bulgaria, he noted, there were peasants in the Caucasus Mountains who lived beyond one hundred years. He observed that the oldest villagers were drinking fermented yogurt containing the bacteria *Lactobacillus bulgaricus*. Metchnikoff suggested that one secret to longevity is consuming healthy bacteria. History would prove him right (and would also see him win the 1908 Nobel Prize for his pioneering work on immunity).

The Science of the Microbiome

Today, the microbiome is recognized as one of the most exciting and disruptive areas of medical research. It's a fast-growing field. In the year 2000, there were only seventy-four articles published on the microbiome. In 2017, more than 9,600 research articles emerged. The science is advancing so swiftly there's no way to boil it all down to a few take-home points. Entire encyclopedias will be written about our bacterial selves, and the knowledge will transform how we understand our health, as well as the practice of medicine, public health policy, and the ways that the food, supplement, pharmaceutical, and diagnostic testing industries produce future products.

I'm choosing to highlight the insights from current cutting-edge research that will help you make better food decisions today. To make things easier, when I describe foods and the bacteria they influence, I'm only going to name a few selected bacteria associated with a health benefit. This deliberate simplification of a highly complicated field will help you become familiar with the microbiome and not be overwhelmed with bacterial taxonomy and the science of metagenomics.

Just as if you were going to the zoo for the first time, my advice is that you focus on getting the main points of the featured attractions rather than trying to memorize the details of every animal on display. Latin names of bacteria are tongue twisting and difficult to remember. But get used to them, because they are actually part of who you are, and it's certain that in the future, the names of helpful bacteria will become so familiar, children in grade school will know them.

Actinobacteria, Bacteroidetes, Firmicutes, Lactobacillus, Proteobacteria… these are some of the names you will read here, but they are just the beginning. The number of bacteria species worldwide is estimated to be more than 1 billion. The vast majority have no direct relationship with humans, but many other varieties have evolved to thrive within our own bodies. There are more than one thousand known species of gut bacteria. More than five hundred species of bacteria have been found in the human mouth, with any individual's mouth commonly containing twenty-five species or more. A milliliter of saliva (about one-fifth of a teaspoon) contains up to 100 million oral bacteria.[9] That's a population almost three times larger than the Tokyo metropolitan area (37 million people) in one swallow.

To unravel the mysteries of the human microbiome, the National Institutes of Health launched the Human Microbiome Project in 2008, inspired by the Human Genome Project.[10] The project published a landmark paper in the prestigious scientific journal *Nature* in 2012 documenting the bacteria of the microbiome of 242 individuals. The study examined multiple sites on the body of each volunteer, over multiple occasions. The body sites probed included mouth, nose, skin, gut, and genital tract. The researchers found that microbial diversity was enormous. Not only did individuals vary greatly in the number and diversity of species in their microbiomes, but the bacteria present in different sites from the same individual's body also varied greatly. No single group of bacteria was universal to everybody, even among healthy individuals.[11]

Microbiome diversity is an important hallmark of health. As with human communities, the diversity of our bacterial ecosystem brings strength and more effective collaborations to protect health. The more numerous and diverse bacteria we have, the healthier we become. Like a dazzling coral reef that thrives with many species living in close proximity, the microbiome is an ecosystem that depends upon the delicate balance of community members tolerating each other and working together on behalf of our health.

Our microbiome influences our health in many ways, including through the substances they produce as they process food passing through our gut. The best-known substances are actually bacterial metabolites known as short-chain fatty acids (SCFAs). These are the byproducts of bacteria digestion of plant-based fiber. (Incidentally, when you hear the term "prebiotic," it's often referring to this dietary fiber that feeds the bacteria that produce SCFAs.) SCFAs have been found to have an amazing array of health functions. They protect the gut as well as your overall health through their anti-inflammatory properties, and they have the ability to improve our body's ability to metabolize glucose and lipids.[12] SCFAs also improve immunity, guide angiogenesis, and aid stem cells, as a connection between four of your health defense systems. Both *Lactobacillus* and *Bifidobacteria* are considered beneficial because they produce SCFAs.

The three major SCFAs—propionate, butyrate, and acetate—each play a unique role in the body. Propionate, for instance, can lower cholesterol, reduce inflammation, protect against buildup of the atherosclerotic plaque in arteries, and improve digestive health.[13] It also activates immune cells.[14] Butyrate is a main form of energy for gut cells in the colon, and it promotes a healthy colon, as well as having anti-inflammatory effects. It also stimulates angiogenesis to nurture wound healing, and it guides stem cells to morph into different types of organs.[15] Acetate is released into peripheral tissues where it stimulates leptin, which suppresses hunger.[16]

Other microbiome metabolites can also foster health. The bacteria *Lactobacillus plantarum*, for example, produces metabolites that stimulate an anti-inflammatory response by intestinal stem cells.[17] This can quiet irritations in the gut and set the stage for intestinal healing. In studies of kimchi, the spicy fermented Korean condiment contains *Lactobacillus plantarum* which has been discovered to produce a bacterial product that protects against influenza A infection.[18] Lignans are plant polyphenols that serve as prebiotics. They are metabolized by the gut microbiome to produce bioactives known as enterodiol and enterolactone. These have been shown to suppress the development of breast cancer.[19] P-cresol and hippurate are also metabolites made in the gut that reduce stress and anxiety (they can be enhanced by eating chocolate).[20] Researchers from the University of Eastern Finland found that a diet rich in whole grains and fiber causes bacteria to produce indolepropionic acid, another metabolite that protects against type 2 diabetes.[21]

There's the flip side. Some substances made by our microbiome can be toxic. So our goal should be to limit their production. For instance, bacteria such as *Desulfovibrio* manufacture hydrogen sulfide, a compound that smells like rotten eggs, which is normally found in volcanoes and hot springs. Hydrogen sulfide is highly toxic to our gut. When it is made by *Desulfovibrio*, it damages the gut lining that normally seals in food and waste contents from the rest of the body. The damage makes the intestines leaky, like perforating a wetsuit, making it easier for food particles and waste from inside the intestines to leak out. Leaking food particles cause an inflammatory reaction around the gut that can generate allergic-like reactions to food and even spark colitis. Not surprisingly, bacteria that produce hydrogen sulfide are found in the stool of patients with inflammatory bowel disease.[22]

Location, Location, Location

Your microbiome is spread all over, especially on the skin and in body cavities. Health-promoting bacteria live on your teeth, gums, tongue, and tonsils and in your nose, lungs, ears, vagina, and especially gut.

The gut is a long tube, approximately thirty feet long, about the length of two pickup trucks. It starts with your mouth and ends with your anus. In between those ends are your stomach, small intestines, and colon. The colon is one of the population centers of your microbiome. Throughout its inside, a layer of sticky mucus protects the gut. This mucus lining forms a barrier to keep any noxious substances you've eaten or generated by digestion or the microbiome inside the gut lining. Both the mucus and the lining can be influenced by gut bacteria. Some bacteria actually thrive in the mucus. Far beyond a simple digestive container, the gut is a command center for your health that is helmed by the microbiome.

Our gut's resident healthy bacteria are put into place before you are born. When I was in medical school, we were taught that the womb of a pregnant mother is sterile, and that healthy bacteria are introduced to a baby only during childbirth as the head is squeezed through the birth canal. The vaginal bacteria are in contact with the baby's lips and bacteria that will colonize the gut is swallowed. The sterile womb idea has been overturned. We now know that healthy bacteria are transferred from the mother to the fetus during pregnancy.[23] Both the placenta and the amniotic fluid in which the fetus floats for nine months contain bacteria that colonize the developing human that contribute to its microbiome and future health.[24] Of course, during vaginal childbirth, bacteria are also transferred to the baby.

Even after the baby is born, the mother is not yet done shaping the microbiome. Newborns are immediately handed to their mother to establish skin contact and closeness with her. The skin-on-skin time puts the infant in contact with bacteria. Then, breastfeeding further loads the baby with microbes.[25] Once again, modern understanding overturns what doctors were once taught in medical school, when they learned that breast milk is a sterile fluid. Wrong. We now know that special cells from the mom's immune system, called dendritic cells, pick up bacteria from her gut and deliver them through lymph channels to the milk ducts of the breast. This means breast milk is chock-full of healthy bacteria destined for the infant's gut. In fact, it's been estimated that almost 30 percent of an infant's gut bacteria comes from its mother's breast milk. Ten percent comes from suckling the nipple and swallowing skin bacteria, and the rest come from other early exposures to the environment.[26] Since an infant consumes about 27 ounces of milk per day, it's estimated that up to 10 million bacteria are swallowed every twenty-four hours. Now, think about the potential impact of antibiotics administered to either the mother or the baby during the period surrounding childbirth. This could diminish critical healthy bacteria in the mother or interfere with their transmission during childbirth and lactation. Infants who are formula fed have substantial differences in their microbiome compared to those who have been breastfed for at least six weeks after delivery.[27]

As an infant switches to a solid food diet, the gut flora change yet again as bacteria and prebiotics in food gain entry into the gut. By the age of three, children have established colonies that will help them defend their health for the rest of their lives. A study of 1,095 "ridiculously healthy people" who have no health issues or family history of serious disease across all age groups (from age three to more than one hundred years old) showed that a common denominator in both young and old is an almost identical microbiome.[28]

The dilemma of how to use antibiotics now faces the medical community. As a doctor, I know the value of antibiotics and know firsthand the benefits of their judicious use. But our growing knowledge of the microbiome is teaching us to think about the consequences of killing the "good guys." Every doctor saw during their training an infection called C. *difficile*. The C stands for *Clostridium*, which, it turns out, is not a foreign invader but a part of the normal microbiome. It is one gut bacterium, however, whose growth needs to be held in check by other bacteria. When sick patients are given antibiotics such as Clindamycin, C. *difficile* can sometimes overgrow and cause an intestinal riot, with severe diarrhea, fever, cramping, and life-threatening complications like bowel perforation and bleeding. But as we learn how our microbiome defends our health, we are rethinking how changing our gut bacteria might contribute to the mysteriously increasing rates of food allergies, diabetes, obesity, cardiovascular disease, cancer, Alzheimer's disease, and even depression. The puzzle is far from solved, but it should make us all the more cautious about the cavalier use of antibiotics and even antiseptics. And it tells us we need to think more about how to keep our gut bacteria in good shape for our overall health. What you eat is one approach.

How Your Diet Affects the Microbiome

How the gut microbiome functions is strongly influenced by our diet. Over the course of your lifetime, sixty tons of food will pass through your digestive tract.[29] What you eat also feeds your bacteria. Prebiotic foods can improve bacterial function. We can also introduce new bacteria into our ecosystem by eating foods that naturally contain healthy microbes. This can be easily achieved by eating some common fermented foods, as you'll see in chapter 8. These are probiotic foods. Other foods modify the environment of the gut, making growth of some bacteria more favorable.

Throughout our lives, we are constantly introducing new bacteria into our body, even exchanging bacteria with friends and family, which then becomes part of our microbiome. A kiss can introduce as many as 80 million bacteria per smooch.[30] But the most common entry point is through eating. Foods that affect the microbiome are either probiotics or prebiotics. Probiotic foods such as yogurt, sauerkraut, kimchi, and cheese contain living bacteria and thus bring their own bacterial contributions to our inner ecosystem. One renowned cheese illustrates this effect: Camembert, a soft, creamy, pungent cow's milk cheese made in

France. Researchers from the French National Institute for Agricultural Research and the Paris Descartes University studied the effects of Camembert cheese on twelve healthy human volunteers who were given three dice-size cubes of cheese (forty grams) cut from the same batch of cheese, to eat twice per day for four weeks.[31] They collected stool samples from the participants once before the study, twice throughout the study, and once more a month following. They examined the cheese samples for microbes, and also checked for any changes in the stool bacteria. The researchers found several organisms of note. One is the fungus called *Geotrichum candidum* that is not normally present in humans but is found in the starter culture for Camembert cheesemaking. This proves that an organism originating in cheese can make it all the way through the gut. The bacteria *Leuconostoc mesenteroides*, used in the starter bacterial culture, was also found in the stool. And *Lactobacillus plantarum*, a bacteria found in both Camembert and healthy human microbiome, was increased in the humans after consuming the Camembert daily. So, not only does eating cheese introduce new bacteria into the gut, but it influenced the bacteria already there.

Prebiotics are nondigestible foods that feed the healthy bacteria in our intestines. They themselves are not microbes, but rather they increase the function of healthy gut bacteria by providing the food they need to thrive and, as a consequence, create healthy metabolites or influence the immune system. Typically, prebiotics are dietary fibers which are metabolized by the microbiota to form a number of beneficial metabolites, notably the SCFAs mentioned earlier. We will discuss different probiotic and prebiotic foods in more detail in part 2.

Other ways that our food can affect the microbiome is by altering the gut environment so that it is favorable to growing healthy bacteria. Think of bacteria species in the gut as competing sports teams. They are each training and preparing to test themselves against each other to gain dominance. Giving one species the food they prefer can fuel their growth over another team, giving them a competitive edge. Researchers are finding out there is a whole subfield of microbiome nutrition, in which the proportion of sugar, fat, and fiber in food can determine which bacteria in the gut wind up becoming dominant.

Small changes in the environment can also favor one species over another. In the tunnel of the gut, the mucus coating the gut wall is home to some bacteria. The mucus contains a gel-forming carbohydrate that helps it maintain its coating property. This carbohydrate is also used by gut bacteria to metabolize food. Certain foods can affect the mucosal lining and help these bacteria by enhancing their environment. *Akkermansia* is one important beneficial bacteria in our microbiome that lives and thrives in the intestinal mucus lining. Eating foods that increase the gut mucus, like cranberries or pomegranates, helps *Akkermansia* grow. These foods will be covered in part 2.

Microbiome and Future Generations

At the same time that we are learning about how bacteria inside you influence your health, other research is revealing how your microbiome can be passed on to future generations, as the legacy of the lifestyle you've led. As mentioned earlier, the more diverse the bacteria in our gut ecosystem, the healthier we are. However, scientists from Stanford, Harvard, and Princeton studying diet and microbiome have shown that, if we're not careful, the way we eat can actually force the extinction of some gut bacteria, which can impact on the health of future generations. The scientists conducted experiments with germ-free mice implanted with gut bacteria obtained from a healthy human. This involved introducing fecal matter from a healthy human volunteer into a mouse's gut, so the bacteria would colonize the mouse and replicate the ecosystem found in the healthy human gut.

In one study, the scientists switched the diet of a group of these mice from a low-fat, high-fiber diet (resembling a plant-based diet that is healthy for both humans and beneficial bacteria) to an unhealthy high-fat and low-fiber diet (Western-like) for seven weeks. This diet switch changed everything in the microbiome. A whopping 60 percent of the diverse bacteria that were originally present in the healthy volunteer reacted to the unhealthy diet by reducing their numbers by half. It gets worse. When the scientists switched the mice back to the healthier plant-based diet, only 30 percent of the decreased bacteria recovered to their previous levels. In fact, the overall microbiome profile remained changed for as long as fifteen weeks (about 10 percent of the life of a mouse) afterward. The scientists concluded that some healthy bacteria are resilient and can bounce back from a dietary insult, while others cannot. They called the persistent defect a "scar" left on the microbiome due to diet.

Here's where it gets interesting in this study. The microbiome scar became larger over generations when the researchers began breeding the mice and exposing each generation of mice to the high-fat, low-fiber Western-style diet. With each generation, more and more of the original bacteria from the healthy human disappeared from their microbiome. By the fourth generation (great-grandchildren of the original), a sobering 72 percent of the microbes from the initial healthy mice were no longer detectable. Generations of eating the same unhealthy high-fat, low-fiber diet killed off healthy gut microbes permanently.[32] They became extinct and could not be regenerated by the healthier plant-based diet as before.

Even in the short term, unhealthy diets wreak havoc on your microbiome and leave a scar that takes time to recover even after you return to eating a healthier diet. These scars can create serious imbalances in your health. Because the microbiome is tied to other health defense systems, an unhealthy diet can by extension damage your angiogenesis defense, disrupt your stem cell function, make it harder for your body to protect its DNA, and compromise your immune system.[33] This is serious because some bacteria activate your immune defenses to protect against cancer and infections. Other beneficial bacteria turn down the immune response, preventing allergic reactions to the foods that enter the gut. I'll provide more details on this when we discuss the immune system in detail in chapter 5.

Microbiome and Disease

Although modern civilization spent most of the twentieth century fighting diseases caused by microbes, in the twenty-first century, we may be fighting disease using bacteria. I began to appreciate the potential of this when I heard a lecture by Susan Erdman, who heads up the Division of Comparative Medicine at the Massachusetts Institute of Technology in Boston. As cochair of an annual wound healing conference, I had invited her to present her research on a bacteria called *Lactobacillus reuteri*, a species that is part of the human microbiome. Erdman described her research showing how this bacteria can make wounds heal faster. Her talk was riveting. She presented convincing data that *L. reuteri*, which is found in some yogurts and as a dietary supplement, could accelerate wound healing in mice if it was put in their drinking water. It also worked in humans when given as a probiotic. Afterward, Erdman and I collaborated on research to understand how these bacteria helped speed up healing. The answer: *L. reuteri*, when swallowed, speeds up angiogenesis in healing skin wounds. Yet another connection was made between the health defense systems.

But wound healing was only the beginning. In the lab, *L. reuteri* also reduced abdominal fat and obesity in mice, even if they ate a junk food diet of potato chips. *L. reuteri* can stimulate the growth of thick, shiny, healthy hair; improve skin tone; boost the immune system; and prevent the growth of tumors in the colon and in the breast. And that's not all. Experiments have shown that in male mice, *L. reuteri* in drinking water increases testicular size, testosterone production, and mating frequency. A truly fascinating finding was that *L. reuteri* stimulates the brain to release the hormone oxytocin, which is the social bonding neurochemical that is released from the brain during a hug or handshake, by close friendship, during kissing, breast feeding, and orgasm. The depth of research conducted with this one bacteria is so impressive it led to an article in *The New York Times* called "Microbes, a Love Story."[34] Needless to say, this is a probiotic worthy of taking because of the scientific evidence for its actions and potential benefits.

Microbiome out of Balance

Dysbiosis is the severe disturbances in the bacterial ecosystem, an imbalance of gut bacteria that is linked to diseases as far ranging as diabetes, obesity, autism, inflammatory bowel disease, infectious colitis, irritable bowel syndrome, cancer, asthma, psoriasis, multiple sclerosis, Parkinson's disease, Alzheimer's disease, atherosclerosis, heart failure, celiac disease, liver disease, chronic fatigue syndrome, cavities, schizophrenia, and depression.[35] The exact microbe or mechanisms of microbial imbalance leading to each of these conditions and whether they are the cause or effect are under investigation by some of the rising stars of scientific research. Meanwhile, the medical establishment is starting to take notice. A once widely used, and now banned, antimicrobial chemical, Triclosan, which used to be in toothpaste, soaps, detergents, and more than two thousand consumer products, was discovered to disrupt the gut microbiome in infants and increase colitis as well as tumor development in mice.[36]

The biotechnology industry is eager to tap into the power of the microbiome. A procedure known as fecal microbial transplantation (FMT) has been developed to treat dysbiosis by replacing unhealthy gut bacteria with beneficial gut bacteria from the stool of a healthy donor. The procedure has been used to treat patients suffering from *Clostridium difficile* colitis, often a complication of antibiotic use, as discussed before. Although the standard of care is to use more antibiotics to kill C. *difficile*, infection recurs in up to 60 percent of people. In those situations, doctors are turning to FMT. A healthy donor is asked to provide a fecal sample, which is mixed with water, and then sprayed along the entire inside of the colon by a doctor using a colonoscope. Despite the ick factor of FMT, its proponents claim the procedure is curative in about 90 percent of the cases after a single treatment. Clinical trials are underway to see if FMT can help prevent or cure recurrent urinary tract infections, chronic constipation, diabetes, ulcerative colitis, and even obesity.

Some biotechnology companies are developing special formulas of probiotics, dietary fiber, and plant bioactives as a smoothie to promote healthy bacteria regrowth in the gut as a means to treat diabetes, obesity, and other conditions. Other companies are taking a diagnostic approach, offering to analyze your stool and give you a report on your microbiota. A stool test called SmartGut sequences the DNA of bacteria in your feces and tells you if there are any bad actors and actions to take. A vaginal microbiota test called SmartJane identifies not only sexually transmitted diseases but twenty-three types of healthy vaginal bacteria.

Probiotic supplements are touted as an easy way to introduce healthy bacteria into our gut, but despite the massive industry that exists—$36 billion in 2016 and expected to grow to $65 billion by 2024—the jury is still out on their efficacy.[37] Probiotic products containing *Lactobacillus* and *Bifidobacteria*, for example, are available at the grocery store and drugstore, and through online shopping. The challenge is that most commercial probiotics are not that well studied compared to the foods you'll learn about in chapter 8. Generally, however, they are accepted as safe in people with healthy immune systems, and potentially helpful for ameliorating diarrhea and other digestive disturbances.

Diet may well be the most powerful tool for influencing our microbiome. Natural foods offer a more diverse source—for instance, yogurt, fermented foods, and some drinks are loaded with bacteria. But even when you aren't directly consuming probiotic bacteria, what we eat has the most profound day-to-day effect on our microbiome defense system. Our diet can shrink or expand the different populations of gut microbiota on an hour-to-hour basis. The foods you eat affect your gut's ability to heal, sometimes in surprising ways. In part 2, I will tell you how eating different types of food can interact with and build your microbiome for the better. For example, you can influence the population of one particular kind of beneficial bacteria in your gut, which in turn has been shown to make some cancer treatments more effective.

But first, I want to share with you another powerful defense system your body possesses to keep you healthy: the body's mechanisms for protecting your DNA.

CONDITIONS WITH DYSBIOSIS OF THE MICROBIOME

Alzheimer's disease	Gallbladder cancer
Asthma	Heart failure
Atherosclerosis	Irritable bowel syndrome
Autism	Leaky gut syndrome
Bipolar disorder	Liver disease
Breast cancer	Metabolic syndrome
Celiac disease	Multiple sclerosis
Chronic fatigue syndrome	Obesity
Chronic obstructive pulmonary disease	Pancreatic cancer
Colorectal cancer	Parkinson's disease
Crohn's disease	Psoriasis
Depression	Rheumatoid arthritis
Diabetes	Schizophrenia
Esophageal cancer	Stomach cancer
Food allergies	Ulcerative colitis

MICROBIOME KEY PLAYERS

Major Bacterial Phyla	
Bacteroidetes	Bacteroidetes make up the second largest portion of the microbiome. Many of them are SCFA-producing bacteria.
Firmicutes	The Firmicutes make up the largest portion of the microbiome, and are the most diverse. The major beneficial SCFA-producing bacterias are within the Firmicutes phylum, but other strains have been shown to be pathogenic.
Proteobacteria	Proteobacteria is generally considered harmful in excess. Several studies demonstrate an increased abundance of proteobacteria in metabolic disorders and inflammatory bowel disease.
Actinobacteria	Actinobacteria is generally considered beneficial. The phylum contains *Bifidobacteria*, which is commonly included in probiotic supplements.
Verrucomicrobia	Verrucomicrobia is a very small, recently discovered phylum. It is notable for containing the beneficial bacteria *Akkermansia*.

Notable Beneficial Bacteria		
Genus/Strain	*Phylum*	
Akkermansia muciniphila (strain)	Verrucomicrobia	Beneficial; increased by certain dietary polyphenols. Helps to control immune system, improves blood glucose metabolism, decreases gut inflammation, and combats obesity. Improves the efficacy of certain cancer treatments.
Bacteroides (genus)	Bacteroidetes	Neutral; associated with higher protein and animal fat consumption. Responsible for glycan-cleavage.
Bifidobacteria (genus)	Actinobacteria	Beneficial; commonly included in probiotic supplements. Produces SCFAs.
L. casei (strain)	Firmicutes	Beneficial; commonly included in probiotic supplements, and found naturally in fermented dairy products. Protective against gastroenteritis, diabetes, cancer, obesity, and even post-partum depression.

MICROBIOME KEY PLAYERS (cont.)

Genus/Strain	Phylum	
L. plantarum (strain)	Firmicutes	Beneficial; commonly included in probiotic supplements. Found naturally in fermented food products such as sauerkraut and Gouda cheese. Produces riboflavin, a B vitamin.
L. reuteri (strain)	Firmicutes	Beneficial; found in probiotic supplements, fermented dairy products, and sourdough bread. Benefits immunity, resists development of breast and colon tumors, influences the gut-brain axis to produce the social hormone, oxytocin, stimulates angiogenesis.
L. rhamnosus (strain)	Firmicutes	Beneficial; found in probiotic supplements and fermented dairy products. Most commonly found in the healthy female genitourinary tract and are helpful supplements in the case of bacterial overgrowth infections.
Prevotella (genus)	Bacteroidetes	Beneficial; associated with plant-rich diets. Produces SCFAs.
Ruminococcus (genus)	Firmicutes	Beneficial; found in probiotic supplements and associated with increased bean consumption. Produces SCFAs.
Harmful Bacteria		
Genus/Strain	Phylum	
Clostridium (genus)	Firmicutes	Harmful; this genus contains several pathogenic bacteria strains, such as C. difficile (causes diarrhea) and C. botulinum (botulism).
C. histolyticum (strain)	Firmicutes	Harmful; pathogenic bacterial strain within the Clostridium genus. Known for causing gas gangrene.
Desulfovibrionaceae (genus)	Proteobacteria	Harmful; sulfate-reducing bacteria. Hydrogen sulfide injures the gut lining. Can result in increased gut permeability and inflammation.

CHAPTER 4

DNA Protection

Picture your DNA as your personal genetic blueprint, twisted into the shape of a spiral staircase (called a double helix) and miniaturized to fit inside a cell. The staircase is made up of the genes you inherited from your parents. This is the source code that every aspect of your health depends upon to keep you alive and able to function normally. Yet, DNA is quite fragile and is the target of vicious attacks throughout your life.

Your DNA sustains more than ten thousand naturally occurring damaging events every single day.[1] Some of the errors are spontaneous breaks that occur as a matter of chance when trillions of cells are working and replicating nonstop, day in and day out. Other errors are a side effect of something destructive that's happening within the body, like inflammation or an infection. And still others are the result of toxic chemicals in the air we breathe, in the foods we swallow, and otherwise absorb through our skin from household products and other environmental sources. However they happen, each error has the potential for derailing our DNA and wreaking havoc on our health. Given this daily onslaught of DNA damage, you might wonder why we don't get sick more often, become mutants, or form deadly cancers every day. It's because our DNA is hardwired to defend and protect itself and thus our health against the consequences of this damage.

Much of what you hear about DNA day to day concerns ancestry, but there are important breakthroughs for genetic screening that aid in detecting your personal risk for hereditary cancers and other diseases.

Genomic testing is also being used to guide cancer therapy in the new era of personalized medicine. You may also have heard about technologies that can be used to edit DNA and replace defective genes with healthy ones. But, the most amazing story of DNA is the one I'm about to tell you: how it works as one of our health defense systems.

When our DNA is damaged for any reason, errors can occur in the way our genetic instructions are followed in the body. When mutations in our genes are inherited, disastrous diseases can result. As we age, our DNA becomes worn down. As we go through life, the choices we make—where we live, what we eat, our lifestyle—either help or hurt our DNA. Protecting our DNA is critical if we want to be healthy. When the human genetic code works perfectly, we are in good health. When it breaks down, or mutates, our health is threatened.

Our DNA uses distinct mechanisms to protect itself. Our cells have evolved with powerful repair processes that constantly monitor our DNA for structural abnormalities. If any are spotted, the repair crew reviews the multiple sets of identical information encoded by the DNA. The damaged sections of DNA are clipped out by molecular scissors in our cells and swapped out with the correct structure and sequence. This prevents the vast majority of abnormalities that might develop on our DNA from being passed on when the DNA replicates itself.

Another way the DNA defense system works is through a response called epigenetic change. This allows DNA to react to environmental and lifestyle exposures, including diet, by amplifying helpful genes and blocking detrimental ones. This makes certain genes more or less available depending on the circumstances.

Telomeres are another key to protecting DNA. Telomeres are like aglets, the caps that cover the tips of shoelaces, sitting at both ends of your chromosomes. They shield your DNA from the wear and tear as you age. A good diet, quality sleep, regular exercise, and other healthy activities can protect your telomeres.

Diet plays an important role in optimizing the power of these DNA protection systems. In part 2, I will share details on which foods have been discovered to support DNA repair, which ones cause health-promoting epigenetic changes, and which protect and even enhance telomeres. Along with the modern progress being made with genomic testing, gene editing, and gene therapy, we are beginning to decipher how diet impacts our DNA health defense system. To see how far we've come, and understand the role of diet, it's helpful to look back, briefly, at the origin story of DNA research.

A History of DNA

Even though grade school children now learn about DNA, remarkably, we've known about DNA for only about 150 years, and cracked its code in the last fifty. The study of inheritance is traced back to a scientist and Augustinian friar from a town called Brno in Moravia (now Czech Republic). His name was Gregor Mendel. Mendel noticed that peas growing in his garden could be crossbred in combinations to achieve certain traits, such as color and shape. In 1866, he published his research showing there were certain rules that applied to the passage of traits from one generation to the next.[2] These are called the rules of Mendelian inheritance—and Mendel speculated that some invisible factors (genes) carried the information that would determine the traits of any organism.

The first actual physical evidence for DNA was discovered in 1869 by Friedrich Miescher, a doctor conducting research in Tubingen, Germany.[3] Miescher was examining wound pus taken from the bandages of soldiers injured in the Crimean War. He found some unusual material that he believed came from the inside of cells. He named it nuclein. Twelve years later, in 1881, Miescher's former professor, the German biochemist Albrecht Kossel, felt it worth examining the findings more closely. Kossel worked out that nuclein was made of deoxyribonucleic acid—and coined the term *DNA*. In 1910, this discovery won him the first of several Nobel Prizes given for research on DNA.

The true nature of DNA, however, remained a black box mystery for another seventy-one years. Then, in 1952, the first high-resolution pictures of DNA were taken by Rosalind Franklin, working at King's College in London. Guided by the images, James Watson and Francis Crick worked out the structure of DNA the following year at Cambridge University, effectively cracking the "code of life," for which they received the second Nobel Prize for DNA in 1962. After this, tens of thousands of scientists rushed into the field of DNA research to unlock the secrets of the source code that makes us human.

In 1990, one of the most ambitious scientific undertakings in all of human history began: the Human Genome Project. The goal of this massive undertaking, which involved more than twenty universities across the United States, France, Germany, Spain, United Kingdom, China, and Japan, as well as the National Institutes of Health and a private company called Celera Genomics—was to map out every gene in the human body. On April 14, 2003, beating its own fifteen-year deadline by two years, the U.S. government announced that the entire human genome had been officially sequenced. This milestone achievement was led by two pioneering scientists, Francis Collins and Craig Venter.[4] Since then, the complete sequencing of the genome has gone beyond humans to include other species, including chimpanzees, dogs, mice, and even frogs.

The Science of DNA

The source code of DNA is written in chemicals with names that begin with one of four letters: A (adenine), T (thymine), C (cytosine), or G (guanine). The steps of the spiral staircase are made of different combinations of pairings of these letters (A-T and C-G). A sequence of these pairings that encodes instructions for a complete protein is known as a gene, which would be akin to a group of steps on the spiral staircase. Collectively, your genes spell out the instructions needed to make the ten thousand proteins your body needs to stay alive.

Amazingly, every cell in your body knows how to read this source code. Cells use the code by downloading it into cellular machinery that acts like a miniature 3-D printer, manufacturing proteins based on the code. The production of these proteins happens behind the scenes, silently, every single second of your life—from the moment you were conceived until the moment you die. When you hear the term *human genome*, it is referring to the complete collection of genes, made up of DNA, that are required to code for what your body needs over the course of your life.

To set the stage for how the genome stays healthy, first consider the mind-blowing amount of DNA inside your body. Each cell contains about six feet of DNA spooled into coils that form tight packages called chromosomes, of which each cell has forty-six inside its nucleus (twenty-three come from your mother, and twenty-three from your father). If you were to pull and straighten out the DNA from all of the cells in your body (current estimate is 37.2 trillion cells) and line them up end to end, you'd have a genetic superhighway extending 42 billion miles long.[5] That's the distance from Earth to Pluto, times ten! Here's the really interesting thing: only 3 percent of this DNA superhighway actually makes up our genes. The other 97 percent of DNA serves as air traffic control to guide the body on how the genes are used.

Just like at a busy airport, where highly trained operators in air traffic control ensure that planes take off and land safely, precision in DNA function is absolutely essential. Errors can have deadly consequences. When the source code is damaged, the 3-D printers in your cells can manufacture too much of a harmful protein or too little of a useful one, or even make the wrong protein altogether, or a defective one. These errors can have dire consequences, just like misdirection by air traffic control can lead to near misses, minor accidents, or total annihilation of a plane and its passengers.

DNA Damage Dangers

Unfortunately, our world is a really dangerous place for DNA. Many external factors pose threats because they can disrupt and damage our source code. Although many dangers are created by industry, not all of the threats are manmade. One of the most harmful factors to DNA is, in fact, ultraviolet radiation. Sunshine. Do you always remember to wear sunscreen when you go outside? Research has shown that the harmful UV radiation from the sun that penetrates our skin is capable of producing 100,000 lesions in our DNA *every hour* if unshielded.[6] And going indoors after lying out on the beach doesn't mean the assault on your DNA is over. Scientists at Yale University have shown that the damage continues even after sun exposure. The melanin pigment in your skin, which tans you and absorbs radiation, actually stores the energy through a process called chemiexcitation. The pent-up energy is released once you are indoors and it continues to cause mutating DNA damage in skin cells for more than three hours even though you are no longer in the sun and cooling off indoors.[7]

Tanning at the beach can be harmful to health, of course, but there are other insidious ways your DNA is damaged by the sun. If you have ever sat in traffic on your morning commute with the sun streaming through your windshield, UV radiation was damaging your DNA the entire car ride. Even more invisible is what happens when you fly in an airplane. Do you wear sunscreen every time you get on a flight? You should. A 2015 study by researchers from the University of California, San Francisco published in the journal *JAMA Dermatology* showed that pilots flying for just one hour at thirty thousand feet altitude receive the same amount of

UV radiation through the cockpit window as they would from a twenty-minute session in a tanning salon.[8] Counterintuitively, cloudy weather makes things even worse. For a pilot and passengers, clouds just reflect the radiation from their tops right back at the airplane, increasing the risk of DNA damage and melanoma.

The sun is not the only threat. Damaging radiation also emanates from the ground. This is in the form of radon, an odorless natural gas that enters homes through basements. Different parts of the earth emit different levels of radon, but it is an invisible home invader that damages DNA. In fact, radon is the number one cause of lung cancer in nonsmokers.[9] If you smoke (you shouldn't), the radon you inhale at home amplifies the lung cancer risk caused by cigarettes.

On its own accord, tobacco smoke is toxic to DNA. There are an estimated four thousand chemicals inhaled in cigarette smoke, of which seventy have been shown to be carcinogenic, including benzene, arsenic, and formaldehyde.[10] There is nothing recreational or calming about inhaling these chemicals. They provoke inflammation throughout your entire body. Even if you are not a smoker, the bad news is that second-hand smoke is equally harmful to the DNA of unwitting friends, family, coworkers, and even pets.

Solvents off-gassing from carpets, new cars, and chemicals in ordinary household products like nail polish remover, shampoo, and paint damage DNA, too. If you drive a car that uses gasoline, when you fill up the tank, you are breathing in fumes containing benzene, which damages DNA.[11] It is wise to stand upwind of the vapor while you are at the gas station.

Research is revealing that these toxic exposures that damage DNA can even affect future generations. For example, the DNA in a father's sperm can be affected by toxic chemicals like bisphenol A (used to make plastic), diethyl phthalate (used to make glow sticks), and cadmium (found in ceramic glazes and cigarette smoke). These exposures alter the genes in sperm through epigenetic mechanisms, and the alterations can be passed onto his offspring.[12] Similarly, noxious chemicals such as benzene (in petroleum), perchloroethylene (used in dry cleaning), and cigarette smoke that a mother may be exposed to during pregnancy can leave its marks on the fetus's DNA, which will persist in the child for the rest of its life.[13]

DNA damage can make you sick or even kill you. But, DNA has one prime directive: to be passed on as intact as possible from one generation to the next. To ensure that it can fulfill this destiny, DNA has defense mechanisms to fight back against harmful exposures. Let's have a look at them, because in chapter 9 we'll see how these defenses can be powerfully enhanced by what we eat.

The First DNA Health Defense: DNA Repair

The amount of DNA damage that occurs every day is staggering, but our DNA has been hardwired to repair most of the damage before it ever becomes a problem. Fewer than one of every one thousand errors introduced to our DNA are estimated to become permanent mutations, thanks to built-in self-repair enzymes. These enzymes perform an intricate dance at the molecular level as they go to work. Their repair ability is perfectly designed to fix DNA's unique structure.

Recall that in every strand of normal DNA, each "step" of the twisted staircase that makes up the double helix contains two molecules. DNA has a strict rule for how the molecules can be paired. Adenine (A) is always paired with thymine (T). Cytosine (C) is always paired with guanine (G). This is called base pairing. Some common forms of DNA damage disrupt these pairings. About one hundred times per day in each cell, cytosine (C) spontaneously transforms into a different chemical compound, creating pairings that don't follow the rules. Exposure to solar radiation is another trigger that can cause two thymine (T) molecules to stick together, creating an abnormal set of chemical conjoined twins that can't function normally. Severe damage can also be caused by free radicals. These natural chemicals contain a highly unstable oxygen atom that can release energy into its surroundings like a chemical grenade, damaging the orderly pairings of normal DNA.

Your cells contain repair enzymes that can spot and fix this kind of damage. The enzymes spring into action when they see deviations from the orderly structure of the DNA double helix. When missing or damaged sections of DNA are identified, they are replaced with normal parts. Like a tailor repairing a damaged garment, the repair enzymes match the material and sew it in to make it as seamless as possible. The material that is matched in DNA repair is drawn from the nucleosides A, T, C or G, and they are replaced in the correct order where they belong in the double helix.

Scientific and clinical research has shown that eating certain foods can reduce DNA damage, either by increasing the speed and efficiency of the repair process after damage or by preventing damage in the first place. Antioxidants are often thought of as protectors of DNA, and their benefits have been heavily marketed by the supplement industry. Yes, antioxidants can help prevent damage by neutralizing free radicals that float around in our bloodstream, but they cannot help DNA after the damage has been done. At that point, DNA repair mechanisms are needed. We will explore the foods that influence DNA protection and repair, including new ways to use antioxidants for health, in chapter 9.

When the DNA repair system springs into action, the cell knows it has to limit the ripple effect of any damage that has occurred. So, it puts the brakes on the cycle of replication, which cells use to copy themselves, including their DNA. This ensures that damaged DNA is less likely to be passed on. If there is just too much damage to fix, a cell can trigger its own demise through a process called apoptosis, a special self-destruct program that leads to a cell's death when it is no longer able to serve its function in the body.

It is worth mentioning that biotechnology companies are exploring ways to tap into the DNA repair process used by bacteria to create new genetic treatments for a whole host of diseases in humans, plants, and even insects. This is known as CRISPR (pronounced like *crisper*), which stands for clustered regularly interspaced short palindromic repeats. CRISPR is naturally found in about 50 percent of bacteria and is used to cut out and remove foreign genetic elements as part of the bacteria's own defense system. Scientists have discovered that this cutting mechanism can be adapted to "edit" human genes—in other words, it can surgically slice out diseased genes to inactivate their abnormal function, so that normal healthy genes can be biotechnologically put in their place. When the CRISPR system was published in 2012, it immediately transformed the genetics industry because it is so much more accurate, adaptable, and nimble than any other known genetic modification system. While the promise of CRISPR for treating human disease is still on the horizon, it is already being used as a powerful tool for studying genetic engineering.[14]

The Second DNA Health Defense: Epigenetic Change

Contrary to popular belief, your genetic fate is not fixed at birth. Quite the opposite. While your DNA code itself doesn't change, specific genes can be turned on or turned off based on influences you encounter in the environment. This includes what you breathe, touch, and eat during the course of your life. Based on this phenomenon, there is another way DNA can protect your health: epigenetics. The Greek prefix *epi* means on or above or nearby, and you can think of these environmental influences as the factors above the genes that control the expression, or protein-making function, of the gene.

Epigenetics answers the question of why every cell in our body has the same DNA but we have so many different cells with different functionality. The tissue environment around each cell is unique from organ to organ. For example, heart cells express the genes that allow them to generate the electrical current that creates a heartbeat and pumps blood to the body. Genes in the heart are influenced by the microenvironment around heart cells. Cells in the human retina, which is located in the back of the eye, use their DNA to produce proteins that recognize light and transmit a signal that our brain interprets as vision. The retina cells are guided by their immediate environment, as well as by the influence of light itself. Remarkably, both heart and retina cells are using the exact same DNA source code, but the parts they use are different, and this is determined by their organ microenvironment and what the DNA needs to be able to accomplish.

Epigenetic expression is not fixed, even in a single organ. Your DNA responds to external influences from inside and outside of the body, depending upon the circumstances. Stress, mindfulness, sleep, exercise, and pregnancy are just a few internal circumstances that have an epigenetic influence. Some of the external influences that can, for better or worse, epigenetically change your DNA's activities are the food you eat and what you drink. Bioactives found in plant-based foods and in tea or coffee can epigenetically influence your DNA in a positive way. Chemicals found in highly processed foods can influence your DNA too, but negatively. Due to epigenetics, helpful genes can be amplified, and detrimental ones can be blocked.

Forms of Epigenetic Change

Diet and the environment can cause epigenetic change, but understanding how this works is tricky. Methylation and histone modifications are two forms of epigenetic change. Through these mechanisms, DNA protects health by making the right genes active or the wrong genes inactive in response to stimuli. Let's first look at methylation.

Remember the spiral staircase description: the two parallel rims of the stairway are DNA's backbone, while the "steps" are made of the letter pairs A-T or C-G that connect the rims. These pairs are like the teeth of a zipper, running along the entire length of the DNA. When DNA is used, specialized cellular machinery unzips the DNA and reads the teeth, which contain the source code instructions for making proteins. A methyl group is a chemical cluster (CH_3 for science junkies) that can be thrown into the zipper as it's being read. This is called methylation. Methylation changes the way cells read the DNA instructions. Hypermethylation occurs when a lot of methyl groups are thrown into the teeth, creating interference, or a form of DNA sabotage. The zipper can no longer be read in that area, so any proteins that section of DNA is responsible for are not made. In the case of a harmful protein, this epigenetic change can stop that protein from being made, which is a good thing. As with most things in biology, an opposite can also happen, called hypomethylation. This is when a methyl group that normally keeps a gene under wraps is removed. Suddenly, that part of the zipper is free and the gene can make lots of the protein. If the protein that is now unleashed is a beneficial protein, such as one that suppresses cancer, that is a good thing.

Histone modification is another form of epigenetic change that scientists are talking about. Like methylation, this modification makes certain genes more or less available. Histones are proteins inside a cell that are folded into ball-shaped structures. DNA coils itself around these histones. A strand of DNA has multiple histones, so that the strand resembles a climbing rope with thick histone knots tied throughout its length. Special enzymes help unwind DNA from the histone knots, so the protein-making machinery can read the source code. Chemical groups called acetyl groups can be added (acetylation) or removed (deacetylation) from the histones, changing their shape.

The result is that different genes can be exposed or hidden, so that more protein or less protein is made by the cell. Neither hiding nor exposing the genes is inherently helpful or harmful to your health. The effect depends on the specific genes and whether they create beneficial proteins or harmful ones. If a gene creates a beneficial protein, such as a tumor suppressor, unwinding the DNA protects your health. If a gene has a harmful effect, then the benefit comes from winding the DNA back up.

A third epigenetic change involves microRNA. While DNA contains the actual source code for proteins, in the process that creates proteins, the code (DNA) is first converted into a template called RNA (ribonucleic acid). RNA does the actual work of making proteins. But there is a special group of RNA called microRNAs, which float around and interact with the main RNA template to control the making of useful proteins. It's thought that microRNAs control at least 30 percent of genes that make these proteins.[15]

Let's summarize epigenetics as simply as possible:

- Methylation silences genes to thwart making proteins; demethylation helps genes make proteins.
- Acetylation uncoils DNA and allows genes to make proteins; deacetylation tightens the coil and hides the DNA, so less protein is made.
- MicroRNA can selectively turn off making specific proteins by interfering with RNA templates.

Epigenetic influences on DNA is a hot area of research especially when it comes to diet, but before I tell you what happens with food, it is instructive to see how other lifestyle activities influence our genes through these changes.

Most healthy activities create positive epigenetic changes, and we now are realizing that this is how they bring us their benefits—through our genes. Exercise, for example, causes epigenetic changes that free up our genes to make useful proteins for building muscles, increasing the pumping capacity of the heart, growing new blood vessels to support muscle expansion, and lowering blood lipids.[16] Other epigenetic changes from exercise can block harmful genes. These are seen after swimming, sprinting, interval training, and high-intensity walking.[17]

Studies in lab rats show that exercise raises DNA activity in the brain. This happens because of epigenetic changes with histone acetylation that free up DNA, so more proteins can be made to maintain brain health.[18] The DNA impact of exercise goes well beyond the health of the person doing the workout. In men, working out affects their sperm in a way that can influence their progeny. A clinical study from the University of Copenhagen studied the epigenetic consequences of a one-hour spin class led by a certified instructor, taken five days a week for six weeks. They looked at the effect of the exercise on the sperm of healthy male volunteers in their early twenties. The researchers collected ejaculate from the men to analyze the sperm before the study, after six weeks of spinning, and then after three months without exercise. The spin class caused a lasting epigenetic change in one genomic hotspot: the specific area of sperm DNA that is responsible for the brain function and nervous system development of the as-yet-unconceived fetus.[19] Thus, a man's workout routine may be beneficial to the brain health of his children, long before they are even conceived.

A good night's sleep causes epigenetic changes in DNA, and so does pulling an all-nighter—but one is good, the other bad. A study by researchers from the University of Iceland and Uppsala University in Sweden studied sixteen young healthy men in their twenties and examined their DNA after a night of sleeping for eight hours (a good night's sleep), followed by a day of total sleep deprivation (all-nighter). Blood was collected before bedtime on the night of sleep and before breakfast the next day after either eight hours' sleep or after total sleep deprivation.

The study showed that eight hours of sleep turns on genes that metabolize fat and prevent obesity, while sleep deprivation interferes with those genes.[20] Inadequate or short sleep duration increases the risk of obesity in children by 45 percent.[21] The epigenetic effect of sleep is profound.

A single night of sleep deprivation can epigenetically interfere with as many as 269 genes, preventing them from being used to make proteins, including one gene that is a tumor suppressor. That's a bad thing. When you silence a gene that blocks cancer, this can increase your risk of developing a tumor.[22]

Meditation causes beneficial epigenetic changes that lower the activity of genes associated with inflammation.[23] On the other hand, stress epigenetically unleashes DNA that is associated with inflammation.[24] People who experienced severe trauma and who have post-traumatic stress disorder (PTSD) have been shown to have many detrimental epigenetic changes in their DNA.[25]

Environmental hazards have been linked to epigenetic changes seen in patients with cancer, autism, depression, schizophrenia, Alzheimer's disease, autoimmune diseases, diabetes, inflammatory bowel disease, obesity, and a host of other serious health problems. Naturally, it is important to reduce your exposure to anything that could have deleterious epigenetic effects. At the same time, dietary interventions can tap into your body's capacity for positive epigenetic change to activate genes that are beneficial to health.

The Third DNA Health Defense: Telomeres

Telomeres are the third part of DNA's defense gear. These are the protective caps at both ends of the DNA in chromosomes that help maintain the structure of chromosomes and keep them from sticking to each other. Telomeres are so vital for protecting our DNA that an enzyme called telomerase is continually at work, repairing the telomeres as they naturally shorten as we age. In 2009, Elizabeth Blackburn of University of California, San Francisco won the Nobel Prize for her work on telomeres, the third Nobel related to DNA research. Blackburn discovered that without telomerase, the telomeres shorten quickly, DNA is unprotected, and cells age quickly and die.[26] Her work is brilliantly described in a TED Talk she gave in 2017.

The groundwork for keeping long, healthy telomeres later in our lives, however, is laid down in our early childhood. A study by researchers at University of California, San Francisco showed that breastfeeding improved the length of telomeres in the child. In a group of 121 children, those who were exclusively breastfed when they were infants had longer telomeres by the time they were of preschool age (four to five years old) compared to children who were formula fed.[27] This shows the durability of the telomere effect—that the benefits of breastfeeding remain years after a child is weaned and eating solid food.

On the other hand, telomeres do inevitably get shorter during aging. Studies of people over sixty-five years old show that those with shorter telomeres die sooner than those with longer telomeres, so research is investigating what behaviors accelerate the shortening of telomeres.[28] Smoking, high stress, poor sleep, and lack of exercise speed up wear on the telomere caps and reduce the activity of telomerase.

What's fascinating is that people that live to one hundred years old have unusually long telomeres.[29] This 2008 discovery has prompted studies of how lifestyle and diet can lengthen telomeres. The findings are conclusive. As to lifestyle, regular exercise is associated with longer telomeres.[30] Relaxation increases telomerase activity and protects telomeres in people who are stressed, and modes of relaxation have even been compared. For example, doing Kriya yoga has a bigger effect on protecting your telomeres than listening to chill out music.[31] Dean Ornish, in collaboration with Blackburn, published their landmark 2008 research in *The Lancet Oncology* showing that comprehensive lifestyle changes can improve telomerase protection of telomeres in men with prostate cancer, with benefits that persisted in a five-year follow-up study.[32] In addition to telomerase effects, lifestyle changes created an epigenetic effect in angiogenesis proteins that favored suppressing cancer, in my collaboration with Dean Ornish in this group of patients. Once again, positive changes in the health defense systems were found to be linked.

Among the influences on telomeres, diet is one of the most powerful. Recall the study of children who had longer telomeres because they were breastfed. When other dietary influences were examined, the researchers found it was possible to shorten telomeres, too. This is a negative effect. They found that telomeres shortened in children who drank soda beginning at age four, and those who drank soda four or more times a week had shorter telomeres than those who drank soda less frequently or not at all.[33] The impact of breastfeeding and soda on telomeres is just the beginning of discoveries on how our diet influences our DNA health defense systems. As we will see in chapter 9, the really interesting reveal is that certain foods, such as soy, turmeric, and coffee, can unleash protective genes while blunting the effects of harmful ones. Some dietary patterns help protect and lengthen our telomeres, including the Mediterranean diet and similar patterns based on it. Before we explore these foods in depth, however, there is one more health defense system I need to introduce to you: the immune system.

SOME CONDITIONS WHERE DNA DEFENSES ARE BREACHED

Alzheimer's disease
Ataxia telangiectasia
Atherosclerosis
Autism
Cancer (all types)
Celiac disease
Cystic fibrosis
Depression
Diabetes

SOME CONDITIONS WHERE DNA DEFENSES ARE BREACHED (cont.)

Inflammatory bowel disease
Li-Fraumeni syndrome
Lynch syndrome
Obesity
Parkinson's disease
Post-traumatic stress disorder
Rheumatoid arthritis
Schizophrenia
Systemic lupus erythematosus

CHAPTER 5

Immunity

Everyone knows a strong immune system helps you avoid the common cold. But did you know that immunity is so powerful it can protect you against cancer? And if you do have cancer, your immune system is capable of eliminating it completely from your body, even if it has spread. Genetics, smoking, the environment, a bad diet, and other factors are often blamed for cancer. But the truth is that regardless of its cause, cancer only becomes a disease once malignant cells escape from being destroyed by our immune system. Indeed, our immune system is one of the best-known health defense systems. It keeps us from becoming infected after we have a cut, fights off viruses, and prevents us from getting sick from harmful microbes coughed into the air by a fellow passenger on a bus. The true power of immunity is being revealed as researchers study how to boost our own immunity to fight cancer. Cancer patients are beginning to survive against overwhelming odds with all signs of their disease melted away using immune-boosting treatments.

As I mentioned in chapter 1, we form microscopic tumors all the time in our body that are invisible to us, and most will never become a problem. One reason is that cancer cells need a blood supply to grow large enough to cause harm. A properly functioning angiogenesis defense system will keep that from happening. But the immune system actually provides the first line of defense. Our immune cells are specifically designed to differentiate friend from foe, including cancer cells. When the earliest signs of cancerous growths are spotted by first responder immune cells, they call in a cellular strike. Special cancer-killing immune cells swoop in and wipe out the abnormal cells before they cause problems.

Sometimes, cancer cells dodge our immune system by camouflaging themselves. They do this by wrapping themselves in "friendly" proteins that fool immune cells into recognizing them as normal cells. This effectively makes cancer cells invisible so they escape detection. By hiding like deadly terrorists blending in with a bustling crowd of ordinary citizens, these cloaked cancer cells have a chance to grow and become dangerous.

Other times, the immune system is weakened and unable to do its job adequately, so cancer cells are missed, and are able to grow. People who suffer from immunodeficiency diseases, like AIDS, or those who have received an organ transplant and have to take lifelong immune-suppressing steroids to prevent organ rejection are at really high risk for developing cancer because their immune defenses are compromised.

New immunotherapy cancer treatments help your immune system do its job to eliminate dangerous cancer cells. This approach is remarkable because it doesn't rely on toxic or targeted drugs to kill cancer cells. Rather, it encourages our own body to rid itself of the cancer. James Allison of MD Anderson Cancer Center in Texas and Tasuku Honjo of Kyoto were awarded the 2018 Nobel Prize in Medicine or Physiology for their pioneering work that discovered how to harness our immune system to fight cancer.

One type of immunotherapy blocks the cloaking proteins that cancers use to hide from the immune system, effectively revealing them. Called checkpoint inhibitors, these treatments allow the patient's own immune defenses to wake up and "see" the cancer. They can then destroy it.

At the age of ninety, former U.S. president Jimmy Carter was diagnosed with a deadly cancer called malignant melanoma. It had spread to his liver and his brain, a situation with a dismal prognosis and usually unsurvivable. Along with some pinpoint radiation to the tumor, Carter received a checkpoint inhibitor called Keytruda (pembrolizumab), which helped his immune system find the tumors. The treatments soon worked. The tumor in his brain disappeared without the need for chemotherapy. My own mother, a musician and professor of piano, was eighty-two when she was diagnosed with endometrial cancer. This cancer develops within the lining of the uterus. Although her cancer was removed by surgery, it came back aggressively and in multiple locations in her body a year later. We performed a genomic analysis on her tumor and discovered the presence of a tumor marker called MSI-H (microsatellite instability-high). This meant that she would likely benefit from Keytruda. Like Carter, with immunotherapy and a tiny dose of radiation, her immune defenses system completely wiped out all trace of cancer.

There are other immune therapy approaches that are game changers for patients with cancer and their oncologists alike. It's possible to collect a person's own immune cells through a process called apheresis, which is similar to blood donation. As blood is collected, the T cells are removed, and the rest of the blood is returned back to the patient. The T cells are then sent to a special center where they are genetically engineered to become CAR-T cells. This procedure reprograms T cells and directs them to target cancers like an immune homing missile. CAR-T cell therapy is effective for treating lymphoma and leukemia. A close friend was diagnosed with an aggressive cancer called diffuse B cell lymphoma. Despite standard treatments the cancer continued to grow and spread. She received an infusion of CAR-T cells made from her own immune cells. After a few weeks, her body showed signs of responding to her souped up immune cells, and in less than two months, all signs of her cancer were eliminated by her immune system. While not all patients who are treated with immunotherapy have their cancer wiped out, those that do have continued to be cancer-free, for years.

Specific foods, and the components within them, can powerfully influence our immune defenses, too. Scientists from the University of Rome in Italy discovered that ellagic acid, a bioactive that is found at high levels in chestnuts, blackberries, walnuts, pomegranates, and straw-berries, blocks production of the same immune-cloaking protein targeted by checkpoint inhibitor drugs (like Keytruda) in bladder cancer.[1] We will talk more about this research in chapter 10.

Clearly, the immune system is one of the pillars of health defense. It is designed to protect the body from invasion by viruses, bacteria, and parasites through an ingenious system of pattern recognition. Immune cells identify and destroy threats, while recognizing healthy cells and leaving them alone. Under normal circumstances in healthy people, the immune system is always on standby, like the fire department, ready to act when an alarm is sounded. Your body automatically knows whether to turn up or turn down its immune response. Neither inactive nor over-active, it operates from a point where all forces are poised and balanced, but in a constant state of alert.

There are many steps you can take to safeguard your immune defenses throughout your life. Exercise, proper sleep, and lowering and managing stress all help your immune system stay healthy. So can your dietary choices. Certain foods boost your immune system and help it fight diseases of aging. And other foods can help calm the immune sys-tem when it is overly active, as seen in autoimmune diseases. Before we discuss these foods, however, I want to tell you about how improving our immunity has played a role in the advancement of the human species and how it's given us a powerful advantage over terrible diseases.

Early Efforts at Immunity Boosting

The disease known as smallpox was once one of the deadliest killers on the planet. This disease scourge dated back to ancient times. Evidence of smallpox was found in Egyptian mummies, including on the head of Pharaoh Ramses V.

Smallpox is an infection caused by a virus called variola. The initial infection starts when the virus is inhaled or touched. Within a week, the virus begins infecting cells throughout the body. Fevers, skin pustules over the entire body, and internal bleeding can occur. Historically, the infection was fatal 30 percent of the time. People who survived smallpox were left with horrible, disfiguring scars and sometimes were blinded when the infection involved the eyes. In the twentieth century alone, smallpox killed more than 300 million people worldwide, equivalent to the entire population of the United States. But in 1980, the World Health Organization issued a history-making declaration: smallpox was officially eliminated and no longer a threat.[2] This achievement was accomplished by mounting a global vaccination program against smallpox that trained the immune systems of people around the world to recognize and destroy the virus before it could cause disease.

The twentieth century was not the first time someone had the idea of priming the body's defenses against smallpox. During the reign of Emperor Kangxi (1661–1722), who ruled China's final dynasty, the Qing Empire, lethal outbreaks of smallpox decimated society. So Kangxi decided to protect his family members and his armies living in the Forbidden City from the deadly epidemic.[3] He ordered imperial doctors to take scabs from the dried pox of subjects dying from smallpox, grind the scabs into powder, and place the powder into the noses of his family and soldiers. When exposed to the pox scab, the immune system began to mount a defense against the smallpox virus, giving the recipients an immunity to the disease. This crude technique was known as variolation (recall that the smallpox virus is called variola), and it later led to what is today known as vaccination.[4] The English family doctor and surgeon Edward Jenner is credited with developing the first vaccine against smallpox in 1796, and he is regarded as the father of immunology.

Over the next two hundred years, medical researchers successfully developed vaccines against diseases like polio, tetanus, rabies, chicken pox, mumps, cholera, diphtheria, and hepatitis to protect the public against once deadly threats. In each instance, the immune system is guided to unleash its defensive might against foreign invaders in the body, so that health is protected and disease thwarted.

In 2006, the vaccine Gardasil was successfully developed to protect women against developing cervical cancer following infection by human papillomavirus (HPV). In 2010, the first vaccine to treat cancer, Provenge (sipuleucel-T), became FDA approved for prostate cancer. The same year, the cancer immunotherapy, the checkpoint inhibitor Yervoy (ipilimumab), was approved to treat melanoma. This set the stage for other breakthrough immune-stimulating cancer drugs like Keytruda, which benefited my mother and Jimmy Carter.

And although it's still early days, it is even possible now to develop a personalized cancer vaccine, in which the DNA from a tumor is analyzed for its unique mutations, and a special protein is made to be injected under the skin of a patient with cancer. The injected proteins train the immune system to search out and destroy the cancer. So, as part of treatment, cancer patients can be vaccinated against their own cancer.

Despite all this progress across history, believe it or not, most of our current understanding of the immune system has come about only in the past fifty years. So, now let's take a look at how our immune system actually works, starting with where it is anatomically located in our body.

Anatomy of Immune Defense

The power of your immune system lies in its military-like capabilities. Similar to the military, your immune system has different branches. Each branch has different types of soldiers with their own specialized training, weapons, and skills for defending their homeland. The central command of the immunity is located in four body sites: your bone marrow, your thymus gland, your spleen and lymph nodes, and your gut.

Bone marrow is the spongy material in the hollow areas of your bones (and as you may recall from chapter 2, bone marrow also plays host to your stem cells). Your bone marrow produces almost all the immune cells in your body, using stem cells called hematopoietic stem cells.

Your thymus gland is an organ located behind your breastbone. It is home to special immune cells called T cells. This gland is where young T cells originally formed in the bone marrow go to mature. The organ is really only active from the time you are born through puberty. It is in this early part of your life that the T cells of your immune system are created and stockpiled. As you get older, the organ atrophies and becomes replaced with fat cells.[5]

Your spleen is a fist-size spongy sack located behind your stomach on your left side. It stores and filters blood. As part of the immune system, the spleen acts like a giant lymph node, where special cells called B cells produce antibodies that recognize bacteria and viruses that invade the body. Some people have had their spleens surgically removed because the organ was ruptured by trauma or abnormally enlarged by disease. They can be more vulnerable to infections and less able to respond to the effects of vaccines, as they are unable to make as many antibodies without their spleen.

The location of the fourth headquarters for immunity, the gut, is critical for understanding the link between diet and immunity. The gut is also home to the microbiome, which, as you saw in chapter 3, can influence the immune system. The importance of the gut for immune defense has been recognized only recently for its profound role in maintaining health. In fact, the immune function of the gut was largely overlooked when I was in medical school. As students, we were taught in histology class there were small patches in the intestines, called Peyer's patches, associated with immune function. We could barely find them under the microscope when we examined slides of the intestines. And our lecturers also told us that the appendix probably had some function, but that it was vestigial, or unnecessary. That was the state of knowledge then—and an underestimation.

We now know the entire gut is an immune organ, with a surface area spanning the size of two parking spots (thirty-two square meters)! In addition to bona fide immune cells that coordinate immune defense, the gut's command center allows healthy bacteria living there to give signals to immune cells elsewhere in the body. Other immune command stations are located in your tonsils, lymphatic vessels, and lymph nodes.

Soldiers of Immunity

As with the other health defense systems I've shown you, the immune system is made up of a number of players that each have a function for protecting your body. I'm going to tell you about the major cells and function, so you will be able to appreciate and better understand the research I'll present about food and immunity in part 2.

The cells of the immune system are known as white blood cells, or leukocytes (the Greek word for white is *leuko*). There are five types of leukocytes, each with a different job description: neutrophils, lymphocytes, monocytes, eosinophils, and basophils. I've listed them here in order from most to least numerous, based on how prevalent they are in your blood. Medical students memorize them by the mnemonic "never let monkeys eat bananas."

Lymphocytes are actually a group of several types of immune cells. The three main types of lymphocytes are T cells, B cells, and natural killer (NK) cells. T cells have three subtypes: helper Ts, cytotoxic Ts, and suppressor T cells. Other immune cells include macrophages, mast cells, and dendritic cells. These are the immune players that defend your health.

All of these cells originate from stem cells in your bone marrow called hematopoietic stem cells. This is why drugs like chemotherapy, which damages bone marrow cells as well as circulating white blood cells, lower your immunity. On the flip side, diet can influence the production of immune cells in the bone marrow. Scientists from the University of Southern California showed that fasting cycles can be used to build a fresh immune system. Remarkably, they showed that fasting two to four days in a row forces the human body to go into a recycling mode, which gets rid of the older, worn-out immune cells. Then, when food is started again, it jump-starts the hematopoietic stem cells in your bone marrow to start regenerating fresh immune cells thus rebuilding the immune system.[6]

A Two-Part Immune System: Fast and Slow

Your immunity is actually made up of two different immune systems, each designed in its own way to protect your body from foreign invaders, whether they are bacteria, viruses, parasites, or cancer cells. One is swift acting, responding immediately to an attack on the body by an invader. It is a blunt instrument, programmed to defend against any invader using the exact same weapons each time. This is the innate immune system. When you have an allergic reaction or inflammation, it is the innate system at work. Ninety percent of all animals species have only this type of immune response.[7]

The second immune system is slower acting, but much more sophisticated. This system takes about a week to assemble its defenses, but when it does, it is very finely tuned to knock out specific targets on invaders in the body. This is the adaptive (or acquired) immune system. It works in two major ways: it can defend by using specialized cells designed for killing, or it can create antibodies that swarm like hornets to surround and attack the enemy. Each system is important for health, and I'll tell you what food can do for each.

Innate Immunity: Master of Inflammation

If you recall the local swelling that happens almost immediately after you cut yourself, you were watching the innate immune system do its job. The innate system is the first responder to any invasion of your body. It acts like a guard dog ready to spring into action the moment a stranger steps into your yard. This system is nonselective and simply blocks and tackles anything in its path. The innate defense includes physical, chemical, and cellular components. Your skin is the physical barrier to intruders. Secretions in your mouth, nose, and airway contain enzymes that wage chemical warfare to kill any invader that you inhale or get in your mouth. If you swallow any microbes, your stomach acid will dissolve them. Coughing and sneezing forcefully ejects foreign invaders that have crawled into your nostrils and lungs.

The cells of the innate system create inflammation, which is the body's response to tissue damage or foreign invasion. Inflammation brings specific immune cells into the injury site to keep the enemy walled off and contained to a specific area, kill invaders, and then dispose of their bodies. Special cells that race to the scene are called phagocytes (*phago* in Greek means "devour"; these cells are neutrophils, monocytes, macrophages, and mast cells), which remove potentially harmful particles and microbes by consuming them. Additionally, phagocytes eat cellular corpses and debris from tissue damage. They make pus in infected wounds, and they can guide other immune cells to the trouble zone.

Swelling, pain, redness, and increased warmth are the cardinal signs that inflammation is taking place. One type of phagocyte, the mast cell, comes on the scene and releases histamine. This chemical causes blood vessels to vasodilate, making the area look red and feel hot. Chemical signals are also released that make the dilated blood vessel leaky. Fluid and proteins rush out of the leaky blood vessels into the hot zone, causing tissue swelling. If you've ever suffered hay fever, this is the same process that leads to the swollen red eyes and runny nose (the antihistamine you take calms this down). The proteins that leak out of the blood vessels help clot blood and any bleeding that might be happening in the scene. But the swelling and chemical signals irritate nerves, causing pain. A similar inflammatory effect takes place in the airways if you have an asthma attack, or in the gut if you have a food allergy.

White blood cells release chemical signals called cytokines that control the intensity of the inflammatory response. One of the most important of these signals is called interferon. This chemical interferes (hence the name) with virus infections and triggers other immune cells to charge into battle, including natural killer (NK) cells. These cells have the ability to distinguish abnormal from normal cells. If an abnormal cell is spotted, the NK cell works with specialized proteins to incapacitate and kill it. Mission accomplished. A cleanup crew of phagocytes then gobble up any debris.

Under normal circumstances, the innate immune response is short lived and subsides within a few days. When it's time to turn down the inflammatory response, a signal called interleukin-10, made by the immune system, shuts down the show and brings the immune defenses back into a normal state of balance in health. If inflammation is not calmed, however, the immune response can become a chronic state and normal cells can become damaged.

You can see at this point how the ability to mount an inflammatory response helps our body repel bacterial invaders. This is an important point, because when you hear about so-called "anti-inflammatory diets" bear in mind that under normal circumstances you don't want to completely wipe out your body's ability to turn on inflammation.

Chronic inflammation, on the other hand, is a whole different situation—and it's a problem. When the foreign invaders don't go away, or when an autoimmune reaction turns the body against itself, the sustained inflammatory response can be devastating. Chronic inflammation is like a campfire that can't be extinguished and that spreads into the surrounding forest, sparking a runaway wildfire that can destroy everything in its path. We will discuss this in greater detail later in this chapter.

The Adaptive Immune System

When you receive a vaccine to prevent a disease, like the polio vaccine, your adaptive immune system is responsible for creating the protection against the disease. The adaptive (or acquired) immune system is the smarter, more sophisticated branch of your immune system. Unlike the innate system, which is a blunt instrument, the adaptive system is very choosy about what it kills. And it has a permanent memory of the invaders it destroys. This memory helps trigger the immune system to deploy a rapid response team should the enemy—be it bacteria, virus, or cancer—rear its head again in the future. You can thank your adaptive immunity for all of the diseases you get only once, like chicken pox, or never at all, after you are vaccinated against it. Once the adaptive immune response learns how to fight off a disease, it protects you for the rest of your life.

As part of its sophistication, adaptive immunity has two strategies. First, it can attack invaders by using cells to kill them. This is called cell-mediated immunity. Alternatively, it can use antibodies as weapons to attack an intruder and mark it for death. Because it takes seven to ten days for antibodies to be made the first time an intruder is spotted, this adaptive immune defense has a slow response time.

Adaptive immunity relies on T cells and B cells, both of which are formed in the bone marrow from stem cells (they are called hematopoietic stem cells). B cells stay in the bone marrow to mature. Once they've matured, they leave the bone marrow and move into lymph organs like the spleen, the gut, and the tonsils. There, they remain on active duty, waiting for an invader to show up. When an invasion occurs requiring immune defense, B cells swarm out from lymph organs to reach the invasion site and defend the body.

T cells, on the other hand, leave the nest early. They exit the bone marrow while they are still young and not yet mature. They travel to the thymus gland, which serves as a boot camp for T cells. There, they are trained to distinguish nonself cells (foreign invaders—the bad guys) from self cells (the good guys). At their qualifying test, T cells that recognize and kill nonself cells are allowed to graduate. They circulate to the peripheral lymph tissues, where they are stationed to wait for the call of duty. During qualifiers, friendly fire is not tolerated, so any T cell that accidentally kills a self cell fails the test and is destroyed. The only T cells leaving the thymus are those that are trained to destroy invaders and will not injure our normal cells.

Both T cells and B cells are skilled intelligence operators. They learn about foreign invaders and tailor their responses accordingly. Once information about an invader is acquired, a counterattack is launched and data about the enemy are recorded for future use. Each of us has an immune filing system in our body containing data on all the bacteria and infections to which we have ever had an exposure. From the battlefront where enemies are invading, special cells known as dendritic cells relay information about what's happening to the adaptive immune system. Dendritic cells record data about the unique protein fingerprints of bacteria, viruses, and cancer cells. On demand, they can present these fingerprints to the proper immune cells that will find, mark, and then kill the invader. T cells and B cells adjust their defense strategies once there's enough intelligence gathered on the front lines. The military analogy is especially appropriate when it comes to coordinating millions of cells to go into battle to defend the body. It's akin to protecting a fortress. If the troops are weak or lazy, the enemies will take over the castle. If they are uncoordinated, undisciplined, or acting without restraint, chaos will ensue. And if the troops turn against the commander, the mutiny can destroy the people they were supposed to protect. Thankfully, our immune defenses are normally well trained, highly disciplined, and dedicated to maintaining peace.

Cell-Mediated Immunity

To understand how foods activate the immune system, you need to know a little more about the chain of command of the immune forces. Different foods influence different parts of the immune system. Some turn up defense, while others turn it down. Diet tends to influence cell-mediated immunity, which involves T cells. Remember, there are three main types of T cells: helper T cells, cytotoxic T cells, and suppressor T cells (also called Tregs because they dampen down the immune system).

Helper T cells have a specific job: they help. They orchestrate an immune attack against invaders by releasing signals that tell other cells what to do. They are called into action when they see red alerts being sent by other parts of the immune system that have been called into battle.[8] Some of the chemical signals released by helper T cells call in the airstrike from other immune cells, while other signals they release instruct B cells to make antibodies against the invader. T cells direct the cellular troops to attack, and they can also bring in reinforcements and new weapons as needed.

Cytotoxic T cells are combat fighters that directly go after and destroy bacteria, infected cells, or cancer cells. They get their hands dirty by making contact with the invaders and annihilating them. Like zombie hunters, cytotoxic T cells recognize and destroy formerly healthy cells that have been infected and are now threats.[9] As I'll show you later, certain foods can activate and increase the numbers of helper T cells and cytotoxic T cells in your bloodstream, as a way to boost your immune defenses.

Suppressor T cells, or Tregs, are another very important regulator of immunity. These cells have the critical job of quelling the immune system when the battle is done. They release chemical signals that turn off helper T cells and cytotoxic T cells, so the immune system can settle back down to its normal, healthy baseline state, where all systems are on standby status. When the immune system isn't quelled, it is overactive. This is seen in autoimmune diseases. Some foods can increase the number of Tregs in your bloodstream, and this can be helpful for preventing autoimmune flares.

Antibodies and a Really Long Memory

When most people think of immunity, they think of antibodies. Antibodies are like bloodhounds that know how to sniff out and find an evildoer lurking in the body. Your B cells give birth to antibodies. B cells are constantly on patrol in the body, like soldiers patrolling the streets. Even when there does not appear to be an infection raging, B cells can take out bacteria and viruses that are silently free-floating in your blood but haven't yet infected your cells. They do this by bodysurfing through your bloodstream to see if they can spot any foreign invaders floating by. The way B cells do this is by displaying antibody receptors on their outer surface, like quills of a porcupine. Each B cell is bristling with up to two hundred thousand antibody receptors. These receptors are made to match up with abnormal antigens from bacteria and virus. Antigens are the pirate flags of foreign invaders.[10] Any invader that has an antigen (flag) matching an antibody receptor (quill) will be snagged and dealt with by the B cell.

B cells also can respond to the signal released by helper T cells that are dealing with a problem. The B cell will float over to the area where the action is taking place and attach its receptors to the antigens of the invader. The name *antigen* is short for "antibody generator." The attachment activates the B cell, and it starts cloning itself over and over, creating more B cells that can make more antibodies designed to attack the specific invader it is seeing. Remarkably, each B cell can make and pump out two hundred antibodies per second, twice the rate of fire of a Minigun, the electric rotary machine gun.[11] The antibodies hit the invaders and mark them for death, and phagocytes swarm in to destroy them. Most of the B cells will die in the battle, but a few of them survive and become memory cells. These memorize the invader's characteristics and then go into hiding. The next time the same invader gets into the body, the memory B cells spring back into action with the know-how of how to make the exact antibody again, next time more quickly, to destroy the enemy. I will tell you later about the foods, like chile peppers and licorice, that activate and increase the number of B cells in your body.

Failed Immunity and Disease

When your immune system fails at its job, your life is in serious jeopardy. True, invading bacteria and viruses do evade our defenses occasionally. That's why you catch a cold or come down with the flu. Massive attacks can come from outside the body or from within. Harmful microbes, for example, can gain entrance to our insides through our nose, mouth, eyes, ears, vagina, or anus—any orifice that is exposed to the outside world. And when you have a laceration, the opening in the skin is a gaping doorway for microbes to crawl en masse into the body. Before antiseptic technique was invented in hospitals, women often died after childbirth from infections transferred by the unsterile hands of doctors and obstetric instruments from one mother to another.[12] If our immune defenses are down, external invaders can have catastrophic consequences.

The best known example of life-threatening collapse of immunity is acquired immune deficiency syndrome (AIDS). AIDS is caused by infection with the human immunodeficiency virus (HIV) which nefariously strips away immunity from within. This leads to a high risk for catastrophic infections as well as for cancers to grow. HIV is an organism called a retrovirus that originated from West African chimpanzees and was transmitted to humans. The retrovirus adapted itself to invade and destroy healthy human T cells.[13] Without adequate T cells, our body's ability to detect and kill all invaders, not just HIV, drops precipitously. The successful control of HIV infection in an infected patient has been one of the most significant accomplishments in modern medicine. Effective treatments can reduce the blood levels of the lethal virus to undetectable levels, allowing an HIV-infected individual to live an otherwise normal life.

There are also a number of inherited immunodeficiency conditions, where patients have defective T cells, B cells, or phagocyte function, or deficiencies in the complement proteins that help activate immune cells. These are known as primary immunodeficiency conditions, and are rare. You may recall the iconic photo of the boy in a bubble, a young child with severe combined immunodeficiency, known as SCID. He essentially had zero immunity and could not survive exposure to the outside world.

Your immune system can be also weakened by cancers, such as multiple myeloma and leukemia; infections, including HPV and hepatitis B and C; medical treatments, such as chemotherapy and radiation; diabetes; malnutrition; and alcoholism. Obesity suppresses the immune system. Studies show that individuals who are obese are at a higher risk for developing an infection after suffering trauma or while being in the intensive care unit compared to non-obese people. This is because their immunity is lowered by their metabolic (obese) state.[14] In fact, simply being obese increases the risk of someone dying in the hospital, regardless of the reason for hospitalization, by as much as seven times.[15] Lowered immunity in obese people also increases their risk of infections of the gums (periodontitis), bladder, skin, and lungs.[16]

Our immune defenses are influenced by our gut microbiota, and this is an important area of research. Just under the surface of our gut lining is an immense immune command center called gut associated lymphoid tissue (GALT). The immune cells inhabiting this layer receive signals from our gut bacteria to "turn on" or "shut down" immune defenses. Specific bacteria have been identified, such as *Lactobacillus, Bifidobacteria, Akkermansia,*

Enterococcus, *Alistipes*, and *Faecalibacterium*, that are beneficial for immunity. If these are deficient or missing, our immune defense is compromised. The Western diet may weaken the immune response because unhealthy foods interfere with the ecosystem of the microbiome, and this can cause miscommunication between the gut and our immune cells.

On the other end of the spectrum, an immune army gone rogue can turn against our health. *Autoimmunity* is the term used to describe an overactive immune system, where normal cells and organs are attacked and their function is destroyed. There are more than forty major disorders falling under the category of autoimmune diseases, including type 1 diabetes, systemic lupus erythematosus, multiple sclerosis, psoriasis, rheumatoid arthritis, and systemic sclerosis. These all share the common feature of chronic inflammation and self-inflicted immune damage to organs.

Autoimmune diseases do not have one cause, but instead are triggered by a number of factors. Genetics, environment, infections, medication reactions, and shifts in the microbiome have all been implicated in autoimmune diseases. The common feature of autoimmune diseases is the breakdown of the normal control that quiets the immune defenses. When the disease flares, the immune attacks can be limited to a specific organ, or there can be a generalized attack throughout the whole body.

Type 1 diabetes is an example of an attack on a specific organ. B cells produce antibodies that target the beta cells in the pancreas, which produces insulin. When T cells destroy those cells, the body is deprived of insulin and becomes unable to metabolize glucose in the bloodstream. This metabolic trip up leads not only to high levels of blood glucose, but also to malfunctions in many different cells and organs, and requires regular insulin injections into the body in order to keep healthy functions going.

In multiple sclerosis (MS), your own antibodies attack the insulation called myelin which coats your nerves. This assault affects your brain and spinal cord, as well as muscles, and is akin to having termites eat away at the electrical insulation within the walls of your house. With badly damaged nerves, people with MS have weak muscles, poor coordination, vision loss, brain deficits, and other serious problems of nerve function.

Yet another example is celiac disease. Individuals with celiac disease have an immune reaction to gluten, a group of proteins found in wheat, barley, and rye. The body's strong immune reaction to gluten causes collateral damage to the wall of the intestines, creating "leaks" in the gut wall. Although the exact mechanism of celiac disease is still a mystery, it is known that autoantibodies damage the small intestines and other organs, causing severe cramping pain.[17] Fortunately, when gluten is avoided, the antibodies wane and the symptoms usually go away.

On the other hand, an autoimmune attack can be generalized and affect virtually every part of the body, a truly dire situation. In the disease known as lupus (systemic lupus erythematosus), an all-out antibody attack is launched against your own DNA, causing body-wide inflammation. The joints, skin, heart, kidney, and even brain can all become inflamed. A classic finding in the blood of lupus patients is the presence of antibodies that attack double-stranded DNA. These lupus autoantibodies tend to cluster together and form immune complexes, essentially microscopic hairballs, that get deposited throughout your organs, causing them to malfunction.

Autoimmune conditions are increasing in modernized societies. While the exact cause is not known, the phenomenon has been linked to unhealthy diets. This may also be tied to dysbiosis of the gut microbiome, which then disrupts the normal control of the immune system.[18]

Other situations with exaggerated immune responses are seen in allergic reactions, such as asthma and food allergies. In severe allergies, the immune system has an overkill reaction to an otherwise harmless allergen (pollen, food) introduced through mucous membranes. The trigger-happy immune system views it as a foreign invader. This leads to the production of antibodies against the allergen and activates T cells to release cytokines. These antibodies and cytokines draw other immune cells to destroy the "invader." In an asthmatic reaction, cytokines are released by T cells in the airway, which causes an overkill response with inflammation. Because of this, asthmatics experience wheezing and difficulty moving air out of the lungs. If unchecked, the inflammation can constrict smooth muscles in the airway, which can tighten up and result in death by suffocation if not treated.

As with the body's other defenses I've described, the immune system can be strongly influenced by what you eat and drink. In part 2, you will learn about the foods that can influence each of the health defense systems, from angiogenesis to regeneration, to the microbiome, to DNA repair and immunity.

CONDITIONS RELATED TO AN ABERRANT IMMUNE SYSTEM

Diseases that Weaken the Immune System	Conditions Resulting from a Weakened Immune System	Conditions with Excessive Immune Response
Acquired immune deficiency syndrome (AIDS)	All cancers	Allergies
Alcoholism	AIDS-related diseases	Asthma
Ataxia telangiectasia		Celiac disease
Chédiak-Higashi syndrome		Crohn's disease
Diabetes		Graves' disease
Hepatitis B		Hashimoto's thyroiditis
Hepatitis C		Multiple sclerosis
HPV (human papillomavirus)		Psoriasis
Human immunodeficiency virus (HIV)		Rheumatoid arthritis
Leukemia		Systemic lupus erythematosus

Malnutrition		Systemic sclerosis
Multiple myeloma		Ulcerative colitis
Obesity		Type I diabetes
Severe combined immunodeficiency disorder		

IMMUNE KEY PLAYERS

Innate Immune System	
Mast cells	Mediate allergic reactions by releasing histamine. Defend against parasites.
Natural killer cells	Can kill abnormal cells by injecting them with an enzyme that dissolves their outer layer. Distinguish between normal healthy versus infected or cancerous cells.
Neutrophils	Accumulate at sites of tissue injury. Form a cluster around the injury and attract macrophages and monocytes to cleanse wounds and clean up cellular debris.
Macrophages	Surround and engulf invading cells to destroy them. Summon many types of immune reactions.
Dendritic cells	Recognize and present antigens of invaders to trigger the T cell response and secrete cytokines to draw immune cells to the problem. Act as messengers between the innate and adaptive immune systems.
Adaptive Immune System	
Helper T cells (Th)	Coordinate immune response by releasing cytokines to recruit other immune cells.
Cytotoxic T cells (Tc)	Recognize virus-infected cells and cancer cells. Initiate programmed cell death by releasing toxins to kill undesirable cells.
Regulatory T cells (Treg)	Monitor and inhibit the activity of other T cells. Maintain immune tolerance of healthy cells. Calm the immune system to restore normal healthy balance.
Memory T cells	Gather data on invading cells and file it away for future reference, which improves the body's defense against future infections.

IMMUNE KEY PLAYERS (cont.)

Natural killer T cells	Recognize antigen-presenting molecules on foreign lipid molecules. Upon activation, they escalate inflammation.
Gamma delta T cells	Found in the lining of the gut and mucous membranes.
B cells	Produce antibodies that mark invader cells. Recognize and present antigens that trigger the T cell response. Some become memory B cells that recall antigens for future antibody production.

PART II

EAT TO BEAT DISEASE

The Evidence for Food as Medicine

Let food be thy medicine and medicine be thy food.
—*Hippocrates*

Each of the five health defense systems in your body are intimately connected to your diet. Research is revealing ever more evidence about how the foods we eat can have powerful influences on these systems that either activate their abilities to keep us in good health or destroy them. In part 2, I will take you on a journey of discovery to learn about the health impact of many foods through the lens of our health defenses.

Research is being conducted on an international scale, so you will learn about the evidence for food and health being generated by scientists and labs in Europe, Asia, Latin America, and North America. I'm focusing mainly on evidence from human clinical trials and epidemiological studies because what matters is how foods influence human health, but I'll also share some exciting laboratory discoveries because they reveal hidden insights that help us understand what happens when people eat certain foods. Much of this data is normally discussed in the corridors of scientific and medical institutions, but I am bringing it to your attention because food has immediacy. Once you learn about it, you can act on the information right away. You don't need to wait for permission or a doctor's prescription. Some of the findings I'm going to tell you about will surprise you, some will delight you (if you are a gastronome), but all will change the way you think about and choose your food. Get ready to open your eyes to a new world of food—seen through the prism of your body's health defenses.

CHAPTER 6

Starve Your Disease, Feed Your Health

Everyone would love to avoid being diagnosed with cancer, heart disease and other killer conditions. Regular exercise, cutting down on red meat and sugar, and not smoking are all solid approaches to dodging diseases, but they are only part of the solution. Using diet to support and amplify your body's angiogenesis defense system can lower your risk for a whole spectrum of feared diseases.

Soybeans were the first food found to influence angiogenesis. In 1993, a seminal paper was published by Theodore Fotsis, a Greek scientist working at the University of Heidelberg in Germany, who discovered that the urine of healthy Japanese men and women eating soyfoods contained a natural substance called genistein with potent anticancer effects.[1] In the lab, Fotsis found that genistein suppressed the kind of blood vessels sparked by tumors. Later it was shown that genistein could directly stop the growth of four different types of cancer cells (neuroblastoma, Ewing's sarcoma, rhabdomyosarcoma, retinoblastoma). Genistein is not made by the body, so its source could only be dietary. The urine had been collected from villagers, mostly farmers who cultivated tea and rice. They were vegetarians and ate a soy-based diet, as is common in Asia. The farmers had thirty times more genistein in their urine than people consuming a Western diet. Fotsis's study was the first report of a food containing a dietary factor that is clearly absorbed in the body and excreted in the urine that could inhibit angiogenesis. The researchers suggested this property of soy might help explain the lower rate of some lethal cancers in people eating an Asian plant-based diet compared to a Western diet.

Another preeminent researcher, Adriana Albini, was working at the National Cancer Research Institute in Genova, Italy, in 2002 when she proposed the term *angioprevention*. Albini conceived that angioprevention could achieve cancer prevention, especially cancer, by interfering with abnormal angiogenesis using compounds that would be safe and well tolerated by healthy individuals.[2] While some medications do fit this bill, food is the safest way to go. Today, angioprevention refers broadly to a health approach that includes using food, medicines, and dietary supplements. Albini and I, along with other scientific colleagues, coauthored a modern review on angioprevention that included diet in the prestigious journal *Nature Reviews Clinical Oncology*.[3] This framework on angiogenesis and disease prevention continues to be developed by the Angiogenesis Foundation and a highly committed international community of scientists and clinicians.

The goal of an angiopreventive diet is to keep the body's angiogenesis defense system in a healthy state of balance. This sometimes becomes a point of confusion among Western-trained doctors, because balance is not typically part of their lexicon for disease treatment. Balance is a more familiar concept in Ayurvedic and traditional Chinese medicine, in which the focus is on balance for preventive health.[4] Health is viewed in those systems as the presence of balanced systems in body and mind. A state of balance is where you want to be at all times. The *Goldilocks zone* is a term used by astrobiologists who use powerful telescopes to hunt for planets that are the perfect distance from their sun to support life: not too close to the sun to burn, not too far away to freeze. The Goldilocks zone for angiogenesis is where there are enough blood vessels to keep every cell in our body well nourished without feeding disease. Not too many, not too few, but just the right amount.

When it comes to preventing disease in healthy people, there's no equal to diet for safety. While some drugs can prevent specific diseases, like colon polyps, pharmaceuticals are always associated with potential side effects of some sort because drugs are never truly about balance. Drugs are created to perform one black-and-white job, usually knocking something out or building something up. For example, the cancer drug Avastin is useful for treatment but not prevention because it can reduce one of the body's angiogenesis signals to almost zero within a few days after an injection. But by mowing down the signal, which is beneficial for cancer treatment, Avastin can disrupt the normal balance of angiogenesis because that same signal is also needed in small amounts for healthy organ function. This disruption in balance can also lead to side effects, such as slower wound healing, a process that needs normal angiogenesis.

By contrast, dietary factors are not so omnipotent and lack destructive power. Bioactives in food and beverages are absorbed in small amounts that can help influence the body's own ability to keep angiogenesis in balance. Antiangiogenic factors in the diet can only prune excessive vessels back to baseline levels. This means that a food that starves a cancer won't starve the heart from getting its necessary blood supply because it's all about keeping the body in a healthy baseline. On the other side of the equation, angiogenesis-stimulating foods also will not cause blood vessels to overgrow their natural boundaries in the circulatory system. Proangiogenic foods and beverages will not put the system into overdrive and provoke cancer. Consistent with the principles of homeostasis, an angiogenesis diet helps maintain the body's state of harmony and balance.

Diseases Driven by Excessive Angiogenesis

Recall that angiogenesis is a common denominator of disease. In chapter 1, I discussed arthritis, blindness, and Alzheimer's disease. Let's look at some other major diseases that could be prevented or made more tolerable by boosting your angiogenesis defense using diet.

There's a little-recognized but important link between angio-genesis and coronary artery disease. The heart is a muscle that needs robust angiogenesis whenever its coronary arteries become clogged by cholesterol-laden plaques. However, these plaques are not just thick lay-ers of sludge that cake themselves onto the walls of a blood vessel. They are actual growths that, like tumors, rely on new blood vessels in order to expand. Coronary plaque neovascularization (another term for angiogen-esis) is deadly. Not only do these microvessels allow the plaque to thicken and block the coronary artery, but like cracks in the pavement, the ves-sels also make the plaque more fragile and likely to rupture.[5] When a coronary plaque ruptures, it is as if a tunnel caves in, the ceiling falls, and the tunnel is suddenly blocked: nothing can get through. When this happens in a coronary artery, blood flow is interrupted and the result is a potentially fatal heart attack. Preventing plaques from developing these dangerous blood vessels is just as important as growing new blood vessels to support the heart muscle itself.[6]

I've already described cancer, but it is worth revisiting because cancer is one of the most feared diseases of all time. Every single type of solid tumor, ranging from breast to prostate to lung to colon, must have angio-genesis to grow beyond a pinpoint size. Without angiogenesis, cancer cells also cannot spread. Even so-called liquid tumors, known as hema-togenous malignancies, like leukemia, lymphoma, and multiple myeloma, depend on angiogenesis. In those conditions, clumps of cancer cells in the bone marrow, lymph nodes, or spleen feed off of growing blood ves-sels that provide survival factors that fuel cancer cell growth.

You can ask your doctor for a testing kit to see if you are at high risk for one of the hereditary cancers. A sample of your saliva or blood can be analyzed to see if your cells carry the mutations that potentially herald heritable cancers, like breast, colon, ovarian, prostate, stomach, mela-noma, pancreatic, or uterine cancer. If your test turns out to be positive for a mutation, you should see a genetic counselor to be advised about how to manage your risks. Other than regular visits to check to see if cancer is already present, or surgery to remove some organs that are likely to develop cancer (such as breasts and ovaries), there's not much else the medical community can advise you on to lower your risk. Taking actions like exercise, sleep, and stress management are definitely important. But dietary antiangiogenesis is a critical opportunity that can help you beat the odds of disease.

Up to 90–95 percent of cancers are linked to exposures from the environment and our lifestyle. Of all cancer deaths, an estimated 30 percent are linked to diet.[7] Most cancer researchers and cancer activists point to harmful dietary factors that should be avoided to lower your cancer risk. But the work of the Angiogenesis Foundation focuses on a completely different opportunity: using foods, beverages, and natural ingredients that can be *added* to your diet to reduce your risk of cancer. As with cardiovascular disease, there's plenty of information about foods to avoid. The Foundation has also been doing the research and analyzing data on foods that can grow life-giving blood vessels to promote healing.

Here's the best part: some of the tastiest foods in the world can keep angiogenesis in balance. Now let's look at the foods and the evidence supporting their benefit. Food lovers take heart: you'll find plenty of items that will surprise and delight you.

Antiangiogenic foods

Soy

After Fotsis's work with urine from Japanese villagers, researchers have confirmed that soyfoods contain potent antiangiogenic properties that can be absorbed by the human body after consumption. Large public studies support the benefits: people who eat more soyfoods have lowered risk for a number of angiogenesis-dependent diseases, from breast and prostate cancer to coronary artery disease.[8]

Soyfoods represent dozens of different kinds of foods made from soybeans, an ancient legume that originated in eastern China three thousand years ago. From fresh soy products, such as edamame, soymilk, and soy nuts, to soyfoods that are fermented, such as soy sauce, tofu, miso, natto, tempeh, and more, soy is encountered in many forms. Asian markets will often have fresh soybeans, but you can also often find them in the frozen section of the grocery store. Fresh tofu is versatile and is a common food in Asia. In Western countries, the best sources to find tofu varieties are Asian markets. Look at the menu of a Chinese, Japanese, Korean, Thai, or Vietnamese restaurant, and you'll find many soy offerings.

Soy contains antiangiogenic bioactives known as isoflavones, specifically genistein, daidzein, equol, and glyceollins. Fermented soy products have higher concentrations of them.[9] A dietary supplement called genistein concentrated polysaccharide (GCP) is a highly concentrated form of genistein and daidzein. At the Angiogenesis Foundation, we tested GCP against human blood vessel cells in the laboratory and found it has potent antiangiogenic activity. GCP can also directly kill prostate cancer and lymphoma cells.[10] Soy bioactives not only suppress cancer growth but they also prevent growth of the atherosclerotic plaque through their antiangiogenic activity.[11] Researchers in Asia have reported that soy consumption can reduce the risk of cardiovascular disease by 16 percent.[12]

There is a widespread misconception that women should avoid eating soy because of a belief that the natural plant phytoestrogens cause breast cancer. It's time to overturn this urban legend. Here's the scientific truth: phytoestrogens in soy do not increase the incidence of breast cancer in human studies. Quite the opposite. Soy phytoestrogens actually act as antiestrogens in humans, interfering with the ability of estrogen to fuel certain cancers.[13] And as you now know, genistein, which is a phytoestrogen, has antiangiogenic, cancer-starving effects.

Among the most convincing epidemiological studies on the benefit, not harm, of soy is the Shanghai Breast Cancer Survival Study, which studied 5,042 breast cancer survivors.[14] During a four-year period, the researchers from Vanderbilt University documented and correlated the amount of soy these women consumed with recurrence of and death from breast cancer. If there were any potential for soy to be truly harmful, it would appear in this population of women. Instead, what was found was that women with the highest level of soy intake had a *reduction* in their risk of cancer recurrence by 32 percent. Their risk of mortality was reduced by 29 percent. This beneficial association with soy was seen regardless of whether the women had estrogen-receptor-positive or negative breast cancer.

The next chance you have, fuel up on soy. The amount that's beneficial to health in human studies is ten grams of soy protein per day, which is found in a cup of soymilk. The human evidence shows that having soyfoods in your diet is associated with a reduced risk of breast cancer. The more soy consumed, the lower the risk. Soy has further benefits, as vegans know, by being an excellent source of protein. Soy is also common in many premade and packaged commercial foods, but it is unclear whether soy used as a filler has the same benefits as fresh or fermented soy products, so I don't recommend choosing highly processed foods simply because soy is listed as an ingredient. Go instead for soybeans, soymilk, tofu, or traditional soy products found in Asian markets and restaurants. If you've never explored soy-related dishes like tofu on the Asian menu, you now have a strong reason to start: soy can starve your cancer and feed your health.

Tomato

Popularly viewed as a culinary vegetable, but technically a fruit, the tomato originated in Mesoamerica, where it was used for traditional cooking in Mexico. Spanish conquistadors brought tomatoes back to Europe and also introduced them to their colonial territories throughout Asia. The Italian word *pomodoro* means golden apple (*pomo d'oro*), so the first tomatoes seen by Europe were most likely yellow-orange colored, not red.

Selective breeding by botanists later generated tomato cultivars that are bright red, perfectly round, and smooth skinned. In the early years, Europeans used tomatoes only for decoration, believing mistakenly the fruit was poisonous because of their association with the deadly nightshade (genus *Solanum*). In Italy, peasants adopted tomatoes in their cooking, where they eventually became one of the essential ingredients in Italian cuisine. When southern Europeans emigrated to North America, tomatoes were also introduced to their new home. Today, tomatoes can be found in markets everywhere. You can buy them fresh, canned, concentrated, dried, powdered, and made into sauces and beverages. Tomatoes are enjoyed in cuisines around the world, from Mediterranean to American to Asian.

Far from being a poisonous fruit, tomatoes contain useful bioactives, especially carotenoids like lycopene, rutin, and beta-cryptoxanthin. Of these, lycopene is the most important because it has been shown to potently inhibit angiogenesis. While all of the tomato contains lycopene, the skin contains three to five times more lycopene than the flesh,[15] so cooking your tomatoes with the skin on is the way to go for health. Cooking is, in fact, an important factor for getting the most out of your tomato. Lycopene in its natural state that occurs in a tomato on the vine exists in a chemical shape called *trans*. Unfortunately, *trans*-lycopene is rather poorly absorbed in the body. By cooking the tomato, though, the heat converts the lycopene structure from the *trans* structure to the *cis* structure, which in fact is readily absorbed by the body.[16] Cooking also releases more lycopene from tomato cells, which increases its concentration in tomato sauce or tomato paste. Lycopene is fat-soluble, which means that it dissolves easily in oil. If you cook a tomato in olive oil, the amount of lycopene absorbed by your blood goes up threefold.

Epidemiological research confirms the health benefits of tomatoes. More than thirty studies have shown the protective effect of tomato consumption on prostate cancer.[17] The Harvard Health Professionals Follow-Up Study examined 46,719 men for lycopene intake and found that consuming two to three cups of tomato sauce per week is associated with a 30 percent decreased risk of prostate cancer, which is consistent with the antiangiogenic effect of lycopene on cancer.[18] In the men who did develop prostate cancer, those who ate more tomato sauce were found to have less angiogenic and less aggressive cancers.[19]

More than one thousand cultivars of tomatoes exist, and the amount of lycopene in each varies greatly. So which ones have the most anti-angiogenic activity? A study of 119 different types of tomatoes showed that cherry tomatoes have 24 percent more lycopene than other types of tomatoes.[20] The San Marzano tomato, an heirloom variety originating from San Marzano, Italy, on the slopes of the volcano Mount Vesuvius, also has one of the highest lycopene levels among tomatoes. It also has a strong distinctive taste, which makes it perfect fresh, canned, and even as a paste used for cooking. A yellow-orange heirloom called the Tangerine tomato is noteworthy because it naturally has high levels of cis-lycopene that is more absorbable in the gut. A clinical trial conducted by researchers at Ohio State University found that tomato juice made from the Tangerine tomato was 8.5-fold better absorbed in the blood than juice from ordinary red tomatoes.[21] The tangy sweet flavor of Tangerine tomatoes makes them worthy for foodies and health seekers alike.[22] Red black-skin tomatoes have more lycopene than red tomatoes, and more than one thousand times more than yellow tomatoes.[23]

Ripe tomatoes should feel heavy in the hand and be firm with a slight give when gently squeezed. They should have a sweet smell. Keep fresh tomatoes at room temperature, away from direct sunlight, and eat them within a few days of picking them off a vine or bringing them home from the market.

Antiangiogenic Vegetables

Broccoli is a cruciferous vegetable and a member of the *Brassica* family of plants. These include broccoli rabe, bok choy, cauliflower, and romanesco. Broccoli originated in Italy. It contains potent antiangiogenic bioactives like brassinin and sulforaphanes. Consuming one to two cups of broccoli per week is associated with a reduced risk of many cancers. Studies from the University of Chicago, the University of Minnesota, Harvard University, and the U.S. National Institutes of Health showed that eating broccoli is associated with a reduced risk of Non-Hodgkin's lymphoma by 40 percent, lung cancer by 28 percent, breast cancer by 17 percent, ovarian cancer by 33 percent, esophageal cancer by 31 percent, prostate cancer by 59 percent, and melanoma by 28 percent.[24]

Kale may be the world's most overhyped healthy vegetable, but it actually deserves its healthy reputation. At least six antiangiogenic bioactives are found in kale: brassinin, indole-3-carbinol, quercetin, lutein, sulforaphane, and kaempferol. Among the many types of kale, there's one that is unusually delicious and available in late fall and winter markets in North America and Europe. It is called cavolo nero (black cabbage), or lacinato, Tuscan kale, or sometimes dinosaur kale. Grown in Tuscany, cavolo nero is a dark-leafed, greenish blue-black varietal that is found in many traditional Italian recipes. It is a key ingredient in original recipes for minestrone and ribollita soups, which are both chock-full of hearty, health-defense-promoting ingredients.

When buying kale, look for bunches with intact leaves and firm stems. Cut the leaves away from the inedible fibrous stem, then chop or shred the leaves, which then can be steamed, blanched, sautéed, used in soup or stew, or mixed into pasta or rice. Properly cooked, cavolo nero is very tender. It turns almost black, and it has a robust flavor with a mild, sweet aftertaste.

Antiangiogenic Fruits

Stone fruit are summer fruits known for sweet flesh bursting with juice, and a pit in the center, the stone. You'll recognize them instantly: peaches, plums, nectarines, apricots, cherries, mango, and even lychee. A host of antiangiogenic (and regenerative as well as DNA protective, which we will discuss later) bioactives, including carotenoids, kaempferol, anthocyanin, quercetin, and chlorogenic acid, are present in stone fruit. Two studies from the U.S. National Cancer Institute and the University of Illinois at Chicago showed that consuming two medium-size stone fruits per day is associated with a 66 percent decreased risk of esophageal cancer and an 18 percent decreased risk of lung cancer in men.[25] When it comes to choosing stone fruit, there are no bad choices, but a useful tip is that plums have three times the amount of cancer-fighting polyphenols compared to peaches. And in the lab, a carotenoid called lutein that is found in apricots, prevents the formation of the brain damaging beta-amyloid fibrils that are linked to abnormal angiogenesis found in Alzheimer's disease.[26] Choose fresh fruits when possible because drying can lower the amount of bioactives, although it may be easier to eat more dried fruits to make up for the loss per fruit.[27]

Apples are good for you, but knowing which type to choose can be confusing. A number of antiangiogenic polyphenols are found in apples, including caffeic and ferulic acid. Two major nutritional epidemiological studies, the EPIC and NIH-AARP Diet and Health Study, analyzed associations between consuming certain fruits and cancer. The results for apples are impressive. Eating one to two apples per day was found to be associated with risk reduction of bladder cancer by 10 percent, colon cancer by 20 percent, and lung cancer by 18 percent.[28]

Of the 7,500 varieties of apples grown around the world, roughly one hundred are available in markets. Except for their taste and texture— firm, crispy, sweet, tart, bland—it's hard to know how they differ from a health perspective. Research is now providing the answer. Of the varietals with the highest levels of defense boosting polyphenols, the top three are: Granny Smith, Red Delicious, and the Reinette (Little Queen).

Whenever apples are in season, so is apple cider. Cloudy apple cider is superior for health because it retains more bioactives.[29] Clear apple juices have been filtered, which can remove many though not all of the healthy compounds. A Mayo Clinic study of 35,159 people showed that drinking two servings per month of apple cider or juice is associated with a 35 percent reduced risk of non-Hodgkin's lymphoma.[30]

Seasonal berries like strawberries, raspberries, blackberries, blueberries, and cranberries can boost your body's angiogenesis defenses. Their intense colors and tartness are a tip-off to the presence of potent bioactives, including anthocyanin and ellagic acid, both of which have antiangiogenic activity. In the European Prospective Investigation into Cancer and Nutrition (EPIC) study, the diet and health patterns of 478,535 people across ten European countries were examined over two decades for their association with cancer and other chronic diseases, including cardiovascular disease. One key conclusion: berry consumption was linked to lower cancer risk. People eating one-fifth cup of berries of any type per day were found to have a 22 percent reduced risk of developing lung cancer.[31]

A special raspberry variant is the black raspberry. The dark color reflects its high bioactive concentrations. Clinical trials with black raspberries have been conducted on patients with Barrett's esophagus, a precancerous lesion, to see their effect. The results show that black raspberries make the lesion less aggressive, reducing the cellular changes that herald the progression to cancer. The same has been seen with precancerous colon polyps. Black raspberries also slow their growth.[32] Blueberries have a dark blue coloration reflecting their antiangiogenic bioactive delphinidin.[33] Studies of 75,929 women showed that those eating one cup of fresh blueberries per week had a 31 percent reduced risk for breast cancer.[34] As I will show you later, blueberries have a remarkable ability to activate multiple health defense systems.

Strawberries are a great source of the bioactive known as ellagic acid, which has potent antiangiogenic activity.[35] The tartness of the berry reflects this acid. High levels of ellagic acid are found in three cultivars: Rubygem (originating in New Zealand), Camarosa (from the Ohio Valley), and Osmanli (from Turkey).[36] These varietals are worth seeking out at the market. Despite their extreme tartness, cranberries actually have low levels of ellagic acid. But what they do have are high levels of bio-active proanthocyanins, which also have anticancer and antiangiogenic effects.[37]

Seafoods

People who eat seafood live longer.[38] The impact of eating fish and shell-fish on angiogenesis provides one explanation. Many seafoods contain healthy polyunsaturated fatty acids (called PUFAs) in their flesh. These healthy fats come from the phytoplankton that fish eat in the ocean. Most people recognize that omega-3 fatty acid is healthy, but there are actually three main forms of this fat that are associated with health benefits: EPA (eicosapentaenoic acid), DHA (docosahexaenoic acid), and ALA (alpha linolenic acid). EPA and DHA can be found in seafood. ALA is found mostly in plant-based foods. Antiangiogenic activity is found in omega-3 PUFAs.[39] However, it's not just the omega-3 PUFAs that play a role in generating health, but the actual ratio between omega-3 and another group of fatty acids called omega-6. The numbers 3 and 6 refer to where the "unsaturated" portion of the fatty acid is located on the molecule. For cancer protection, researchers have found that the higher the overall intake of marine omega-3 in the diet, the greater the benefit. In contrast, higher omega-6 PUFA consumption in relation to omega-3 PUFA (the omega 6:3 ratio), which comes from vegetable oil, for example, is linked to unhealthy inflammation and an increased risk of disease.[40]

Large population studies such as the Singapore Chinese Health Study and the EPIC study have found an association between seafood intake and a reduced risk of cancer. The Singapore study examined the health of 35,298 women and found that eating three ounces of fish or shellfish per day was associated with a 26 percent reduced risk of breast cancer.[41] The EPIC study showed that eating three ounces or more of fish daily was associated with a 31 percent decreased risk of colon cancer.[42]

The benefits of fish extend way beyond cancer prevention. In the Women's Health Study of 38,022 middle-aged women, Harvard researchers found that those who consumed one or more servings of fatty fish per week over a ten-year period had a 42 percent decreased risk of developing age-related macular degeneration (AMD), the most common cause of vision loss in the elderly, associated with leaky blood vessels caused by destructive angiogenesis in the back of the eye.[43] A large meta-analysis conducted by the Changshu No. 2 People's Hospital in China involved 128,988 people across eight different studies in Iceland, the Netherlands, United States, and Australia. The analysis showed that eating fish, ranging in frequency from less than once a month to three to four times per week, was associated with a decreased risk of AMD by 24 percent.[44] The study found differences in protection based on the type of fish consumed. Mackerel, salmon, sardines, bluefish, and swordfish were beneficial and linked to 32 percent reduction of AMD. Eating tuna was linked to a 42 percent risk reduction. While they are delicious, the danger with eating tuna, swordfish, bluefish, and other large fish high up on the food chain is that they often contain high levels of mercury, so consume these fish with caution and only in moderation.

Fatty fish should not be an optional food if your goal is better health. If you live along a coast, you probably are eating fresh seafood already. But, even inland folks can buy seafood that has been flash frozen at sea. This captures the beneficial omega-3 fatty acids, which are still present when the fish is thawed at home. How to choose the best seafood is the big question. If you visit the world's top fish markets, such as Japan's Tsukiji market, Barcelona's Mercat de Sant Josep de la Boqueria, or Venice's Mercato del Pesce, your jaw will drop when you see the dazzling array of fresh, edible creatures that are pulled from the sea every day—amazing fish, crustaceans, and shellfish of a diversity unmatched anywhere else.

To help you navigate the assortment of seafood you encounter in a fish market, I've compiled a list of frequently encountered seafoods based on their level of omega-3 PUFAs and their common appearance in markets and on restaurant menus. To generate this list, I surveyed the world's top fish markets, restaurant menus, and fisheries sustainability charts, then cross-referenced items with reputable databases for nutrient composition across eight countries (Denmark, France, Iceland, Italy, Japan, Norway, Spain, United States) to extract information on the products with the highest levels of omega-3 PUFAs (EPA + DHA) per 100 grams of the seafood. Food lovers rejoice (I've got your back): delicacies like bottarga, squid ink, and sea cucumber are among those with potent antiangiogenic activities.

Here are the top selections for seafood with antiangiogenic omega-3s:

HIGHEST LEVEL (3–30 grams/100 gram of seafood): Hake, sea cucumber, manila clam, big eye tuna, yellowtail, sea bass, bluefin tuna, cockles, bottarga (roe of the gray mullet), caviar (sturgeon), fish roe (salmon).

HIGH LEVEL (>0.5–2.44 grams/100 gram): salmon, red mullet, halibut, Pacific oysters, gray mullet, sardines, arctic char, bluefish, sea bream, Mediterranean sea bass, spiny lobster, anchovies, pompano, redfish, black bass, swordfish, John Dory, eastern oysters, squid, rainbow trout.

MEDIUM LEVEL (>0.2–0.5 grams/100 gram): crab, mussels, striped mullet, octopus, scallops, cuttlefish, shrimp and prawns, whiting, dried cod (bacalao), striped bass, sole, Atlantic lobster.

LOW LEVEL (<0.2 grams/100 gram): cod, grouper, brown shrimp, periwinkle, whelk, abalone, skate.

One final note on fish: be careful of tilapia. This domesticated freshwater fish is found on many menus, and its white flesh has a mild flavor, but there's a hidden threat. Tilapia has a high unhealthy ratio of omega-6 to omega-3 PUFAs, making it a less desirable fish from a health perspective.

Chicken Thigh

Among meats, chicken is one of the healthier choices. Most of us are used to thinking of breast meat as the best part of the bird, because white meat has less fat, but dark meat offers other unique health benefits, especially if you trim off the fat. Research has revealed that thighs and drumsticks are especially healthy choices. Dark chicken meat contains vitamin K2, or menaquinone, a naturally occurring fat-soluble vitamin.[45] Unlike vitamin K1, which is made by plants like spinach, K2 is made by bacteria. It has antiangiogenic properties.

At Hiroshima University in Japan, scientists studying vitamin K2 discovered that it potently suppresses angiogenesis and growth of colon cancer cells.[46] Researchers at the University of Illinois showed that vitamin K2 could inhibit both angiogenesis and prostate cancer growth.[47] K2's benefits extend to heart disease as well. People who ate more K2-containing foods had more than a 57 percent reduction in the chance of dying of heart disease, and a 52 percent reduced risk for severe hardening of the arteries due to plaque buildup.[48] Remember that plaque growth requires angiogenesis, so this association makes sense. Researchers have discovered that menaquinone also interferes with the body's ability to make cholesterol and can prevent hardening of the arteries as well.[49] So, even though you may have grown up accustomed to choosing the chicken breast meat, when it comes to health, it's a no brainer: choose the flavorful legs and thighs.

Air-Cured Ham: the Good, the Bad, and the Ugly

Processed meat is considered a carcinogen by the World Health Organization (WHO). But two meats merit a mention because many people do not know they contain beneficial fats. These are prosciutto di Parma from Italy, and jamón Ibérico de bellota, from Spain. These two hams come from a different breed of pig than typical factory farm pigs. They are bred to have fat streaking throughout their muscles, which makes their meat exceptionally tasty.

Parma pigs are raised in traditional fashion where they are fed the whey of Parmigiano-Reggiano cheese as youngsters, giving the flesh a nutty flavor, and then they finished with a diet of omega-3 PUFA-rich chestnuts. The PUFAs make their way into the fatty streaks of the meat, and the finished product contains healthy PUFAs, just like seafood. Spanish Ibérico pigs are a black-footed species that are free range.[50] They are later fed a diet of omega-3 PUFA-rich acorns, which provides a high level of oleic acid, like in olive oil. Oleic acid facilitates the generation of HDL, the good cholesterol, while it lowers LDL, the bad cholesterol. These hams are air cured, and no artificial preservatives are used. Carved into wafer-thin slices on demand, both hams are a source of omega-3 PUFAs. In fact, nine slices of prosciutto di Parma or jamón Ibérico di bellota will give you the same amount of omega-3 PUFAs (fourteen grams) as a three-ounce serving of salmon.

Is calling prosciutto and jamón healthy too good to be true? Yes, just because they contain beneficial omega-3 PUFAs does not override their downsides. Cured ham is not a health food. Keep in mind that both meats have about twice as much saturated fat as salmon. Both prosciutto and jamón are very high in sodium. They have about twenty-five to thirty times as much sodium as a serving of salmon (which actually lives in salt water). Jamón has about 30 percent less sodium than prosciutto. High sodium intake is linked to hypertension and an increased risk of stomach cancer, and as you'll see in the next chapter, salt harms your stem cells. Compared to salmon, prosciutto also has a higher ratio of omega-6 PUFAs, which is pro-inflammatory, so caution is definitely indicated. Use these facts if you like these hams. If you must, be like the Italians and the Spanish, and eat just a little to enjoy the taste.

Beverages

Tea is the second most popular beverage in the world after water, and it has been brewed for more than four thousand years. Tea leaves contain more than two thousand bioactive compounds like catechins

(EGCG), gallic acid, and theaflavins, many of which end up in the tea-cup when you steep leaves in hot water. At the Angiogenesis Foundation, we began studying teas for their biological properties using lab testing sytems originally designed to evaluate antiangiogenic cancer drugs. We found that tea extracts had really exceptionally potent angiogenesis inhibitory effects, indeed comparable to that of drugs. What was interesting was that different varietals of teas exhibited different potencies. We found Chinese jasmine tea to be more potent than Japanese sencha tea, and Earl Grey tea was even more potent than jasmine tea. The most remarkable finding was that when we crossed cultures and mixed sencha (Japanese) with jasmine (Chinese) tea, the resulting tea blend had a synergistic effect on blood vessel growth that was more than twice as potent against angiogenesis than either one alone.

Of course, green tea is the type of tea most people commonly associate with health benefits. One of the best studied bioactives in green tea is the polyphenol called EGCG (epigallocatechin-3-gallate). Green tea has six-teen times the level of EGCG compared to black tea. EGCG reduces harm-ful angiogenesis and cancer growth, lowers blood pressure, improves blood lipids, restores homeostasis of immune cells, and has antioxidant and anti-inflammatory properties.[51] Green tea technically covers a wide range of beverages, from sencha to jasmine to oolong tea. Drinking two to three cups of green tea a day is associated with a 44 percent reduced risk of developing colon cancer.[52]

Chamomile tea is a popular herbal tea made with the dried petals of the chamomile flower. Chamomile contains bioactives like apigenin, caffeic acid, and chlorogenic acid that have antiangiogenic activity. Researchers at the University of Minho in Braga, Portugal, found that chamomile tea could inhibit angiogenesis by interfering with the signals needed to activate vascular cells to start developing blood vessels.[53]

The varietal, time of harvest, and processing can affect the level of bioactives in tea. White tea is green tea picked early in the season, and it has little to no caffeine. As tea leaves mature over the season, the bioactives in the leaves, including caffeine, increase in their levels. One way to control the potency of the tea you drink is to buy loose-leaf tea, because this allows you to control how much tea leaf is placed in each cup. Bagged teas allow you to dunk the tea in the cup repeatedly, which helps to extract the bioactives into the hot water. Buy only enough tea to last for a month or two to keep you going back to the tea shop for more fresh teas, which are picked and made seasonally. The bioactives and flavor of tea are generally stable for about two years, if the tea is kept dry and stored in a dark place.

Red Wine

Red wine is associated with cardiovascular benefits and anticancer activity. Although wine contains several hundred bioactive compounds, the best known one is resveratrol. But red wine also contains beneficial polyphenols common in other foods, such as catechins, gallic acid, rutin, quercetin, and caffeic acid, among others that are known to be antiangiogenic.[54] Not all wine is created equal, due to the differences in grape varietal and quality, as well as vintage, all of which can affect its antiangiogenic properties. At the Angiogenesis Foundation, we conducted research on the antiangiogenic activity of six different wines made by different grape varietals from the same winery (Vintage Wine Estates) and the same vintage, grown on the same terroir. Among the six, we identified the most potent antiangiogenic wines as Cabernet Sauvignon, Cabernet Franc, and Petit Verdot.

Epidemiological research supports the antiangiogenic effect of wine on cancer. The EPIC-Norfolk study followed 24,244 people for eleven years and found that drinking one glass of wine per day was associated with a 39 percent decreased risk of colorectal cancer.[55] The North Carolina Colon Cancer Study, which followed 2,044 people, found similar results, specifically that drinking less than a full glass of red wine per day was associated with a 27 percent reduced risk of colorectal cancer.[56] Note that high levels of alcohol intake, including wine, are hazardous and can cause atrial fibrillation, hemorrhagic stroke, and cardiomyopathy, as well as esophageal and liver cancer. Everything in moderation is key, because when it comes to wine, it's not the alcohol itself that confers health—the benefits come from the bioactives in the drink.

Beer

Beer hops contain xanthohumerol, which is an antiangiogenic bioactive.[57] A large study undertaken by the U.S. National Cancer Institute was the Prostate, Lung, Colorectal and Ovarian Cancer Screening Trial, which enrolled 107,998 people. An analysis was conducted of the link between beer consumption and kidney cancer, also known as renal cell carcinoma. The study found that drinking approximately five beers per week was remarkably associated with a 33 percent reduced risk for kidney cancer.[58] The North Carolina Colon Cancer Study of 2,044 people found that moderate beer intake (slightly less than one beer per day) was associated with a 24 percent reduction in risk of colon cancer.[59]

Beer consumption has also been linked to cardiovascular benefits. A study from Instituto di Recerche Farmacologiche Mario Negri in Santa Maria Imbaro and Catholic University in Campobasso, Italy, examined fourteen research studies across ten countries and found that drinking one beer per day was associated with a 21 percent reduction in the risk of coronary artery disease.[60] One German study suggests a benefit of beer for the prevention of dementia. The study, led by the Central Institute of Mental Health in Mannheim, was conducted across six German cities (Bonn, Dusseldorf, Hamburg, Leipzig, Mannheim, and Munich) and evaluated 3,203 elderly people over the age of 75. The researchers correlated the intake of different types of alcoholic drinks with the incidence of dementia.[61] Individuals who drank one and a half to two beers per day were found to have a 60 percent reduction in the risk of dementia and an 87 percent reduced risk of being diagnosed specifically with Alzheimer's disease. The same caution for wine goes for beer: high intake levels are dangerous to your health. Be a light or moderate drinker. Alcohol itself is a brain toxin and can increase the risk of dementia at high doses.

Cheese

Cheese as a food predates recorded history. There are more than nine hundred different kinds of cheese, but you'll find only a fraction of them in any given market or grocery store. Although cheese is high in sodium and saturated fats, it also contains antiangiogenic vitamin K2 as a by-product of bacterial starters used in cheese making. A study conducted by Maastricht University profiled vitamin K2 levels in cheese and reported the highest levels to be found in Munster, Gouda, Camembert, Edam, Stilton, and Emmenthal. Jarlsberg cheese also contains high levels of a form of vitamin K2. Cheeses can contain K2 levels comparable to those found in chicken thighs.[62]

The EPIC-Heidelberg study examined the link between vitamin K intake and cancer. The researchers studied 23,340 people for up to fourteen years and found that cheese was the major source of vitamin K2 (menaquinone) in this group. An association was found between consuming the amount of vitamin K2 found in one to three slices of cheese per day and a 62 percent reduction in the risk of lung cancer.

A similar analysis was conducted for men only, and consuming the K2 found in the equivalent of two slices of cheese per day was associated with a 35 percent reduction in the risk of prostate cancer.[63]

Cheese typically contains saturated fat, cholesterol, and high sodium, which are unhealthy factors, so moderation is important. But the evidence allows us to rethink cheese as a food with the potential for some health benefits rather than a food we should categorically rule out as unhealthy.

Olive Oil

Olive oil has been in human use for as long as four thousand years, and its origins stem from Asia Minor and the Mediterranean. Once used as lamp oil and for rituals, olive oil eventually became incorporated into cooking. Spain, Italy, and Greece are the major producers of olive oil today, and all three countries grow olive varietals that contain high levels of bioactive polyphenols. These include oleic acid, oleuropein, hydroxytyrosol, tyrosol, and oleocanthal. These compounds have anti-angiogenic, anti-inflammatory, antioxidant and, as you'll see in chapter 7, unique anticancer properties. Extra virgin olive oil (EVOO) is made from pressed olives without any chemicals or refinement and contains the highest level of bioactives, as well as best taste. It has a shelf life of about two years.

A study conducted by the Instituto di Ricerche Farmacologiche Mario Negri and the University of Milan examined twenty-seven thousand subjects in Italy for their consumption of extra virgin olive oil, butter, margarine, and seed oils.[64] Their consumption was analyzed for links to different type of cancer. They found that three to four tablespoons per day of olive oil was associated with a reduced risk of esophageal cancer by 70 percent, laryngeal cancer by 60 percent, oral and pharyngeal cancer by 60 percent, ovarian cancer by 32 percent, colorectal cancer by 17 percent, and breast cancer by 11 percent. These benefits were not seen with any of the other fats. Butter, in fact, was associated with an increased risk of esophageal, oral, and pharyngeal cancer by twofold. There was no cancer-risk-reducing benefit seen with seed oils.

When buying olive oil, always look for the extra virgin cold-pressed product. To find the oil with the highest levels of health-generating polyphenols, look carefully at the label and see if the type of olive used is identified. By choosing monovarietal olive oils, which are made with only one type of olive, you can choose a product made from olives best for health: Koroneiki (from Greece), Moraiolo (from Italy), and Picual (from Spain). The oils from these olives have great flavor profiles that work well for cooking, salad dressings, or mopping up with bread.

Tree Nuts (Walnuts, Pecans, Almonds, Cashews, Pistachios, Pine Nuts, Macadamia) and Beans

Nuts not only are a popular snack food, but they also contain potent anti-angiogenic omega-3 PUFAs. Thus, nuts are an antiangiogenic food.

A multicenter study led by Harvard Medical School examined 826 patients with stage 3 colon cancer who underwent surgery two months before entering the clinical trial.[65] Participating centers included Duke University, the Southeast Clinical Oncology Research Consortium, Memorial Sloan Kettering Cancer Center, Toledo Community Hospital, Hôpital du Sacré-Coeur de Montréal, Loyola University, Northwestern University, University of Chicago, Virginia Oncology Associates, University of California San Francisco, and Yale University. Patients received standard-of-care chemotherapy, and their intake of nuts was measured and correlated with their clinical outcomes from cancer treatment. The results showed that two servings of tree nuts per week were associated with a remarkable 57 percent reduced risk of death. The amount of nuts in one serving required to achieve this effect are: seven whole walnuts, or eighteen cashews, or twenty-three almonds, or eleven macadamias.

For cancer prevention, the EPIC study examined nut intake in 478,040 people and found an association between women consuming one and a half servings of nuts and seeds per day and a 31 percent reduced risk of colon cancer.[66] For this effect, the dose of nuts would be one of the following: eleven whole walnuts, twenty-six cashews, seventeen macadamia nuts, or four tablespoons of pine nuts. Another study from the University of Toronto studied 1,253 men from Toronto and Quebec and evaluated their intake of nuts, seeds, and beans, among other foods.[67] In relation to nuts or beans, those men who consumed one serving per day had an associated 31 percent reduced risk of prostate cancer. In terms of beans, the serving size would be only two tablespoons per day.

Dark Chocolate (Cocoa)

The health benefits of cacao are emerging to the delight of chocoholics. Scientists at the University of California at Davis have shown that bioactives called procyanidins in cocoa have potent antiangiogenic effects through their ability to stop the signals activating blood vessel cells.[68] Research my group has conducted on cocoa powder showed that not all chocolate is the same. When we studied the antiangiogenic effect of cocoa from two different suppliers of the powder, one of the samples had twice the potency of the other.

Spices and Herbs

Although epidemiologic studies have not yet been performed on spice intake, a large body of lab research shows that common herbs and spices in your kitchen contain antiangiogenic bioactives and antitumor activity. The benefits are seen in both fresh and dried product. Rosemary, oregano, turmeric, licorice, and cinnamon all have antiangiogenic effects.[69] In cells and in lab animals, these have been shown to have potent effects in suppressing tumor angiogenesis. Sprinkling antiangiogenic herbs and spices into your food is a good idea and flavor-enhancing addition to any meal.

Diseases in Need of More Angiogenesis

On the other side of the angiogenesis defense equation, boosting blood vessel growth with diet can help feed your organs and stave off disease. You may be wondering, *Can I safely eat foods that promote angiogenesis without provoking cancer or other diseases that have excessive blood vessels?* The answer is yes. Remember that foods cannot override the body's own normal setpoints for angiogenesis. This means that antiangiogenic foods can't reduce the number of blood vessels in the body needed to maintain the health of your organs. And it also means that angiogenesis-stimulating foods can't shut down your body's defensive ability to keep excessive blood vessels pruned back so they cannot cause disease. Diet can only help enhance the natural state of balance. By nourishing your angiogenesis health defense on both sides of the equation, you can eat to beat many diseases simultaneously.

Dietary angiogenesis can help your organs thrive in a number of situations. Your cardiovascular system needs blood vessels to function at its optimal level. When there are not enough vessels to meet the circulatory demand of your heart, brain, legs, or internal organs, the cells become oxygen starved and are crippled. Eventually, they will die.

Ischemic heart disease is caused by the narrowing of the coronary arteries that bring blood to your heart muscle. Ischemia occurs when there is an inadequate blood supply. As cholesterol-laden plaques grow in your blood vessel walls over your lifetime, they can choke off a part of your circulation and lead to chest pain, known as angina. Some people have inherited conditions like familial hypercholesterolemia in which the body can't remove harmful cholesterol (low-density lipoprotein) from the blood. If you have this condition, your risk of a heart attack is five times that of someone with average blood lipid levels. As a response to blockages, the heart opens up collateral blood channels at the same time as it valiantly tries to grow new blood vessels to improve its blood flow and oxygen levels.

Unfortunately, angiogenesis is often insufficient or occurs too slowly to meet the high blood flow demands of the compromised heart. The ischemia gets worse, and eventually the heart muscle weakens and heart failure results. Heart attacks are caused by a sudden rupture of a coronary plaque that closes off the vessel like a trapdoor, sealing off blood flow and killing the heart muscle beyond the blockage. If you survive the event, your heart will grow new blood vessels to repair the damage and bypass the blockage to limit further cell death—but as we touched on before, if the angiogenic response had been more effective before the crisis, the damage may never have happened.

Your brain can suffer the same type of crisis. When the brain blood vessels become narrowed, brain cells become oxygen starved. This can also happen when the carotid arteries, the major trunks of blood vessels coursing through your neck to your brain, become blocked. The brain tries to form natural bypass channels by mounting an angiogenic response. If this is inadequate, and no bypasses form, the brain tissue slowly dies. A blood clot can also be sent to the brain, causing an ischemic stroke. There are other causes of stroke, too, such as bleeding in the brain, but in each situation, there is the need for robust angiogenesis to avoid severe disability or death.

The same narrowing that can occur with atherosclerosis in the heart and brain can also occur in your legs. This is called peripheral artery disease, and it leads to inadequate blood flow to the lower limbs and feet. Poor blood flow makes it difficult to do any sort of exercise, including walking. The lack of oxygen in the muscles causes severe cramping. If the blockages become more severe, the leg tissues will eventually start to die. Insufficient angiogenesis prevents the leg from compensating under these conditions.

Chronic wounds begin as skin ulcers, usually on the legs and feet, which do not heal. People with diabetes are especially prone to foot ulcers because the blood supply to the nerves in the foot is insufficient, and the nerves suffer ischemia and can die. Many people with diabetes do not have sensation in their feet. So, small injuries to toes or to the sole of the foot, from even a pebble in the shoe, can wear a hole in the foot without the person even feeling it. These wounds have trouble healing because diabetes interferes with wound angiogenesis. Non-healing wounds easily become infected, and this can insidiously lead to gangrene.

Problem wounds occur even in people who do not have diabetes. Venous leg ulcers are the most common wounds in aging people because the valves in their veins malfunction. This leads to the backup of blood in the lower leg, causing massive swelling. This back-pressure eventually stretches the skin of the calves to the point of blistering and bursting, creating a shallow wound. Healing can be extremely slow due to insufficient angiogenesis that occurs in these types of wounds.

Similarly, pressure ulcers (or bed sores) can occur in anyone who puts inordinate and unrelieved pressure on any one spot on the body. People who are bedridden and unable to move can develop these ulcers on their buttocks and near their tailbone. People who are amputees put a high degree of pressure on their stump when they wear a prosthesis. Unrelieved pressure impairs angiogenesis, and the sores are slow to heal, often becoming infected.

Erectile dysfunction is a serious problem for many men. It has many underlying causes, but insufficient angiogenesis to help bring blood to the pudendal nerve will definitely knock out function of the penis. Erectile dysfunction is common in men with poorly controlled diabetes, and the same type of impaired angiogenesis seen in the diabetic foot also occurs in the penis.

Alopecia, or hair loss, can be due to inadequate blood vessel growth. Hair follicles require new blood vessels for their nutritional needs. When this is compromised, hair is not replaced as it naturally falls off the scalp. Poor circulation in the scalp compromises the ability of hair to grow normally and can contribute to baldness.

Angiogenesis-Stimulating Foods

Until a few years ago, no one knew that foods can stimulate angiogenesis and improve blood flow. But the scientific evidence is now very clear that your diet can help increase your circulation. Here's a list of the currently identified proangiogenic foods.

Grains and Seeds

Barley is an ancient grain commonly used for making soups, stews, and beer. It is high in dietary fiber and has been shown to lower blood cholesterol. The bioactive in barley is beta-D-glucan, which activates angiogenesis and grows new blood vessels in oxygen-starved organs.[70] Researchers at the Institute of Life Sciences—Scuola Superiore Sant'Anna in Pisa, Italy, studied barley's effects on human blood vessel cells growing in culture, as well as in the hearts of mice that had suffered a heart attack.[71] They developed a pasta enriched with barley beta-D-glucan and fed it to the mice. The mice that ate the beta-glucan from barley had double the survival after a heart attack, compared to those who did not consume it. The scientists found the barley beta-glucan increased angiogenesis in the heart. The new blood supply protected the heart and decreased the amount of damage caused by the heart attack. The researchers also found adding barley beta-glucan to the mice's drinking water could similarly protect the heart from damage.

Seeds like flaxseed, sunflower seeds, sesame seeds, pumpkin seeds, and chia seeds are nutrient-dense snacks that contain bioactives called lignans. One such lignan, secoisolariciresinol diglucoside (SDG), has been shown to stimulate angiogenesis in the heart after a heart attack. Researchers from the Molecular Cardiology and Angiogenesis Laboratory at the University of Connecticut Health Center fed lab rats a high-cholesterol diet and then induced an experimental heart attack.[72] The rats were divided into two groups, and one was also fed a diet that contained SDG. After the heart attack, recovery and mortality of the animals was assessed. The animals fed the seed bioactive had a twofold increase in the angiogenic growth factor VEGF. Their hearts had 33 percent more new blood vessels, and their hearts pumped blood 22 percent more efficiently compared to mice who did not have the seed bioactive. The size of the tissue damaged by the heart attack was also 20 percent smaller in these animals. Seeds containing SDG have another benefit:

they are high in dietary fiber, which can lower cholesterol as well as feed the gut microbiome. This adds other useful layers of benefit that can protect your heart and your health.

Foods Containing Ursolic Acid

Ursolic acid is a powerful bioactive known as a triterpenoid that is found in ginseng, rosemary, peppermint, and in fruit skins, including apple peel. In the lab, ursolic acid stimulates beneficial angiogenesis and can grow new capillaries and enhance blood flow in mice with compromised leg circulation.[73] Remarkably, it also inhibits harmful angiogenesis that feeds cancers.[74] Thus, this bioactive is one of the unique factors that can work both sides of the angiogenesis equation at once, helping to ensure balance of this health defense system. A number of dried fruits, such as sultana raisins, cherries, cranberries, and blueberries, contain ursolic acid because they are dried with the fruit skin or peel intact.[75]

Foods Rich in Quercetin

Quercetin is a bioactive that stimulates angiogenesis in the face of oxygen deprivation of tissues, yet it does not provoke growth of cancers.[76] In fact, quercetin inhibits inflammation and tumor angiogenesis in animals with lymphoma and breast cancer, thus also working both sides of the angiogenesis equation.[77] This double-barreled approach can defend against cancer and heart disease. Foods that contain quercetin include capers, onions, red-leaf lettuce, hot green chile peppers, cranberries, black plums, and apples.

Putting It All Together

Specific foods and beverages can activate your angiogenesis defense system and help maintain a healthy state of balance. Eating the right foods can beat back and prune away excessive blood vessels to thwart diseases like cancer, endometriosis, vision loss, arthritis, Alzheimer's disease, and even obesity, because these conditions all involve abnormal new blood vessels growing in your body. Foods and beverages containing a rich supply of natural antiangiogenic substances can boost your body's own natural defenses against pathological blood vessel growth and help keep these diseases from gaining a foothold. On the flip side, food and beverages with natural angiogenesis-stimulating factors can aid your body's natural abilities to keep up a robust circulation where it is critically needed, such as your heart, brain, skin, nerves, and even hair follicles. Healthy growth of blood vessels allows your organs to maintain their form and function.

The angiogenesis dietary approach is easy to adopt into everyday living. All you need is to know how your blood vessels influence your health, and then be able to identify foods and beverages and ingredients that can keep your healthy circulation flourishing and not growing out of control. The growing number of foods that are being discovered to help your body control angiogenesis means you have many choices to select from and match with your own personal dietary preferences. If you are a health-minded person who just wants to optimize their defenses, you can keep a supply of these fresh angiogenesis-influencing foods at home. You can look for them at the market, and on the menu when ordering at a restaurant. And, importantly, if you are in the midst of battling an angiogenesis-dependent disease, know that your diet is one health intervention that you can prescribe to yourself.

KEY FOODS AFFECTING ANGIOGENESIS

Antiangiogenic			
Almonds	Caviar (sturgeon)	Lychee	Red black-skin tomatoes
Anchovies	Cherries	Macadamia nuts	Redfish
Apple Cider	Cherry tomatoes	Mackerel	Romanesco
Apples—Red Delicious, Granny Smith, Reinette	Chestnuts	Mango	Rosemary
Apricots	Chicken (dark meat)	Manila clam	Salmon
Arctic char	Cinnamon	Muenster cheese	San Marzano tomatoes
Beer	Cockles	Navy beans	Sardines
Big eye tuna	Cranberries	Nectarines	Sea bream
Black bass	Dark chocolate	Olive oil (EVOO)	Sea cucumber
Black beans	Eastern oysters	Oolong tea	Sea bass
Black raspberries	Edam cheese	Oregano	Sencha tea
Black tea	Emmenthal cheese	Pacific oysters	Soy
Blackberries	Fish roe (salmon)	Peaches	Spiny lobster
Blueberries	Gouda cheese	Pecans	Squid
Blue fin tuna	Green tea	Pine nuts	Squid ink
Bluefish	Grey mullet	Pistachios	Stilton cheese
Bok choy	Hake	Plums	Strawberries
Bottarga	Halibut	Pomegranates	Swordfish
Broccoli	Jamón iberico de belotta	Pompano	Tangerine tomatoes
Broccoli rabe	Jarlsberg cheese	Prosciutto di Parma	Tieguanyin tea
Camembert cheese	Jasmine tea	Rainbow trout	Tuna
Cashews	John Dory	Raspberries	Turmeric
Cauliflower	Kale	Red mullet	Walnuts
Chamomile tea	Licorice root	Red wine	Yellowtail
Angiogenesis Stimulating			
Apple peel	Cherries (dried)	Ginseng	Sesame seeds
Apples	Chia seeds	Onions	Sultana raisins
Barley	Chile peppers	Peppermint	Sunflower seeds
Black plums	Cranberries	Pumpkin seeds	
Blueberries (dried)	Cranberries (dried)	Red-leaf lettuce	
Capers	Flaxseed	Rosemary	

CHAPTER 7

(Re)generate Your Health

We all want to remain youthful and keep our vitality as long as possible so we can truly enjoy everything life has to offer. Even if you are not interested in living until you are one hundred, you still always want a spring in your step and to be sharp of mind. Science is telling us that we can counteract the effects of aging through foods that stimulate our stem cells to act like they once did in our youth. Plain old aging makes our stem cells wane in number and potency, and it slows down your body's ability to regenerate. Selecting the right foods can help you kick your stem cells into action to help grow muscles, maintain vigor, and slow the ravages of aging.

Not only do stem cells keep you youthful, they can also regenerate tissues damaged by aging. Recall the study from Homburg, Germany, showing that patients who suffered heart attacks or strokes had poorer survival if they had low baseline levels of circulating stem cells. We know that a specific type of stem cell called the endothelial progenitor cell (EPC) supports the creation of new angiogenic blood vessels, as we saw in the last chapter. But these stem cells also repair and regenerate damaged blood vessels caused by aging and high cholesterol, protecting cardiovascular health. Lifestyle changes, such as quitting smoking, exercising, or taking medications such as statins, recruit more EPCs into the bloodstream to enhance this effect. So can some foods and beverages.

While it may seem counterintuitive that eating chocolate could lower the risks of having coronary artery disease, chocolate is a stem cell–recruiting food. Cocoa powder contains bioactives called flavanols. Epidemiologists have long established a connection between the consumption of foods with flavanols and lower incidence of death from cardiovascular disease.[1]

At the University of California, San Francisco, researchers explored whether a chocolate drink made with cocoa containing high levels of flavanols could influence stem cells and blood vessel health.[2] They recruited sixteen patients with known coronary artery disease and divided them into two groups. One group received hot cocoa with a low flavanol content of only nine milligrams per serving. The other group was given hot cocoa with a high flavanol content of 375 milligrams per serving (42 times more flavanol), made with a powder called CocoaPro. Both groups drank the hot chocolate twice a day for thirty days.

At the end of the study, the researchers compared bloodwork from before and after the experiment. Amazingly, participants who drank the high-flavanol hot cocoa had twice as many stem cells in their circulation compared to the people who drank the low-flavanol cocoa. The researchers wanted to see if there was any improvement in blood flow from the cocoa. So, they used a test called flow mediated dilation, in which a blood pressure cuff and an ultrasound scanner measure how quickly blood vessels dilate to restore blood flow after they are constricted. High dilation indicates less damage to the blood vessel walls and overall better health. The high-flavanol cocoa group's results in this test were two times better than at the beginning, demonstrating a functional benefit of the cocoa to circulation. In fact, the beneficial effect on stem cell levels was reported by the researchers to be comparable to that seen from taking statins, common cholesterol-lowering drugs also known to improve stem cell levels.[3]

Chocolate is just one of the foods that is being revealed to increase our body's regenerative power. The stem cells in bone marrow, skin, the heart, and other organs can be called into action by what and how we eat. Eating regenerative foods makes you more fit from the inside out, and keeps rebuilding your organs so they are in their best possible shape. Foods that mobilize stem cells help counteract and prevent the organ damage that inevitably develops with aging. Stem cells can also help reverse the ravages of diabetes, cardiovascular disease, smoking, high cholesterol, and obesity. Imagine if patients recovering from heart attack or stroke, for example, could dine on a menu at the hospital or at home designed to activate stem cells to repair their hearts and brains and speed recovery. Imagine if they had started with a regenerative diet as children or young adults. They might have been able to dodge the disease altogether.

You will hear in the news how exciting feats of engineering are being accomplished to develop regenerative therapies using 3-D printed organs or genetically engineered cells that can be injected or implanted. But here's what you need to know: Mother Nature has already beaten these efforts to the punch with foods and beverages that can mobilize our stem cells. There are also some foods and dietary patterns you should avoid or minimize, because they can actually harm your stem cells and weaken your regenerative defenses. Then there's a twist in the story: while most stem cells are helpful, some special types of stem cells are harmful, and can form cancers. These are cancer stem cells, and they need to be destroyed. Some foods can do that, too.

Diseases of Importance: Conditions Where Increasing Stem Cells Can Help Heal

There are many conditions for which your body could use a boost of stem cells to improve health. This includes any condition associated with aging, including Parkinson's disease and Alzheimer's disease.[4] Many cardiovascular diseases share as a common feature damage to the inner lining of blood vessels that are in need of repair and regeneration. In heart failure, the weakened heart tries to call in stem cells to regenerate the heart muscle, but usually it is too little, too late. In the brain, stem cells can regenerate brain cells after an ischemic stroke. They also help regenerate new blood vessels to restore blood flow in struggling brain tissue. When the muscles, tendons, and nerves of your legs start dying in peripheral artery disease, the body calls in stem cells to try to reverse the damage. Chronic wounds in the feet, ankles, and lower legs need stem cells to regenerate healthy tissue and close the injury, in order to avoid infection and deadly gangrene.

Diabetes is a multiheaded dragon of a disease where metabolism is deranged and organs become damaged. The high levels of blood sugar seen in people with diabetes damage their stem cells and lower their numbers, reducing the body's ability to repair organs. This can lead to many of the destructive consequences of diabetes: diabetic cardiomyopathy (heart failure), diabetic nephropathy (kidney failure), diabetic neuropathy (nerve death), diabetic foot ulcers (chronic wounds), diabetic retinopathy (vision loss). Speaking of eye disease, ophthalmologists have shown the benefits of delivering stem cells in early clinical trials of regenerative therapy in age-related macular degeneration.[5]

Osteoporosis has been shown in lab research to improve after injecting bone-building stem cells.[6] Stem cells can regenerate skin after reconstructive and plastic surgery following trauma or after surgery for cancer. They can regenerate and rebuild cartilage in osteoarthritis.[7] They also grow new nerves after spinal cord injury and peripheral nerve injury. Stem cells are being explored for growing hair in alopecia, and for restoring penile function in erectile dysfunction.[8] There is even compelling evidence that stem cells can be useful for treating some forms of autism, Parkinson's disease, and acute brain injury.[9]

Stem Cell–Boosting Foods

A wide variety of foods, including cocoa, are being studied for their beneficial effects on our stem cells. By supporting the body's regenerative defense system, these foods can help influence everything from repairing damaged organs to counterbalancing the effects of eating too much fat.

Fish Oil

As we saw in chapter 6, the omega-3 polyunsaturated fatty acids (PUFAs) found in fish benefit the heart and brain by reducing the damage caused by vascular inflammation and atherosclerosis. Some of the highest levels of marine omega-3 PUFAs are found in fish like hake, tuna, and amberjack (yellowtail) as well as shellfish like Manila clams and cockles. A delicacy of Asia, the sea cucumber, is also high in omega-3 PUFAs.

Scientists at the University of Montreal discovered that a diet rich in fish oil increases production of endothelial progenitor stem cells that can regenerate oxygen-deprived muscles.[10] In the lab, they studied mice with ischemic limbs that are in danger of severe muscle damage from poor blood flow, similar to what happens in humans with severe peripheral artery disease. The mice were fed either a 20 percent fish oil diet (high omega-3 fatty acids) or a corn oil diet (more pro-inflammatory omega-6 fatty acids) for twenty-one days. The results showed that those fed with fish oil had 30 percent more endothelial progenitor cells produced in their body than those who were fed corn oil, resulting in a better circulation and less muscle damage in their legs.

The researchers also directly tested the two oils on isolated stem cells. They exposed some cells to the omega-3 rich fish oil and others to the corn oil and then looked for the stem cells' ability to migrate across a surface, a function needed for regeneration. The stem cells exposed to fish oil could migrate 50 percent better than cells exposed to corn oil. This study suggests that consuming fish oil may help your stem cells improve circulatory function.

Squid Ink

Squid ink, which actually usually comes from cuttlefish, contains bioactives that not only inhibit angiogenesis, but also can protect stem cells.

Scientists at Ocean University of China fed the ink to mice who suffered radiation injury to examine its effects on bone marrow stem cells.[11] The radiation caused suppression of the bone marrow and damaged the stem cells contained within it. One group of mice received ink daily for a total of 40 days. The other group received only saline. The results showed that ink-fed mice had significantly protected stem cells in the bone marrow, so the mice were able to regenerate more blood cells, including immune cells, compared to those who did not have any ink. This study showed squid ink has the ability to protect and increase the regenerative capacity of stem cells following radiation injury.

Whole Wheat

Food made with whole grain is healthier because it includes the grain's outer shell, which contains fiber, as well as the inner core that contains bioactive polyphenols. Common wheat (*Triticum aestivum*) is an ancient domesticated cereal crop dating back at least twelve thousand years and is used for making bread and other baked goods. Epidemiological studies have shown that eating a whole grain diet is associated with the reduced risk of many diseases, including cardiovascular disease and diabetes.[12] Scientists at the University of Pisa in Italy have found that whole-wheat extracts make endothelial progenitor cells live and function longer.[13]

Green Beans

A component of green beans (specifically the Lady Joy varietal *Phaseolus vulgaris*, the common green bean) has been shown to protect endothelial progenitor cells against oxidative damage from free radicals and improve their survival.[14] Green beans can be eaten fresh or dried, and there are many varieties that are grown and used in cooking.

Black Chokeberry

The black chokeberry is a dark-colored, blueberry-size fruit from a hardy bush (*Aronia melanocarpa*) growing in North America and Europe. Its color tells you it is packed with polyphenols. Sometimes called aronia, these berries are traditionally used in Eastern Europe for jams and juices, but they have become more popular worldwide for their healthful properties. Scientists at the University of Warsaw in Poland examined endothelial progenitor cells in the blood of healthy young individuals and found that exposing them to chokeberry extracts could protect the stem cells against stress. The exposure to chokeberry also improved the ability of the stem cells to migrate and participate in regenerating blood vessels.[15]

Rice Bran

Rice grains come from the field covered with a hard, edible, vitamin-packed layer called the bran. The bran is often removed and discarded during refining to convert brown rice into white rice, but it actually contains many health-promoting bioactives, including beta-glucan and the polyphenol ferulic acid. Rice bran is also a good source of dietary fiber.

Researchers from the University of Seville and the University of Lleida in Spain, the University of Saarlandes in Germany, and the University of Leipzig in Germany showed that the ferulic acid from rice bran can protect and improve the activity and survival of endothelial progenitor cells. They gave five healthy human volunteers ferulic acid extracted from rice bran to consume for fifteen days. The researchers took blood samples from the volunteers before and after the study, isolated their stem cells, and grew them in plastic dishes. They then exposed the stem cells to hydrogen peroxide, which creates cell-damaging oxidative stress.

For stem cells taken before the exposure to rice bran extract, the hydrogen peroxide caused the stem cells to die through a process called apoptosis, a form of cell suicide, at a rate 4.7 times their normal rate.

However, the stem cells taken after rice bran exposure were completely protected against this biochemical stress and survived normally.[16]

Eating a diet high in saturated fat damages the lining of blood vessels and leads to the formation of the vessel-narrowing plaques causing cardiovascular disease. In the lab, scientists showed that adding rice bran to the diet of mice eating a high-fat diet reduced the incidence of arteriosclerosis.[17] By protecting the blood vessel lining from damage, a job of stem cells, the formation of the atherosclerotic plaque was reduced by 2.6-fold. Taken together, these studies suggest that rice bran can protect the stem cells involved in repairing the damage in blood vessels caused by eating a high-fat diet.

One important caution about brown rice: some fields where it is harvested have high levels of arsenic. Brown rice has more of the exposed shell of the rice, so it can contain 80 percent more arsenic than white rice. According to a study by *Consumer Reports*, the safest sources of brown rice are California, India, and Pakistan, which has about a third less arsenic than brown rice from other sources.[18]

Turmeric

Turmeric is a root in the ginger family, commonly used in Southeast Asian cuisine. It can be eaten fresh but more commonly is dried and ground into a bright orange powder used as a spice, and as a traditional medicine. The main bioactive in turmeric is curcumin, which has anti-inflammatory, antioxidant, antiangiogenic, and pro-regenerative properties. A study conducted by Soochow University in China examined mice with diabetes whose legs had poor circulation.[19] As known to occur in diabetes, the mice had a significantly reduced number—only half—of endothelial progenitor cells in their circulation compared to mice without diabetes. The diabetic mice were given curcumin dissolved in olive oil by mouth for two weeks. After receiving curcumin, the endothelial progenitor cells in the diabetic mice increased twofold, or back to normal levels seen in nondiabetic mice. Blood flow in the leg also improved dramatically, by as much as eightfold, after curcumin was consumed. Considering this is spice that also adds flavor to many dishes, people with diabetes may wish to incorporate turmeric into their diet.

Foods and Beverages High in Resveratrol

Resveratrol is a bioactive well known to be in grapes, red wine, and grape juice. But resveratrol is also present in blueberries, cranberries, peanuts, and even pistachios, as well. In nature, resveratrol acts as a natural fungicide to fight fungi that could destroy the plant. So this is a bioactive that is first and foremost part of a plant's health defense system.

When humans consume resveratrol, different types of human cells are stimulated and the bioactive influences their behavior. For example, resveratrol activates cardiac stem cells that usually lie dormant in your heart but are capable of regenerating heart tissue under stress. Scientists at Soochow University, the Third People's Hospital in Kunshan, and Nanjing Medical University in China studied the effect of resveratrol on stem cells in the hearts of mice. They gave resveratrol each day to normal, healthy mice for a week and found that even in the absence of disease, it caused the number of cardiac stem cells to increase in the heart tissue by 1.7-fold.

In mice that had suffered a heart attack, the researchers injected 1 million cardiac stem cells therapeutically to see if they could rescue the heart. Animals given resveratrol in addition to the injection had an increased number of blood vessels in the heart and almost a doubling of the survival of cardiac stem cells.[20]

The practical challenge with resveratrol is that it is present only in small amounts in red wine and most foods, so it would require a huge intake of wine to match the amounts used in most research studies. Because of this, resveratrol may be one of the few exceptions where the bioactive may be better obtained through a concentrated supplement rather than the actual food.

Foods High in Zeaxanthin

Zeaxanthin is a bioactive known as a carotenoid. It is a pigment that gives corn and saffron their yellow-orange color, but it's also common in leafy green vegetables, like kale, mustard greens, spinach, watercress, collard greens, Swiss chard, and fiddleheads. Zeaxanthin is also found in high concentration in goji berries, the dried flat elliptical red berries used in Asian herbal teas, soups, and stir-fried dishes. This bioactive is very important for eye health. After foods containing zeaxanthin are eaten, it accumulates in the retina, the layer in the back of the eye where light is sensed and relayed to the brain. Clinical studies have shown that consuming zeaxanthin can help to protect the eye against the blinding condition age-related macular degeneration.[21]

Scientists from Jinan University in Guangzhou, China, and Shenzhen Third People's Hospital have examined the impact of zeaxanthin on stem cells. They obtained stem cells from human fat using liposuction, and exposed them to zeaxanthin. Those stem cells survived better and showed less evidence of inflammation than stem cells that did not have any exposure to zeaxanthin.

The scientists then tested whether zeaxanthin could help stem cells rescue an organ damaged by disease. They injected mice with failing livers with 2 million mesenchymal stem cells obtained from human fat tissue so the stem cells could regenerate their livers. Some of the mice received stem cells that had first been exposed to zeaxanthin, and the rest received untreated stem cells. After seven days, the plain stem cell therapy had decreased the liver damage by roughly half. However, in mice who received stem cells that had been treated with zeaxanthin, the stem cells reduced liver damage by an impressive 75 percent in the same period of time.[22]

The results of this study suggest that eating zeaxanthin-containing foods may help the performance of our stem cells for organ regeneration.

Foods High in Chlorogenic Acid

Chlorogenic acid is another powerful bioactive found in high concentrations in coffee and also present in black tea, blueberries, peaches, fresh and dried plums, eggplants, and even bamboo shoots. It has anti-inflammatory, antiangiogenic, and blood-pressure-lowering effects.[23] Stem cell protection can now be added to its benefits. Researchers at Nanchang University in China studied how chlorogenic acid can influence the survival of mesenchymal stem cells that are involved with organ healing and regeneration. They found that when stem cells were exposed to chlorogenic acid, they became more resilient against stress and this doubled their rate of survival, which extended their ability to participate in maintaining organ health in the body.[24]

Black Raspberries

Their dark color and tartness reveal that black raspberries contain many potent bioactives like ellagic acid, ellagitannins, anthocyanins, and quercetin. In fact, a dietary supplement made from black raspberries has shown clinical benefits in patients with colon cancer, and in pre-diabetes.[25] The ellagic acid of the black raspberries activates stem cells.[26] Researchers working at the Korea University Anam Hospital in Seoul studied the effect of the berries in fifty-one patients who had metabolic syndrome.[27] This is a cluster of dangerous health conditions such as obesity, elevated blood sugar, hypertension, high triglycerides, and low HDL (good cholesterol) that puts anyone with them at high risk for developing cardiovascular disease. Their blood was drawn at the beginning of the study, and the number of circulating stem cells was measured. The patients were then given black raspberry powder or a placebo to consume daily for twelve weeks.

Here's what they found: individuals eating the black raspberry powder had a 30 percent increase in their circulating endothelial progenitor cells, while those taking a placebo actually had a 35 percent *decrease* in their stem cell levels due to their metabolic syndrome. When the researchers measured the blood vessel stiffness of people who consumed black raspberry powder, they found there was a reduction in the stiffness over the twelve weeks, reflecting healthier blood vessels and the beneficial effects of more circulating stem cells.

Chinese Celery

Chinese celery is a common vegetable in Asia, with thinner stalks and a stronger flavor than Western celery. You might have eaten it as part of a stir-fry because it is commonly used in dishes on the menu of authentic Chinese restaurants. The leaves, stalks, and seeds of Chinese celery are all edible and contain a number of health-promoting bioactives, including a tongue twister: 3-n-butylphthalide (NBP).[28] NBP is important because it was approved as a pharmaceutical drug in 2002 by regulatory agencies in China for doctors to use as a neuroprotective treatment in patients who have suffered a stroke.[29] NBP, also found in supplements containing celery seed extract, improves brain circulation, lowers brain inflammation, grows nerves, and limits brain damage from stroke.[30]

Researchers from Soochow University in China studied how NBP helps patients recover from a stroke. They recruited 170 individuals who had suffered an acute ischemic stroke, meaning a blood clot caused an interruption of blood flow and killed part of the brain.[31] In the trial, some patients took oral NBP, and some received only standard care. The researchers drew blood seven, fourteen, and thirty days after treatment. In all patients, the number of stem cells in the bloodstream increased immediately after the stroke, which is the expected response from the regenerative health defense system, but in patients who received only standard care, the stem cell levels declined after day 7. In contrast, in patients who received NBP, their circulating stem cells steadily increased. By day 30, NBP-treated patients had circulating stem cell levels 75 percent higher than the patients who received only standard care. Brain CT scans showed that those who took NBP also had improved blood flow in the area of the stroke, which is explained by the greater stem cells homing to the injured site in the brain.

While these results are from a drug form of NBP, it shows that a bioactive present in Chinese celery has stem cell–activating properties that may help heal and regenerate organs after a medical catastrophe like a stroke.

Mangoes

Mangoes are a stone fruit with an intensely sweet, orange-colored, edible flesh that is eaten raw, cooked, dried, or pickled. They can also be cooked with other ingredients, and are commonly found in the cuisines of Southeast Asia and Latin America. Although they have many bioactive carotenoids that give the flesh its orange color, mangoes contain a unique bioactive called mangiferin that has antitumor, antidiabetic, and pro-regenerative properties.[32] In lab animals, mangiferin has been shown to improve blood sugar control by actually regenerating the beta-islet cells of the pancreas that produce insulin.

Scientists from the Sichuan Academy of Medical Science, the Sichuan Provincial People's Hospital, Sichuan University, and the People's Hospital of Leshan in southwestern China found that mangiferin could increase insulin secretion in mice by increasing the number of beta-islet cells in the pancreas by 67 percent and by activating genes for regeneration and insulin production.[33] Other scientists have shown mangiferin can stimulate bone regeneration.[34] These experimental studies injected mangiferin, so the doses cannot be directly translated to mango consumption, but the results demonstrate the remarkable activity of the bioactive.

Stem Cell–Stimulating Beverages

Red Wine

Moderate consumption of red wine is beneficial for health. Researchers from the Taipei Veterans General Hospital in Taiwan studied the stem cells of eighty healthy people, in their mid-thirties, who were given either red wine (half glass),[35] beer (one can), vodka (one shot), or water each day for three weeks.[36] They were not allowed to drink tea, grape juice, or any other alcoholic beverages other than what was specified during the study period. All individuals had similar blood pressure, stem cell levels, and other physical parameters at the beginning of the study.

After three weeks, the bloodwork showed that red wine drinkers had a twofold increase in the levels of endothelial progenitor cells in circulation. The same benefits were not seen with the subjects who drank beer, vodka, or water. When these stem cells were exposed to red wine or resveratrol, they had an even greater ability to migrate, form blood vessel tubes, and survive. Moreover, the red wine drinkers had a 35 percent improvement of their blood vessels' ability to dilate, a reflection of vascular health. Red wine drinkers also had a 50 percent increase in blood levels of a powerful signal called nitric oxide, one of the body's most fundamental signals that control health. Nitric oxide not only helps blood vessels dilate, but it stimulates angiogenesis for healing, and it signals for stem cells to be activated.

When it comes to red wine, more isn't better. Researchers have reported that the benefits are seen with up to one to two glasses of wine a day, but with more wine, there is less benefit. It's important to know that high levels of alcohol actually damage stem cells and interfere with their ability to regenerate organs. So, as with most things in the diet, moderation is key.

Researchers from the Instituto di Richerche Farmacologiche Mario

Negri in Italy analyzed thirteen clinical studies of red wine and its effects on cardiovascular disease. The combined studies involved 209,418 people. Their analysis concluded that red wine intake was associated with an overall 32 percent reduced risk of atherosclerosis.[37]

Beer

Beer is made with yeast, and the hops from beer production contain bioactive polyphenols such as xanthohumol, that wind up in the beverage itself. These bioactives may explain the 25 percent reduction in risk of death from cardiovascular disease with moderate (one to two drinks per day) alcohol consumption of beer.[38] In contrast, cocktails like gin or vodka are distilled alcoholic beverages and do not contain polyphenols. Not surprisingly, these drinks are not associated with health benefits.

Researchers from the University of Barcelona in Spain examined the effect of beer on endothelial progenitor cells in thirty-three men between the ages of fifty-five and seventy-five who had diabetes and other cardiovascular risk factors, like smoking, obesity, high cholesterol, or a family history of premature heart disease.[39] They gave the men either two regular beers containing alcohol, a beer with its alcohol removed, or two shots of gin to drink each day for four weeks. Blood was drawn at the beginning and at the end of the study to count the number of circulating stem cells. The results showed that men drinking alcoholic beer had an eightfold increase in circulating endothelial cells, and those drinking nonalcoholic beer had a fivefold increase. Gin drinking did not increase stem cells. The beer also increased blood levels of a protein that recruits stem cells, called stromal cell derived factor-1 (SDF-1).

The researchers then compared the effect of beer versus gin and found that men drinking gin had a *decrease* in their circulating endothelial progenitor cells and also had less stem cell recruitment protein in their blood compared to beer. Clearly, beer is a better choice than hard liquor if you want to protect your stem cells. But remember, as with wine, more is not better, due to alcohol's toxic effects on stem cells at high levels.

Green Tea

Green tea has many well researched health benefits, and now among them is activating the regenerative system. This has been studied in people who smoke. Cigarette smoking chemically scorches the blood vessel lining, which leads to increased risk of atherosclerosis and cardiovascular disease. Cigarette smoking is also damaging to stem cells, and reduces the number of circulating stem cells. People who smoke have 60 percent fewer stem cells in their bloodstream compared to nonsmokers—another reason not to smoke.[40]

Researchers from Chonnam National University Hospital in Korea and the Nagoya University Graduate School of Medicine in Japan examined the effects of drinking green tea on the stem cells of smokers.[41] They enrolled twenty young men in their late twenties who had smoked for six years and gave them four cups of green tea to drink each day for two weeks (a total of 56 cups). Their blood was drawn at the beginning and at the end of the study to count the number of circulating endothelial progenitor cells present. The results showed that drinking green tea increased the number of circulating stem cells by 43 percent over two weeks.

The health of the smokers' blood vessels was also improved by green tea over the study period. Their vascular dilation response was improved by 29 percent. In the lab, scientists have discovered that green tea and its catechins can stimulate regeneration of brain, muscle, bone, and nerves and can promote wound healing.[42] Green tea offers benefits for the regenerative system across the entire body, another reason to drink this beverage.

Black Tea

Black tea was once thought to be devoid of health benefits because it is fermented and has fewer polyphenols than green tea. But researchers at the University of L'Aquila in Italy have shown that black tea can, in fact, mobilize stem cells.[43] To study this effect, they recruited nineteen individuals in their fifties who had recently been diagnosed with mild to moderate hypertension but who had not yet been treated with any medication. The subjects had no other diseases and were not taking any medications. They were given a cup of black tea or a placebo beverage to drink twice per day for one week. Instructions were given for them not to add any milk, sugar, or other additives to their tea. The researchers measured the number of circulating endothelial cells in the blood. After one week, drinking black tea increased the circulating endothelial progenitor cells by 56 percent. The health of the vascular system was also improved with two cups of black tea per day, as seen by the ability of the blood vessels of black tea drinkers to dilate better. To see if black tea would protect the circulation against the effects of dietary fat, the researchers then asked the subjects to consume high-fat whipped cream, and then drink black tea. Eating whipped cream had a surprisingly swift negative effect on blood flow. Vessel dilation actually *decreased* by 15 percent within two hours after eating whipped cream. However, drinking black tea protected the blood flow of tea drinkers against this impact and preserved the ability of blood vessels to dilate.

Stem Cell–Boosting Dietary Patterns

While we have been focusing on the evidence for specific foods and beverages to influence stem cells, the overall pattern of eating can have its own beneficial effect on the body's regenerative capacity.

Mediterranean Diet

The Mediterranean diet was not originally a formal diet but rather a broad dietary pattern consumed by people living in Mediterranean countries. Data on this style of eating was first collected from Italy and Greece by Ancel Keys at the University of Minnesota and his colleagues conducting the famous Seven Countries Study, started in 1958. The study examined and compared food and health associations of twelve thousand men living in Italy, Greece, Yugoslavia, the Netherlands, Finland, Japan, and the United States. It was one of the first studies to show the link between saturated fat intake and heart disease. The diet of the Mediterranean region has been long associated with comparatively better outcomes for heart health. Now, we know from many different clinical and epidemiological studies that the Mediterranean diet lowers the risk of developing many different types of chronic health ailments. The hallmark of this dietary pattern is that it comprises fruits, vegetables, whole grains, legumes, nuts, olive oil, and fish—diversity is a characteristic, and each food contains its own trove of health-defense-activating bioactives.

The beneficial impacts of the Mediterranean diet include stimulating stem cells to help the body regenerate. Researchers at the University of Cordoba in Spain examined twenty healthy elderly people (ten men and ten women older than sixty-five years) who consumed either a Mediterranean diet containing extra virgin olive oil; or a diet high in saturated fatty acids (38 percent fat with butter); or a low-fat, high-carb diet (walnuts, biscuits, jam, bread) over the course of four weeks. They measured circulating endothelial progenitor cells in the blood at the beginning and end of the study. The results showed that people who consumed the Mediterranean diet had a fivefold increase of circulating endothelial progenitor cells compared to the less healthy diets containing saturated fats or high in carbohydrates.[44]

To test whether the diets affected blood flow, the researchers performed a test called the ischemic reactive hyperemia test. This test uses a laser to measure how well blood vessels recover from a four-minute period of constriction using a standard blood pressure cuff on the upper arm. The cuff is inflated to temporarily cut off blood flow. How well the blood flow returns to normal after the cuff is released reflects the general state of circulatory health in the subject. In the Spanish study, the people who consumed a Mediterranean or low-fat, high-carb diet had a 1.5-fold improvement of blood flow recovery compared to the saturated fat diet, correlated with the higher levels of endothelial progenitor cells seen. These stem cells protect the blood vessel lining leading to better vascular health.

This research into the Mediterranean diet's effect on stem cells adds a whole new dimension to understanding its heart-healthy benefits.

Caloric Restriction and Fasting

Caloric restriction is not a fad diet but a condition that has been experienced throughout human evolution. Especially during the hunter-gatherer period, finding food was an unpredictable event. As a result, our metabolism not only evolved to tolerate caloric restriction, but also in fact functions perfectly well under these conditions. It's become well known that caloric restriction, defined as reducing intake of calories by 20–40 percent, can increase longevity and reduce the risk of chronic diseases. Scientists at the Massachusetts Institute of Technology have discovered that caloric restriction activates stem cells in the intestines, which helps regenerate cells of the gut.[45] Other studies have shown that reducing calories in mice increases the production of the regenerative protein SDF1 and its receptor CXCR4, which together recruit and attract stem cells from the bone marrow into the bloodstream.[46]

Kicking things up a notch, an amazing discovery was made in a joint study by scientists from the Shanghai Jiao Tong University School of Medicine and the Second Military Medical University in China. They showed that fasting can stimulate brain regeneration. Unlike caloric restriction, in fasting, food is completely restricted for a sustained period of time. The scientists studied mice suffering from acute stroke. They fasted a group of mice for forty-eight hours and compared them to mice that had access to a normal unrestricted diet. They then removed endothelial progenitor cells from the mice four days after their stroke and found that the stem cells from the fasted group were superior in their ability to regenerate both the brain and blood vessels needed to bring blood flow to help stroke recovery. When the fasted stem cells were later injected into the bloodstream of other mice suffering from stroke, the fasted stem cells also gave a superior performance. They migrated right to part of the brain affected by the stroke, and created a 50 percent better than usual angiogenic response to restore blood flow and a 32 percent reduction in the size of the damaged area of the brain. The mice treated with fasted stem cells also had better neurological recovery, including improved balance and walking speed, when compared to mice receiving stem cells obtained from mice that did not fast.[47]

Dietary Patterns That Impair Beneficial Stem Cells

It probably won't surprise you to learn that the foods with a reputation for being unhealthy also damage your stem cells. Staying away from these types of foods will protect your regenerative health defense system. A well-functioning set of stem cells will not only help you keep your organs in good shape, but they will also help slow down the aging process.

High-Fat Diet

A high-fat diet containing unhealthy saturated fats is very damaging to stem cells.[48] The damage is bodywide but it's worthwhile noting what this can do to your brain. This can lead to problems with neurogenesis, the process that regenerates neurons in the hippocampus region of the brain responsible for forming new memories.[49] Avoiding a high-fat diet helps maintain cognitive health, which is important at any age, whether you are in grade school or a nursing home.[50]

High-fat diets also hurt your circulatory system by damaging endothelial progenitor cells. Scientists from Chang Gung University College of Medicine in Taiwan looked at the impact of a diet containing high levels of saturated fat on the body's response to ischemia in mice.[51] In their study, the researchers fed a high-fat diet to mice with high blood cholesterol and high fasting blood sugars, which mimic a prediabetic state in humans. The number of stem cells were measured in the blood. On the high-fat diet, mice had 41 percent lower levels of circulating endothelial progenitor cells compared to a normal diet. Then, the mice underwent a procedure to lower blood flow to their limbs. The normal response to this would be a wave of stem cells surging out from the bone marrow to the limb. These stem cells help regenerate the circulation and dying muscle. However, in mice who ate the high-fat diet, the researchers found blood flow was diminished by 75 percent and there were 55 percent fewer capillaries growing in their limbs. The reduced stem cells, poor blood flow, and diminished angiogenesis reflect the negative impact on regeneration caused by a fatty diet.

Unfortunately, high-fat diets do not impair fat stem cells, which are the source of more fat cells in adipose tissue. Scientists from the University of British Columbia showed that mice fed a high amount of saturated fat actually had a 42 percent enhancement of the growth of fat stem cells under the skin.[52] Even worse, a lab study conducted at the Massachusetts Institute of Technology showed that a high-fat diet can influence normal intestinal stem cells in a dangerous way: by increasing their tendency to develop tumors.[53] To be clear, these studies use saturated fats in their diets, so you can assign these stem cell problems to "bad" saturated fats rather than "good" polyunsaturated fats.

By avoiding saturated fats in your diet, you may improve your ability to regenerate your circulatory system, improve your cognition, and help stop your stem cells from generating new fat cells or tumor cells.

Hyperglycemic Foods

Add this to the sugar rap sheet: high levels of sugar incapacitate our regenerative defense system. Food and beverages that raise blood sugar block the production of stem cells, lowering your body's ability to repair organs. It gets worse. Elevated blood sugars have been shown to cripple and kill important stem cells across the board, from endothelial progenitor cells to bone progenitor cells to cardiac stem cells.[54] If you need your stem cells to be at their best, take a low glycemic index approach to your diet. This means minimizing or avoiding altogether sugary, processed foods containing little or no fiber that can cause blood sugar to spike, such as sugar-sweetened beverages and many packaged snack foods.[55]

High-Salt Diet

Salt makes food taste good, but chronic high salt intake is linked to a slew of health problems ranging from high blood pressure, to cardiovascular disease, to stripping away the protective mucus lining of your stomach and increasing your risk of stomach cancer. Scientists at the Medical College of Wisconsin studied salt's impact on stem cells by feeding rats different diets containing varying amounts of salt. One group was given a normal diet (0.4 percent salt), and another group a high-salt diet (4 percent salt), with ten times more salt.[56] The scientists collected stem cells from the bone marrow of rats in both groups after seven days of feeding the diet. Then, they injected these stem cells coming from normal or high-salt diets into a new group of rats whose legs had damaged blood flow to test their regenerative capability.

The results showed that stem cells from rats fed a normal salt diet could improve the leg circulation in the recipient rat by 24 percent. However, the stem cells exposed to a high-salt diet were crippled and could barely participate in regeneration, with only 6 percent improvement in blood flow. Highly salted stem cells did not survive long, with a 50 percent increase in cell death after they were injected as treatment compared to normal salt stem cells. Patients with cardiovascular disease who are told by their cardiologists to avoid excessive salt in their food because of the risks of high blood pressure now have another even more compelling reason to stay on a low-salt diet.

Diseases of Importance: Cancer and Its Dangerous Stem Cells

Cancerous tumors contain a tiny but deadly population of stem cells, known as cancer stem cells. These stem cells were discovered in 1994 and they are dangerous. They are mutations of normal stem cells. This means they are capable of regenerating tissue like normal stem cells, but the tissue that is created is cancerous. Cancer stem cells also help grow tumors that have metastasized to other organs.[57]

Foods That Kill Cancer Stem Cells

Finding ways to kill cancer stem cells has been one of the holy grails in cancer research. While this is a target of biotechnology companies working on cancer treatment, scientists have already discovered dietary factors that have the ability to kill them, at least in some forms of cancer. Cancer stem cells are responsible for initiating many cancers, as well as igniting the recurrence of cancers after treatment.[58]

Green Tea

Green tea has many useful functions, including the ability to kill cancer stem cells. Scientists at Nanjing Medical University and Sun Yat-Sen University Cancer Center in China studied the effect of the green tea polyphenol, epigallocatechin-3-gallate (EGCG), in the lab and found that it could reduce the growth of colon cancer stem cells by 50 percent.

In addition, EGCG forced the cancer stem cells to commit cell suicide through the process of apoptosis.[59] Another study from the University of Salford in England showed that matcha green tea, a form of powderized tea leaf, can interrupt the metabolic pathway of breast cancer stem cells, depriving them of energy and causing them to die.[60] The effect of the EGCG in green tea on targeting cancer stem cells may help explain the protective effects of tea against colon and other cancers.

Purple Potatoes

Originating from Peru, purple potatoes were prized by the ancient Inca for their nutritive benefits. They contain the bioactive anthocyanin, a blue-purple pigment that also gives many dark berries their hue. Scientists at Penn State University explored the effect of purple potatoes on cancer stem cells.[61] In the lab, they fed mice that are at high risk for developing colon cancer the dietary equivalent of one purple potato (Purple Majesty variety) each day for a week. They compared the effects of the potato with that of an anti-inflammatory drug called Sulindac, which is known to suppress colon polyps and colon cancer development.[62] After one week, the colons of the mice were examined. The mice fed purple potatoes had 50 percent fewer tumors. When the colon tissues were more closely examined under the microscope, there was a 40 percent increase in the killing of colon cancer stem cells compared to the group that did not eat purple potatoes. They found that the cancer stem cells in mice fed purple potatoes were deprived of key survival factors. When the scientists removed the cancer stem cells from the mice and exposed them to a purple potato extract, they found the extract caused a twenty-two-fold reduction of aggressiveness in the behavior of the cancer stem cells.

The scientists prepared the purple potato in different ways, including baking, dicing, and freeze-drying, yet the bioactive cancer stem cell-fighting components appear to be stable even under different conditions and preparation techniques. Given their effects, purple potatoes may have in addition to their marvelous color features unique cancer-fighting properties that traditional white potatoes do not.

Walnuts

Walnuts are popular tree nuts that are eaten raw, roasted, candied, or even pickled. They are nutrient dense and contain bioactives like gallic acid, chlorogenic acid, and ellagic acid. As described earlier, eating walnuts is associated with a reduced risk for developing colon cancer and also improves survival in patients who have colon cancer. Scientists from Ewha Womans University, Seoul National University, and Sungkyunkwan University in South Korea studied a walnut extract for its ability to kill cancer stem cells.[63] In the lab, they grew colon cancer stem cells isolated from a patient, and exposed the cells to a walnut extract. After two days of exposure, the number of cancer stem cells treated with walnut extract declined by 34 percent. By six days, there was a stunning 86 percent suppression of cancer stem cell growth. The potent effect of walnuts on cancer stem cells might help explain the results of the study of 826 patients with stage 3 colon cancer who had a 57 percent lower chance of death, and a 42 percent lower chance of cancer recurrence associated with eating nuts.[64]

If you have colon cancer, eating walnuts may literally save your life.

Extra Virgin Olive Oil

Extra virgin olive oil contains a class of bioactives known as secoiridoids, which represent up to 46 percent of the total polyphenols present in olive oil. These natural chemicals are absorbed in the small intestines and can be detected in the blood plasma and in urine, proving their presence and availability in the body.[65] Scientists from Spain showed in the lab that olive oil secoiridoids could dramatically reduce the growth of breast cancer stem cells.[66] When mice were injected with breast cancer stem cells that were exposed to secoiridoids, as many as 20 percent of the mice did not develop tumors. In the 80 percent that did develop tumors, the tumors were fifteen times smaller and grew at a much slower rate than untreated breast cancer cells. This result is consistent with the suppression of breast cancer stem cells.

The power of the olive oil secoiridoids on stem cells was evidenced at the genetic level: after the breast cancer stem cells were exposed, the bioactives changed the activity of 160 genes involved with controlling stem cells. One gene was reduced in its activity fourfold, while the activity of another gene that antagonizes cancer stem cells was increased thirteenfold. The health-protective power of extra virgin olive oil now extends to targeting dangerous stem cells.

Other Foods That Target Cancer Stem Cells

Other noteworthy bioactives found in foods can suppress cancer stem cells. Genistein is found in soy. Luteolin occurs in celery, oregano, and thyme. Quercetin is found in capers, apples, and peppers. All three of these compounds kill prostate cancer stem cells.[67] Luteolin is especially potent and can shut down the activity of prostate cancer stem cells twentyfold. The bioactive of green tea, EGCG, has also been shown to work together with the bioactive quercetin to inhibit prostate cancer stem cells, as well.[68]

Some bioactives play dual roles. They can promote healthy functions in a defense system while combating the opposite effect in the same system. As we saw in chapter 6, chlorogenic acid helps maintain normal circulation through angiogenesis in healthy tissues, while it can simultaneously starve dangerous tumors by cutting off their blood supply. Similarly, chlorogenic acid enhances normal stem cell function for organ regeneration, but it also cripples cancer stem cells. In fact, scientists at Nihon University in Japan found that chlorogenic acid blocks the genes supporting lung cancer stem cells, and it increases the activity of genes that kill cancer cells by one-thousand-fold.[69] How the bioactives work in dual fashion is not well understood. Foods high in chlorogenic acid include coffee, carrots, and stone fruit, like apricot and plums.

Scientists at Seoul National University in Korea discovered that resveratrol, the bioactive found in red wine, grapes, peanuts, pistachios, dark chocolate, and cranberries, could interfere with the growth of breast cancer stem cells by 60 percent.[70] Ellagic acid is another bioactive that has been discovered to target breast cancer stem cells.[71] Foods high in ellagic acid include chestnuts, blackberries, walnuts, and pomegranates.

Ketogenic Diet

The ketogenic diet involves eating a high-fat, very low-carbohydrate diet that mimics fasting for the purpose of generating ketones in the body. Ketones are created from fat stored in the body when carbohydrates are not available for metabolism to make glucose. The ketones are used as an energy source by cells in place of glucose. This dietary strategy, although difficult to sustain, has been used for decades to help control epilepsy and is being explored to help treat glioblastoma, a deadly brain tumor.[72]

While normal healthy cells can adapt to use ketones as an energy source, cancer cells cannot adapt the same way because they rely on glucose to keep up with their high energy demands. When glucose is low, tumors have difficulty growing. Ketones also interfere with the ability of cancer cells to obtain energy, making tumors more likely to respond to treatment when the patient is adopting a ketogenic diet. In lab mice with brain tumors, the ketogenic diet can shrink tumors by 50 percent and lengthen survival.

To explore the impact of a ketogenic diet on glioblastoma stem cells, researchers at the University of Florida in Gainesville obtained cancer stem cells from patients with glioblastoma whose tumors had been surgically removed.[73] The cells were grown in incubators with normal glucose, low glucose, or ketogenic conditions. In low-glucose conditions, brain cancer stem cells were stunted in their ability to grow compared to normal glucose conditions. This supports the idea that high sugar consumption, which may stimulate cancer stem cell growth in cancer patients, should be avoided. When the cells were exposed to ketone bodies in addition to low glucose, there was a more than twofold suppression of glioblastoma stem cells.

Glioblastoma was used to study the ketogenic effect, in part because of the importance of cancer stem cells in this disease. Even if this cancer is successfully removed or treated initially, the glioblastoma stem cells help it return aggressively. Avoiding added sugar and adhering to a ketogenic diet are strategies that may be helpful in fighting brain tumors.

Putting It All Together

Your stem cells are always at work, but as you age, they slow down and can use some help. Eating foods that mobilize your stem cells can boost your body's intrinsic ability to protect and maintain your organs. Regenerative eating, which stimulates stem cells from within, is a whole new way to think choosing which foods and beverages to consume every day.

Keep in mind that Mediterranean and Asian dietary patterns commonly contain ingredients that have been shown to help your stem cells. And be aware that other patterns, such as high-fat, high-salt, or high-sugar diets, can stun them—not something you want to do frequently.

If you are fighting a chronic disease, activating your stem cells may be important for helping you overcome the damage it does to your tissues. If you've had a heart attack or a stroke, your stem cells can help save your heart and rebuild your brain. In these situations, powering up your stem cells is a way to fight for your health, regain your strength, and keep your body functioning the way it needs to for a long life.

If you want to improve fitness, eating regenerative foods will help you improve blood flow, and have more energy and better endurance. If you are an athlete or in training for physical performance of any kind, you'll want to recruit those stem cells to build muscle. If you are middle-aged and want your body to stay youthful, if you've had surgery and need to heal fast, or if you are recovering from an illness and want to bounce back to health quickly, eating foods that increase your circulating stem cells may be one way to achieve your goals.

Finally, not all stem cells are your friend. Cancer stem cells are extremely dangerous. If you have cancer, or have ever had it, your number one focus should be to kill those cancer stem cells. There's no medicine that can do this yet, but there are a growing number of foods, and their bioactives, that are being studied for their suppressive effects on cancer stem cells. Fortunately, foods that target cancer stem cells do not harm beneficial stem cells.

KEY FOODS AFFECTING REGENERATION

Stem Cell Boosting		Cancer Cell Killing	
Bamboo shoots	Green tea	Apple	Plums
Beer	Kale	Apricot	Pomegranate
Black chokeberry	Mango	Blackberries	Purple potatoes
Black raspberries	Mustard greens	Capers	Red wine
Black tea	Peaches	Carrots	Soy
Blueberries	Peanuts	Celery	Thyme
Chinese celery	Pistachios	Chestnuts	Walnuts
Coffee	Plums	Coffee	
Collard greens	Red wine	Cranberries	
Cranberries	Rice bran	Dark chocolate	
Dark chocolate	Seafoods high in omega-3	Grapes	
Eggplants	Spinach	Green tea	
Fiddleheads	Squid ink	Olive oil (EVOO)	
Goji berries	Swiss chard	Oregano	
Grape juice	Turmeric	Peanuts	
Grapes	Watercress	Peppers	
Green beans	Whole grain	Pistachios	

CHAPTER 8

Feed Your Inner Ecosystem

When an expectant mother at the dinner table says she is eating for two, she's almost certainly going to think about making better food choices because of the baby growing in her womb. But we should all make these better choices when we sit down to feed ourselves, because we are never eating for just one, or even two, but for 39 trillion. This is the number of bacteria making up the microbiome in our body.[1]

Properly feeding our gut bacteria starts a biochemical domino effect that influences not just our digestion but also our overall health. A well-cared-for community of gut bacteria will affect your ability to resist diseases like cancer and diabetes, influence your ability to heal wounds, and instruct your brain to release chemicals that make you more social. We are just beginning to learn how our microbiome helps our body resist diseases ranging from inflammatory bowel disease, depression, obesity, cardiovascular disease, and even Alzheimer's and Parkinson's disease.

Let's look at just one example of how powerfully our microbiome can influence health. A gut bacteria called *Akkermansia muciniphila* makes up 1 to 3 percent of all the bacteria in the gut microbiome. But this small population has a mighty impact. *Akkermansia* can help control the immune system, improve blood glucose metabolism in the body, decrease gut inflammation, and combat obesity.[2] Its impact on the immune system is especially startling. Patients with some forms of cancer are now receiving breakthrough immunotherapy cancer treatments called checkpoint inhibitors. These inhibitors are an entirely new way to treat cancer.

Unlike chemotherapy, which damages the immune system, these treatments specifically harness a person's own immune system to wipe out their cancer. The way they work is by ripping off the biochemical cloak cancer cells hide behind in order to stay undetected by our immune system.

In 2015, researchers led by Dr. Laurence Zitvogel at the Institut Gustav Roussey in Paris showed that making even small alterations to the gut microbiome of mice could affect how well they responded to immunotherapy treatment. They found the same connection in human cancer patients, identifying *Akkermansia* as one of the key healthy gut bacteria present in the microbiome of people who benefit from this type of cancer treatment.[3] If patients had the bacteria present in their gut, they are more likely to respond to treatment and are able to call their own immune system in to fight the cancer. If patients lacked the bacteria, their immune system did not respond to the checkpoint inhibitor, and the cancer would still escape the immune system and continue to grow. Out of 39 trillion bacteria in the microbiome, the presence of *Akkermansia* predicted a better response to a cancer immunotherapy.

Here's the thing: diet can be used to increase *Akkermansia* in your gut. Certain fruit juices influence the gut's environment to become one in which *Akkermansia* likes to grow. Pomegranate juice, for instance, is high in ellagitannins, a specific group of bioactives that about 70 percent of people can metabolize into urolithin-A, yet another bioactive. Urolithin-A has antioxidant, anti-inflammatory, and anticancer activity. It is thought that *Akkermansia* is responsible for this metabolism. Perhaps not surprisingly, ellagitannins have been shown to encourage growth of *Akkermansia*. Cranberries also improve conditions in the gut that help *Akkermansia* thrive.

The data on cranberry and pomegranate juice show how powerfully our diet can influence our microbiome, which can in turn influence our immune response to cancer therapy, literally with life-and-death implications. This kind of research into the connections between specific foods, the good and bad bacteria they influence, their metabolites, and associated health outcomes is changing our approach to human nutrition, and these discoveries will profoundly influence what your doctor or dietitian recommends that you eat.

You can immediately benefit from a healthier microbiome by eating foods and using dietary patterns known to influence members of your 39 million resident bacteria. Anything you swallow that is not fully absorbed in your small intestines trickles down to the tail end of your gut. There, the bacteria in your microbiome await their meal. They, too, digest and metabolize proteins, carbohydrates, fats, bioactives, and even additives and the synthetic chemicals in food. Scientists are discovering how diet can help maintain a healthy bacteria ecosystem, and even help reshape the ecosystem. A microbiome with too few useful bacteria can be enriched with those bacteria, and a system with too many harmful bacteria can have those reduced. In this way, adjusting the microbiome can restore optimal balance, in essence raising our shields and boosting our microbiome's ability to defend our health. On the other hand, some foods can lower our shields by changing our bacteria negatively, which can promote disease. Before we look at microbiome-influencing foods, let's have a look at the diseases linked to imbalances of microbiome.

Diseases That Matter: Where the Microbiome Is Disturbed

Disturbances of the microbiome, called dysbiosis, are now being discovered in serious health conditions ranging from obesity to metabolic syndrome to type 2 diabetes, and more. These conditions have abnormalities and damage to gut bacteria that are associated with unhealthy eating patterns, as well as environmental factors and antibiotic use. In inflammatory bowel diseases, such as Crohn's disease and ulcerative colitis, researchers are finding pro-inflammatory bacteria dominating the colon. These bacteria strip away the protective mucus layer in the intestines, making the gut lining more vulnerable to inflammation and toxins. Food allergies are now linked to dysbiosis. Children with less diversity in their microbiomes are more likely to develop long-term food allergies.[4] The microbiome of children who suffer from food allergies is different than that of their siblings who don't have food allergies.[5]

Cancer, especially in the organs in the gastrointestinal tract (esophagus, stomach, pancreas, gallbladder, colon, and rectum) is associated with microbiome disturbances.[6] When beneficial bacteria are absent, the immune system's ability to detect and fight cancer cells is disarmed. The wrong bacterial residents interfere with the body's ability to defend itself. Bacteria influence our body's ability to manage blood cholesterol. Dysbiosis is also associated with atherosclerosis and cardiovascular disease.[7] When the bacteria in your mouth, the oral microbiome, are disturbed, hypertension and heart disease can result.[8] An overabundance of certain bacteria can cause your body to produce higher levels of a toxic substance called trimethylamine N-oxide (TMAO) when red meat is consumed. TMAO damages the lining of blood vessels and makes it easier for dangerous atherosclerotic plaques to form inside your arteries, which we know can lead to fatal heart attack and stroke.[9]

Disruptions of the gut microbiome are also observed in people with Parkinson's disease and Alzheimer's disease. There is emerging evidence that harmful bacteria growing in the gut can produce neurotoxins that provoke brain inflammation.[10] Altered microbiome is seen in major depressive disorder, bipolar disorder, and even schizophrenia.[11] People suffering from asthma and chronic obstructive pulmonary disease (COPD) have different bacterial profiles in their sputum compared to those without lung disease.[12]

Dysbiosis in the gut also generates abnormal proteins that trigger the body to produce antibodies that cause autoimmune diseases.[13] Reduction of healthy bacteria is observed in multiple sclerosis, rheumatoid arthritis, celiac disease, and inflammatory bowel diseases. All of these conditions are associated with abnormalities in the microbiome. It is very likely that many of the most serious diseases of our time share an altered microbiome as a "common denominator," and conversely the right constellation of beneficial bacteria is a requisite feature of good health.

The good news is we know that eating certain foods can help shape the bacterial population of our microbiome health defense system, increasing good and reducing bad bacteria.

Foods Containing Healthy Bacteria

One way to help our microbiome is to actually eat bacteria.[14] Many foods contain healthy bacteria that are used to ferment foods and keep them from spoiling. It's not as gross as it might sound. Preserving foods with edible healthy bacteria dates back to ancient societies in Greece, Rome, China, and India. Even today, live cultures of bacteria are central to making many common foods. Eating fermented foods can increase the diversity of your gut microbiome, which improves your health defenses. Here are just a few of the foods that are made with bacteria and their health benefits.[15]

Sauerkraut

Sauerkraut is a slightly sour, tangy, savory accompaniment to many a traditional meal, and it is sometimes used as a condiment similar to relish. It is incredibly microbe-rich, made by fermenting very thinly sliced cabbage with lactic acid-producing bacteria (*Lactobacilli*).[16] A single one-cup serving of sauerkraut can have up to 5 trillion bacteria.[17] Sauerkraut actually originated in China, and through trade routes early merchants brought it to both Eastern and Western Europe, where it became incorporated into Slavic and German cuisine. The shredded cabbage is salted, and airborne *Lactobacilli* in the environment are allowed to settle on and grow in the mix. Many different types of bacteria initially colonize and contribute to fermenting the sauerkraut. As the mash becomes more sour over time, the change in acidity alters the makeup of the bacterial population until it stabilizes at the point of sauerkraut maturity.

A substantial body of research has been conducted on sauerkraut and health.[18] Scientists from North Carolina State University profiled changes in the bacterial population of sauerkraut during fermentation. They found while many different bacteria are initially present, the bacteria that eventually dominates is *Lactobacillus plantarum*. This important gut microbe is often found in commercial probiotics. *L. plantarum* has been associated with a number of health-promoting actions, including stimulating an anti-inflammatory response by intestinal stem cells.[19]

The bacterial fermentation of shredded cabbage also releases new bioactive compounds.[20] As one example, fermentation releases glucosinolates from the plant. Bacterial enzymes then break these down into smaller fragments called isothiocyanates. These last products have anti-angiogenic properties and they can kill cancer cells directly. Remarkably, food scientists from the Natural Resources Institute of Finland found that levels of isothiocyanates are actually higher in sauerkraut than in raw cabbage.[21]

In addition to the probiotic bacteria and the bioactives generated, sauerkraut is also a good source of dietary fiber, which feeds the microbiome.

Kimchi

Anyone who has enjoyed Korean cuisine has probably eaten kimchi, a tasty, spicy staple of salted and fermented vegetables such as napa cabbage, radishes, scallions, chile peppers, garlic, ginger, and a fermented seafood product called jeotgal. The name *kimchi* comes from the Korean word *gimchi*, which literally means "submerged vegetable." The traditional way to make kimchi is to prepare the vegetables in a ceramic pot and bury it in the ground to ferment. More than 160 varieties of kimchi exist, generally served as a side dish to accompany meals. You can find kimchi on every Korean restaurant menu and on the shelves of Asian grocery stores.

Kimchi is, in essence, a probiotic. Like yogurt, it delivers a load of healthy bacteria and bioactives to your gut. Many of the bacteria involved with fermenting the kimchi are the same ones found in a healthy human microbiome: *Bacteroidetes*, *Firmicutes*, and *Lactobacillus*, among others.[22] Scientists from the World Institute of Kimchi in Korea have even discovered a new species of bacteria named *Lentibacillus kimchi* that produces vitamin K2, or menaquinone. Recall from chapter 6 that vitamin K2 is an antiangiogenic bioactive found in chicken dark meat and cheese.[23] Another bacterial product in kimchi is propionic acid, one of the short-chain fatty acids that lowers cholesterol, reduces inflammation, prevents buildup of atherosclerotic plaque in arteries, and improves digestive health.[24] Extracts from kimchi have been found to kill cells from colon, bone, and liver cancer, as well as leukemia.[25] The *Lactobacillus plantarum* growing in kimchi makes a bacterial product that is protective against influenza A.[26]

Researchers from Ajou University in Korea studied twenty-one middle-aged individuals with prediabetes and metabolic syndrome, the term used to describe a perfect storm of maladies that set up an individual to develop cardiovascular disease: abdominal obesity, elevated blood lipids, high blood pressure, and elevated blood glucose. Each participant had blood glucose levels below the strict criteria set for diabetes, but higher than normal (fasting glucose levels between 100 and 125 mg/dl on a blood test). The purpose of the study was to determine if kimchi could improve their metabolic status and see if there are differences between fresh versus fermented kimchi.[27]

The participants were divided into two groups. One group ate freshly made kimchi, and the other ate fermented kimchi for eight weeks. All the kimchi was made in the same factory. The fresh kimchi had 15 million *Lactobacillus* per milliliter of material, while the fermented kimchi contained 6.5 billion bacteria per milliliter, or 433 times more than the fresh. During the experiment, the researchers measured total fat mass, body fat percentage, and blood pressure of the participants, and they ran blood tests to check for inflammation and determine glucose levels. After eight weeks, the researchers asked the participants not to eat any fermented food for four more weeks, in order to "wash out" their systems.

Across the board, fermented kimchi, which had more bacteria, had a greater effect than fresh kimchi. Eating fermented kimchi significantly lowered body fat mass by 6 percent compared to 3.9 percent for fresh kimchi, meaning the fat loss was 1.6 times better. The fermented kimchi-eating group also had a 2 percent decrease in body fat percentage, while there was no significant change in the fresh kimchi group. The group eating fermented kimchi also experienced a significant lowering of their blood pressure.

The participants also underwent an oral glucose tolerance test to see how efficiently their body processed glucose after eating kimchi. They were given a drink containing an amount of sugar equivalent to forty-two jelly beans. The researchers checked their blood glucose levels before the drink and two hours later. The participants eating fermented kimchi had a 33 percent improvement in their glucose tolerance test, compared to their response prior to eating kimchi. The improvement in glucose tolerance was 3.5 times better in the group eating fermented kimchi versus the group eating fresh kimchi. So, while eating any kind of kimchi has benefits for body fat, blood pressure, and glucose sensitivity, fermented kimchi had greater benefits than fresh.

Another study by Dongguk University in Korea examined twenty-four women classified as overweight with their BMI greater than twenty-five.[28] They were given 1.2 cups of fresh or fermented kimchi to eat daily for eight weeks, with measurements related to obesity, blood biomarkers, and fecal microbiome. Similar to the Ajou University study, there was significant improvement in the group that ate fermented kimchi, including a 5 percent decrease in body fat.

A word of caution: kimchi is very high in salt. Be careful eating it if you have hypertension or are at high risk for stomach cancer.

Pao Cai (Chinese Fermented Cabbage)

Pao cai (pronounced "pow tsai") is a traditional fermented vegetable dish in China that is often found in Chinese restaurants as a cold appetizer. Like kimchi, pao cai is prepared by pickling healthy vegetables: cabbage, radish, mustard green stems, carrots, and ginger. The bacteria involved in pao cai fermentation are many of the same ones in the healthy human microbiome.[29] These include *Firmicutes* and *Lactobacillus*, which are the dominant species in the pickle. A scientific study conducted by Shaanxi Normal University in China found as many as thirty different bacteria species, making pao cai a rich probiotic food.[30] The cabbage in pao cai is also a source of dietary fiber, and one cup contributes to 9 percent of the daily recommended fiber intake. In China, these pickled vegetables are often eaten as a condiment with rice.

Cheese

When it comes to the microbiome, cheese is good for your gut. Cheese is made with milk, an enzyme called rennet, and a starter culture. The starter is composed of different types of bacteria, depending on the type of cheese being made. These bacteria create lactic acid and together with the enzyme convert the milk to curds and whey, which then undergo various steps to generate the unique flavors and textures of traditional and commercial cheeses.

Each cheese has its own microbiome, which is the result of its starter culture and is established by the region where the cheese is made and the environment where the cheese matures (think: cheese cave). Over the course of weeks, months, or even years that a cheese ages, many organisms ranging from bacteria to molds and yeasts settle on and invade the cheese, contributing to its flavor and its own "cheese microbiome." When we eat cheese, we are ingesting live bacteria as well as the products made by the bacteria, both of which can benefit our health.

Parmigiano-Reggiano is a delicious traditional hard cheese from Parma, Italy, made in the shape of giant disks that are aged for one to two years before being sold and eaten. Although diverse bacteria are present during the first few months of cheese making, the acidity changes as the cheese matures, and many bacteria disappear by the time the cheese is ready for market.[31] Among the surviving bacteria are *Lactobacillus casei* and *Lactobacillus rhamnosus*. Both have been observed to have beneficial activity against gastroenteritis,[32] diabetes,[33] cancer,[34] obesity,[35] and even postpartum depression.[36] Parmigiano-Reggiano is a natural source of probiotic bacteria.

Gouda cheese, made from cow's milk, is another cheese that has been studied for its probiotic properties. Recall from chapter 6 that Gouda contains vitamin K2 (menaquinone), which has antiangiogenic activity. It also has diverse microbiome of more than twenty species, including *Lactobacilli plantarum* and *Lactobacillus casei*, whose populations change while the cheese is aging. Gouda found in Europe is made from raw milk, but it is a pasteurized product in the United States. Research from Ghent University and the Institute for Agriculture and Fisheries in Belgium showed that Gouda made with raw milk has greater diversity of bacteria, a beneficial trait, than pasteurized cheeses.[37] While cheeses made from raw milk are prized in their countries of origin, in the United States, the Food and Drug Administration mandates that milk products must be pasteurized in the package of their final form.[38] This federal protection aimed at food safety emerged in 1949 after outbreaks of disease associated with consuming raw milk cheese, and in 1987, the FDA prohibited all raw milk product sales. Although a few cheeses aged more than sixty days may be exempt from this regulation, it means that cheeses available in the United States will not have the full microbiome portfolio of the same type of cheese from Europe.

Recall from the experiment described in chapter 3 that Camembert cheese contributes to a healthy gut microbiome. Camembert also has a prebiotic effect, which influences levels of bacteria in the gut that aren't part of the cheesemaking starter culture. A clinical study from the French National Institute for Agricultural Research showed that people who eat Camembert cheese have increased numbers of a gut bacteria called *Enterococcus faecium*. This bacteria is not present in the cheese, but the prebiotic effect of the cheese fuels the growth of this natural gut bacteria.[39]

So we can see cheese is a food containing its own microbiome that influences the human gut microbiome through both pre- and probiotic effects. Cheese bacteria survive digestive enzymes. They make their way through the entire digestive system and can be found in the stool of cheese eaters. Keeping in mind the qualifying warnings about its salt and saturated fat content, add to the health influence of cheese its ability to contribute to the human microbiome.

Yogurt

Yogurt is made from milk that is heated, cooled, and then mixed with bacteria for fermentation. It is an ancient food dating back at least five thousand years, and its health benefits were described in the writings of ancient Greece. Natural yogurt came into existence when milk was accidentally contaminated by bacteria, and the resulting product was discovered to be edible. But, the actual presence of a bacteria, *Lactobacillus*, was not known until it was discovered by a Bulgarian medical student studying the microbiology of local yogurt.[40] Later, the Nobel laureate Ilya Metchnikoff observed the longevity of Bulgarian peasants and attributed it to their eating yogurt, which was a staple food. Today, yogurt in its pure form (without added sweeteners) is considered a healthy food, and its benefit may be due its probiotic benefits.

Researchers from Youngstown State University in Ohio conducted a small study of six healthy volunteers who were given one cup of yogurt to consume, about the same amount commonly ingested in yogurt-loving

Europe and Australia, for forty-two consecutive days.[41] The yogurt was provided every three to four days throughout the six-week study. Each dose contained approximately 1 billion bacteria. Subjects were asked to provide fecal samples every seven days, for a total of seven samples over the course of the study. The researchers found an overall increase in different health promoting *Lactobacillus* species after yogurt consumption. The bacterial changes were highly variable among individuals (a different study even showed that the microbiome's response to yogurt varies between men and women[42]). But the Youngstown study did detect increases in *Lactobacillus reuteri*, *Lactobacillis casei*, and *Lactobacillus rhamnosus*, which are often found in commercial probiotics, showing that eating yogurt can influence the gut microbiome.

A much larger study of yogurt was conducted in Spain as part of the PREDIMED study of the Mediterranean diet.[43] The researchers studied 7,168 participants and examined their consumption of yogurt along with their consumption of lignans. Lignans are plant polyphenols that are metabolized by gut bacteria into the bioactives, enterodiol and enterolactone, which lower the risk of heart disease.[44] The source of lignans in the diet of these participants was mostly from olive oil, wheat products, tomatoes, red wine, and asparagus. The PREDIMED researchers were interested in seeing if eating lignans and yogurt would feed the bacteria present in yogurt and lead to a greater health benefit.

The results showed that those who consumed the most lignans had lower blood glucose levels, and that participants who ate high levels of both lignan and yogurt had lower levels of total blood cholesterol, including reduced levels of harmful LDL cholesterol. The *Lactobacillus* found in yogurt can increase the elimination of cholesterol from the body, so the researchers speculate that the lignans have a prebiotic effect and feed gut bacteria. At the same time, yogurt has a probiotic effect, supplying the bacteria itself. Eating yogurt along with a plant-based diet rich in lignans can offer protective benefits against cardiovascular disease and better blood glucose control.

Sourdough Bread

Bread is a staple food worldwide, and archeologists have discovered that early humans were baking it as long as fourteen thousand years ago, before the dawn of agriculture, making it a bona fide "Paleo" food.[45] Made only with flour and water, and leavened with yeast or bacteria, bread can be baked, steamed, or fried. Traditional sourdough bread is made with a starter containing *Lactobacillus* bacteria. *Lactobacillus* makes lactic acid, which gives sourdough its classic mildly sour taste. Sourdough starters, along with the original bacteria, are passed on in traditional bread making from generation to generation through a process called back slopping. To do this, small pieces of bacteria-laced dough are pinched off and reserved from each time the bread is made and saved to make the next batch.

One type of sourdough bacteria, *Lactobacillus reuteri*, has remarkable health functions. It has been shown to improve immunity and suppress tumor development.[46] *L. reuteri* also reduces weight gain and can speed wound healing. The bacteria also activates the gut-brain axis by stimulating the brain to release the social hormone oxytocin.[47]

Scientists at the University of Alberta in Canada working with colleagues from Huazhong Agricultural University and Hubei University of Technology in China studied this bacteria in commercial sourdough bread starter. They found that one strain of *L. reuteri* in a sourdough starter that had been handed down from one baker to another since 1970 had actually evolved to live and thrive in bread dough.[48] To dominate in their new turf, some *L. reuteri* strains in the starter actually developed the ability to produce a natural antibiotic called reutericyclin that kills other harmful bacteria growing around it. While the bacteria itself does not survive the high oven temperatures used for baking, scientists from Massachusetts Institute of Technology have shown that the benefits may not require live bacteria at all when it comes to *L. reuteri*. In the lab, scientists completely pulverized the bacteria so no live *L. reuteri* survived, but they found that substances coming from the particles of dead bacteria could create the same benefits as the live bacteria. This is a complete surprise, because it's always been assumed that the benefits of gut bacteria require them to be alive. Discoveries like this show us how much there is to learn about the microbiome and our health. So, even when *L. reuteri* in sourdough bread is killed in the hot oven, the bacterial fragments that remain in the finished bread may still be able to offer health benefits when consumed.[49]

Foods That Have a Positive Influence on Your Microbiome

By eating probiotic foods like the ones we've just discussed, you can introduce beneficial bacteria into your body. But even foods that don't contain live and active cultures can influence your microbiome for the better, by creating conditions that allow helpful bacteria to thrive. Research has indicated specific foods that can have this effect, but before we dig into this science, it's important for you to know the general dietary principles that will keep your helpful bacteria happy.

Caring for Your Microbiome

The guiding principles for taking care of your gut microbiome follow three basic rules of thumb: Eat lots of dietary fiber from whole food. Eat less animal protein. Eat more fresh, whole foods and less processed food. I'm going to present you with the data that illustrates why these rules are important in your life.

First principle: eat lots of dietary fiber from whole food. Dietary fiber comes from whole plant-based foods and is health food for your microbiome.[50] Since the dawn of *Homo sapiens* three hundred thousand years ago, fiber was the core of human sustenance. Fibrous foods like ancient grains, nuts, legumes, and fruits were foraged and eaten.[51] Animal protein was only rarely consumed. Moreover, the food was hand-picked from bacterial-laden soil and vegetation, so what our remote ancestors ate was loaded with not only fiber but also microbes. This dietary pattern, containing fiber and bacteria, shaped the way our bodies evolved for survival. Our bodies are still built for this original pattern of eating, which is still best for our microbiome and our general health. The heavily processed food of today is a recent development, emerging only in the mid-twentieth century. This means that the modern dietary pattern of eating industrialized food has been around for only 0.02 percent of human existence, and is a relatively unfamiliar pattern for our bodies in terms of how they were designed to function nutritionally.

Second principle: eat less animal protein. Eating meat is hard on your microbiome. After the first Agricultural Revolution of 10,000 BC, humans moved away from hunting and gathering, which was slow going, to rely on cultivated crops, which could scale up the availability of food. Still, people ate mostly plant-based foods. Livestock was at that time a local food resource. But by the eighteenth century, agricultural advances led to improved crop and livestock management, increasing food availability. Both plant-based foods and meat became more plentiful. By the latter half of the twentieth century, agriculture inverted the model of food from local to global. Human dietary patterns centered themselves on a high intake of animal proteins and became less focused on plant-based foods, resulting in less consumption of dietary fiber needed by your microbiome. Less fiber leads to an unhealthy ecosystem of gut bacteria, and less production of anti-inflammatory short-chain fatty acids. At the same time, more animal protein shifts the bacteria to behave in ways that generate more inflammation in the gut.[52]

Third principle: eat more fresh, whole foods, and less processed food. Along with more meat consumption, modern chemistry has made its way into the food industry. Heavily processed foods contain synthetic food additives, preservatives, and flavors. Industrialization made food less expensive, more available, shelf stable, and, through flavor manipulation and marketing, even more seductively appealing than traditional fresh foods. At the same time, sanitary conditions, food industry regulation, and public health efforts reduced human exposure to all bacteria in our environment. Pasteurization and improved sanitation led to less exposure to disease-causing bacteria, but also to health-promoting bacteria as well. Our modern industrialized dietary practices have changed our relationship with our microbiome—and our health.

Let's take a look at some of the scientific evidence that supports these rules of thumb. Researchers from the University of Florence in Italy conducted a deeply telling study in the late 2000s that illustrates the importance of these principles. Specifically, researchers examined in detail the diets and microbiome of children from two contrasting cultures: a rural village in Burkina Faso, West Africa, and the city of Florence, Italy.[53] The people of Burkina Faso live in a rural agrarian society. They eat largely a grain-, legume-, and vegetable-based low-fat diet. Meat is a rarity. By contrast, people living in Florence eat an industrialized, urban diet. The rural Burkina Faso diet was low in fat and animal protein, while the European diet was higher in both.

The researchers collected and analyzed fecal samples from children in both areas in the morning, after their first meal. Not surprisingly, the researchers reported that the children of Burkina Faso consumed 1.8 times more dietary fiber than the Florentines. Analysis of the fecal microbiome revealed that 90 percent of the bacteria of both groups of children belonged to four major categories, or phyla, of bacteria: *Actinobacter*, *Bacteroides*, *Firmicutes*, and *Proteobacteria*. In the African children, *Bacteroides*, which breaks down plant-based foods, was 2.5 times more predominant than in the Florentine children.

The researchers examined fecal matter for the production of beneficial short-chain fatty acids (SCFAs), the byproducts of bacteria digestion of plant-based fiber. Recall from chapter 3 there are three types of useful metabolites SCFAs that are generated by gut bacteria: acetate, butyrate, and propionate. These protect the gut and overall health by decreasing inflammation, improving immunity, inhibiting angiogenesis, aiding stem cells, and improving insulin sensitivity. Correlating with their increased intake of dietary fiber, the children from Burkina Faso had threefold higher levels of SCFAs compared to European children. Analysis of the fecal bacteria found that the Burkina Faso children had greater diversity of bacteria in their feces than their European counterparts. Microbiome diversity is an important hallmark of health, and a plant-based, low-fat diet is associated with a more diverse, healthier microbiome that can produce higher levels of protective SCFAs.

The modern industrial food consumed in most of the developed world has shifted the human microbiome inexorably toward a less healthy profile. Because the microbiome influences our immune system, the medical community is now seeing alarming connections between the microbiome and rising ailments like food allergies, obesity, diabetes, and other chronic diseases that begin in childhood and plague us as adults. And remember, the study I just described involved Italy, the home of the Mediterranean diet, and still considered to be among the healthiest in the modern world. You can imagine the impact of a less healthy Western diet.

Now that you understand the importance for your microbiome of eating a diet high in fiber, low in animal protein, and based primarily on unprocessed whole foods, let's look at some of the specific foods that can have a beneficial effect.

Foods with a Beneficial Effect on Your Microbiome

Pumpernickel Bread

One bread with microbiomic benefits beyond the actual bacteria itself is pumpernickel bread. Originating in central and northern Europe, pumpernickel in its traditional form is made with a sourdough starter and whole rye flour. Rye is a kind of cereal that contains dietary fiber, polyphenols, and lignans. These bioactives are prebiotics that influence your microbiome as well as your metabolism.

A team of international researchers from Universite Joseph Fourier, Universite Grenoble, and University of Auvergne in France, from the University of Parma in Italy, and from the University of Almeria in Spain examined the effects of whole rye consumption on the microbiome. In the lab, they fed healthy rats chow made with either whole or refined rye for twelve weeks and studied the effects on their microbiome.[54] The results found that animals consuming the whole rye had 60 percent lower levels of *Desulfovibrionaceae*, a bacteria that generates a toxin called hydrogen sulfide, which injures the gut lining. When the gut is damaged in this way, it is easier for food particles to leak out from inside the intestines, causing an inflammatory reaction. This can potentially generate allergic and even autoimmune reactions (this is the phenomenon popularly known as "leaky gut"). The whole rye of pumpernickel bread has a prebiotic effect that may decrease the population of toxin-generating bacteria in your gut, resulting in an overall healthier gut and body.

Kiwifruit

The fruit we call "kiwi" has a proper name: kiwifruit. It's actually a large berry that originated in China, where it was once collected from the wild for medicinal purposes. Now found in markets all around the world, kiwifruit is egg-size and has a fuzzy brown skin surrounding intense green flesh dotted with tiny black seeds. The fruit (once called Chinese gooseberry) was brought to New Zealand in 1904, where it was later cultivated. In 1959, the fruit was first exported to the United States and commercially named kiwifruit, referring to a furry brown flightless bird that is the national icon of New Zealand.

Researchers from the National University of Singapore conducted a study to examine the effect of kiwifruit on the gut microbiome.[55] They fed six female volunteers the equivalent of two kiwifruits a day for four days (total of eight fruits) and looked at changes in their fecal microbiome. The differences appeared rapidly. They found that the presence of *Lactobacillus* was increased by 35 percent within twenty-four hours of eating kiwi. Another bacterium, *Bifidobacteria*, increased gradually by 17 percent over four days in most (83 percent) of the subjects. Both *Lactobacillus* and *Bifidobacteria* are considered beneficial gut bacteria that produce SCFAs, which help lower inflammation. The SCFAs help to maintain the integrity of the gut lining to prevent digested food from leaking out, and they improve glucose and lipid metabolism.[56] Eating kiwifruit thus has prebiotic effects that shape beneficial gut bacteria and lower inflammation.

Brassica

Brassica is a family of vegetables with a well established reputation for being healthful. These include broccoli, cauliflower, bok choy, cabbage, kale, rutabaga, turnips, and arugula. As we saw in chapter 6, these plants contain bioactives with antiangiogenic benefits. They also modify the microbiome by *decreasing* the presence of harmful bacteria in your gut.

Researchers from the Institute of Food Research in Norwich, United Kingdom, conducted a clinical study of brassica vegetables (broccoli, cauliflower) in ten healthy adults in their thirties to examine changes in their microbiome over two weeks.[57] Subjects were given either one cup per day of brassica foods (broccoli, cauliflower, broccoli-sweet potato soup) or they ate a diet with only 10 percent of the brassica (one-tenth of a cup) compared to the other group. Examination of their stool at the end of the study revealed that those eating the high brassica diet lowered the number of toxin-producing bacteria by 35 percent. This toxin, hydrogen sulfide, damages the gut lining and is found in high levels in the stool of patients with inflammatory bowel disease.[58] Like rye bread, brassica vegetables may protect against the development of colitis and gut inflammation by reducing the harmful bacteria that produce hydrogen sulfide.

Bamboo Shoots

Many people know that bamboo is the food of pandas. But throughout Asia, the shoots of bamboo plants are a popular vegetarian dish that is extremely high in dietary fiber and bioactives. They are found cooked, canned, and dried in the cuisine of China, Japan, Korea, and throughout Southeast Asia. In Western countries, sliced bamboo is sometimes found as a topping at the salad bar.

A study by the Chinese Academy of Sciences looked at how eating bamboo shoots affects the gut microbiome and obesity.[59] In the lab, researchers fed mice either a low-fat or a high-fat diet. They then added bamboo fiber (the equivalent of eating one-third cup of bamboo shoots daily in humans) into their food for six weeks and measured the weight, glucose tolerance, adipose (fat) tissue, and microbiome of the mice. The bamboo had a significant impact.

In mice eating a high-fat diet, adding bamboo *decreased* the amount of weight gain by an impressive 47 percent. Fat development was reduced by 30–50 percent in their abdomen and pelvis and under the skin with bamboo. When the researchers looked at the microbiome, the mice eating bamboo shoots had a 45 percent increase in bacterial diversity in their gut. Remember, more bacterial diversity is better for your health. The microbiome changes were substantial after eating bamboo. There was 300 percent more *Bacteriodetes*, one of the core bacteria important in a healthy gut microbiome. One interesting finding: eating bamboo shoots led to a decline in the family of bacteria to which *Akkermansia* belongs. Although these findings were in mice, *Akkermanisa* is so important for treatment response in cancer patients receiving immunotherapy (specifically, checkpoint inhibitors like atezolizumab, avelumab, durvalumab, nivolumab, and pembrolizumab), it might be wise to avoid bamboo shoots if this is your situation.[60]

An important health tip: fresh, raw bamboo shoots harvested from the forest contain small amounts of a toxin related to cyanide. Cooking the shoots by boiling for 10–15 minutes removes most of the toxin.[61] Don't go foraging in the jungle to find and eat raw bamboo.

Dark Chocolate

Along with its antiangiogenic and stem cell–stimulating benefits, the cacao used to make chocolate has positive effects on gut microbiota. A study by researchers from Louisiana State University found that fiber found in cacao feeds healthy gut bacteria such as *Bifidobacteria* and *Lactobacilli*. The bacteria use the fiber to generate acetate, proprionate, and butyrate, the useful SCFAs with anti-inflammatory properties that also improve glucose and lipid metabolism.[62]

Remember from chapter 3 that many lifestyle factors beyond food affect your microbiome, including stress. Researchers at the Netherlands Organization for Applied Scientific Research designed a study to test whether eating chocolate could mitigate stress-related effects on the microbiome.[63] They recruited thirty healthy individuals between the ages of 18 and 35 and first established their self-reported stress levels using a survey. Their results divided them into high-anxiety and low-anxiety groups. The researchers tested the blood and urine of both groups for stress markers at the start. Then, participants received forty grams—the equivalent of a medium-size chocolate bar—of a commercially available dark chocolate (Noir Intense, 74 percent dark) to eat every day for two weeks. The researchers monitored the stress markers in both their blood and urine.

When high-anxiety subjects ate dark chocolate for two weeks, the researchers found that levels of the stress markers cortisol and adrenaline decreased in their urine, as well as two markers called p-cresol and hippurate, which are metabolites of gut bacteria. Chocolate reduced these biomarker levels in high-anxiety subjects down to levels seen in the subjects reporting low anxiety.[64] This study showed that for stressed-out individuals, eating dark chocolate for only two weeks can influence gut bacteria and reduce stress markers in the body.

To study the specific bacteria affected by chocolate consumption, researchers from the University of Reading in the United Kingdom recruited twenty-two healthy volunteers in their thirties and gave them a beverage containing either high-cocoa flavanols or low-cocoa flavanols for four weeks.[65] The high-cocoa beverage was made from a cocoa flavanol-enriched powder (CocoaVia). The researchers took blood and fecal samples before and after the four weeks and found that the high-cocoa flavanol drink strikingly improved the ratio of good to harmful bacteria. There was an increase of beneficial *Lactobacillus* (by 17.5 times) and *Bifidobacteria* bacteria (3.6 times), and there was a decrease in harmful *Clostridium histolyticum* (by 2 times), a bacteria best known for causing gangrene. All of these studies offer evidence that cacao can boost good bacteria while controlling bad bacteria, and it may even help correct disruptions to the microbiome caused by chronic stress.

Walnuts

Walnuts are a good source of omega-3 PUFAs and dietary fiber. Eating walnuts lowers your risk of many conditions, from cardiovascular disease to cancer. Along with other mechanisms, their benefits are linked to the microbiome. Researchers from the University of Munich studied 135 healthy people over the age of fifty and divided them into groups that were fed a walnut-enriched diet (roughly twenty-one walnut halves per day) or a nut-free diet for eight weeks.[66] When comparing fecal samples from before and after the study, walnut eaters had significantly increased numbers of beneficial *Bifidobacteria* and *Firmicutes* bacteria, which produce anti-inflammatory SCFAs (butyrate, priopionate, acetate). At the same time, eating walnuts decreased the numbers of harmful *Clostridium* bacteria. Another study from the University of Illinois at Urbana-Champaign corroborated these walnut-led changes. Individuals who were fed a similar number of walnuts per day for three weeks had a 60–90 percent increase in beneficial butyrate-producing *Firmicutes* bacteria.[67]

By eating walnuts, you can make changes that optimize the balance between beneficial and harmful bacteria in your microbiome.

Beans

Bean are good for your gut bacteria because they are high in fiber. A study by the University of Guelph in Ontario and Agriculture and Agri-Foods Canada studied the effect of two kinds of beans, navy beans and black beans, on the gut microbiome.[68] In the lab, they fed mice with either standard chow or chow made with cooked navy beans or black beans for three weeks. The amount of beans used was equivalent to a human dose of 1.6 cups of navy beans or 1.2 cups of black beans per day. At the end, comparing the groups, they found the mice who ate beans had a seventy-one-fold increase in a healthy bacteria called *Prevotella*, which makes the anti-inflammatory SCFAs (acetate, proprionate, butyrate). There was also a 2.3-fold increase in another bacteria called *Ruminococcus*, which breaks down plant cells as another way to create SCFAs.

The researchers also examined the effect of the beans on the protective mucus lining of the intestines, as well as gut barrier function, both of which are linked to gut bacteria. More mucus protects the gut, and a strong gut lining forms a barrier to inflammatory substances that can leak from the gut. The bean eaters had an 81 percent decrease in harmful bacteria that break down the protective mucus in the gut. When the scientists actually examined the gut of the bean eaters, they found that the protective mucus-secreting cells of the upper colon increased by 60 percent in mice fed navy beans, and by 120 percent in the mice fed black beans. In the lower colon, mucus cells increased by 57 percent with black bean chow. These studies showed how both black beans and navy beans can contribute to healthy conditions in the gut. Chickpeas, lentils, and peas are all in the bean family and would be expected to have similar types of benefits.

Mushrooms

Mushrooms are fungi that grow in bacteria-rich soil and, like cheese, they possess their own microbiome.[69] They contain bioactives like beta-glucan that are antiangiogenic and activate the immune system. Mushrooms are also excellent sources of dietary fiber, which acts as a prebiotic.

Mushrooms increase the diversity of our microbiome, a sign of a strong microbiome health defense. Scientists from Penn State University studied this effect by feeding healthy mice chow made with a small amount of white button mushroom (1 percent by weight) or just normal mouse chow for six weeks. In the mushroom chow group, each mouse ate the equivalent of only one five-hundredth of an average-size white button mushroom each day. Researchers collected and analyzed blood, urine, and fecal samples throughout the experiment.

Urine tests showed that mice eating white mushrooms had a sevenfold increase in levels of an acid called hippurate, an indicator of microbiome diversity and health.[70] Mushroom consumption also both increased protective gut bacteria (*Bacteroidetes* and the bacteria phylum Verrucomicrobia, which includes the desirable *Akkermansia*) while decreasing harmful species from the *Firmicutes* phylum. At the end of six weeks, the researchers challenged the mice by exposing them to a harmful bacteria *Citrobacter rodentium* that infects the gut. The scientists found that mice who ate white button mushrooms had less gut inflammation and less damage from the infection, demonstrating the gut protective effect of eating mushrooms.

Scientists at the South China Institute of Technology and the Treerly Women's Nutrition and Health Institute in China studied the effect of shiitake mushrooms on the aging microbiome by feeding adult and elderly mice shiitake extracts for four weeks.[71] Aging mice have lower levels of *Firmicutes* and *Bacteroidetes*, but shiitake consumption increased amounts of these bacteria in aging mice by 115 percent. In humans, an interesting study of centenarians, or so-called super-agers, showed these same patterns of gut microbiota.[72] In both mice and people, shiitake mushrooms may be able to reverse the changes to the microbiome that typically accompany old age.

The Lion's mane mushroom, renowned for its culinary and medicinal properties, was the subject of a study by scientists at Jiangnan University in China to test its effects on the microbiome.[73] In the lab, they fed mice with severe gut inflammation the human equivalent of one tablespoon of Lion's mane mushroom. The results showed that Lion's mane could decrease the symptoms and the proteins associated with gut inflammation by as much as 40 percent. The mushroom increased the healthy bacteria *Akkermansia* while decreasing the harmful sulfur toxin-producing *Desulfovibrio*.

Beverages

Fruit Juices: Pomegranate, Cranberry, and Concord Grape

Drinking certain fruit juices have a positive impact on the levels of *Akkermansia muciniphila*, which is associated with decreased gut inflammation and the ability to combat obesity, as well as antitumor responses to some types of cancer immunotherapy.[74]

The microbiome benefits of drinking pomegranate juice are linked to its bioactives, the ellagitannins. As we saw in chapter 3, pomegranate is abundant in ellagitannins. These can be metabolized by *Akkermansia* into a metabolite called urolithin-A, which is excreted in the urine.[75] Studies suggest that about 70 percent of people can metabolize ellagitannins in this way. Researchers at the University of California Los Angeles studied twenty healthy volunteers and relied on urine tests to identify those who could make urolithin-A. In those patients, drinking one cup of pure pomegranate juice per day for four weeks increased the presence of *Akkermansia* by 71 percent.[76]

Cranberries contain proanthocyanins that increase the mucous layer in the gut where *Akkermansia* live. In a mouse study, scientists at Laval University and the University of Quebec at Montreal tested the effect of a cranberry extract equivalent to humans drinking about one cup per day of cranberry juice. They fed healthy mice either a standard diet or a high-fat diet. The cranberry extract could increase the levels of *Akkermansia* by 30 percent after nine weeks, and also protected the animals from weight gain.[77] Eating whole fresh or frozen cranberries is the best way to get their benefits, because the commercial processing of cranberries for juice removes some of the bioactives that are in their skin and seeds.[78]

The dark blue and purplish Concord grape was developed by a farmer named Ephraim Bull in Concord, Massachusetts as the "perfect" grape. It is the grape used to make classic grape jelly. Scientists from Rutgers University and the University of California San Francisco studied the effect of a Concord grape extract in mice that were fed a high-fat diet for thirteen weeks.[79] Mice that consumed extracts each day equivalent to that found in a one-third cup of Concord grape juice had less weight gain and five times more *Akkermansia* than in mice that did not consume the grape extract. The mice fed Concord grapes also had 21 percent less weight gain on a high-fat diet compared to mice eating just the high-fat diet.

Fruit smoothies are a way of getting the benefit of fruit bioactives in a beverage. Stone fruits like peaches, apricots, and mangoes contain chlorogenic acid, a bioactive that also promotes the growth of *Akkermansia*.[80] Cherries contain anthocyanins, and they promote *Akkermansia* growth in the colon. Scientists at Michigan State University fed freeze-dried cherries to lab mice that naturally develop colon tumors and found that eating cherries mixed in their chow reduced the number of tumors that developed by 74%.[81]

Red Wine

The benefits of red wine can now be extended to improving the gut microbiome and reducing inflammation in the body.[82] Wine polyphenols are not well absorbed in the small intestines, meaning they continue through the gut to reach the colon where they feed the gut bacteria. The bacteria convert the polyphenols into bioactive metabolites that can be measured in the feces. Researchers at the Institute of Food Science Research at Autonoma University in Spain studied the effect of drinking a large glass of red wine (250 milliliters) on red wine polyphenols in the stool.[83] They found that four weeks of drinking the equivalent of a large glass of red wine every day led the bacteria to create metabolites from wine polyphenols, specifically propionic acid, benzoic acid, and valeric acid. These have beneficial anti-inflammatory properties.[84] So whether or not you are a wine connoisseur, when you drink a glass or two of red wine, the benefits are not only the enjoyment experienced by your palate, but also the bacterial metabolites of the wine at the other end of your digestive tract.

In a different study from Spain, researchers from the University of Oviedo and the Instituto de Productos Lacteos de Asturias–Consejo Superior de Investigaciones Cientificas found that drinking only two-thirds of a glass of red wine daily correlated with lower blood levels of a DNA-damaging toxin called malondialdehyde, a marker of aging, oxidative stress, and cellular damage in the body. The researchers attributed this to shifts in fecal microbiota they observed in these subjects.[85, 86]

Teas

In addition to their antioxidant, anti-inflammatory, and antiangiogenic properties, the health-promoting polyphenols in tea help make a more favorable microbiome in our gut. As we've seen, green tea has star power when it comes to health, but it is not the only tea that promotes the health defenses.

A study by scientists from Ninbo University and Wenzhou Vocational College of Science and Technology in China tested green, oolong, and black teas for their effects on gut bacteria, and all three generated beneficial effects.[87] The researchers found that the bioactives in all three types of tea passed through the small intestine, where they were not completely absorbed, and made it to the colon, where they influenced the microbiome. Researchers incubated the tea polyphenols from green, oolong, and black tea separately with fecal samples taken from young, healthy volunteers and observed the microbiome in the lab. The researchers found that teas could generate a 3 percent increase in the beneficial bacteria *Bifidobacterium* and *Lactobacillus* and a 4 percent decrease in the harmful *Clostridia histolyticum*. Oolong tea had the greatest effect. The researchers also examined the concentration of the antiinflammatory SCFAs in the feces after thirty-six hours of exposure to the teas. Each tea substantially increased the three SCFAs acetate, propionate, and butyrate. Surprisingly, black tea polyphenols had an overall better increase compared to green or oolong tea. Thus, in addition to its benefits relating to stem cells, black tea is especially good for the microbiome and is now emerging to be a healthful tea in its own right.

Tea saponin, a natural chemical that has soaplike properties, is one of the hundreds of bioactives found in tea. Scientists from the University of Wollongong in Australia and Xuzhou Medical University in China have shown that tea saponins influence the microbiome.[88] They fed mice a high-fat diet, which caused an impaired gut microbiome as well as obesity, brain inflammation, and poor memory in the mice. But when the mice were fed tea saponin in addition to the high-fat diet, their guts grew 40 percent less *Desulfovibrio*, the bacteria that makes toxic hydrogen sulfide. The mice taking tea saponin also had less weight gain, less brain inflammation, and better memory compared to the mice eating a high-fat diet alone.

Overall, drinking black, oolong, and green tea can increase good bacteria, decrease bad bacteria, and helps the microbiome produce beneficial health promoting short-chain fatty acids.

Avoid Artificial Sweeteners

So far, I have focused primarly on foods you can add to your diet that actively make you healthier, rather than on foods you should eliminate, but when it comes to the microbiome I want to address one substance that may be best to avoid altogether: artificial sweeteners. The artificial sweeteners that are currently approved for human consumption are: saccharin, aspartame, sucralose, acesulfame, and neotame. They do the job they were designed for extraordinarily well—they taste very, very sweet.[89] Saccharin is 300–500 times as sweet as sugar, aspartame 180 times, and sucralose 600 times. Their advantage is that they satisfy the sweet tooth without delivering the calories of sugar. One of the ways they achieve this is having low absorption in the gut. But this means they are delivered right to the gut bacteria. So the big question is, how do these sweeteners affect the microbiome?

Scientists at the Weizmann Institute of Science and Tel Aviv University in Israel have examined the impact of three of these sweeteners—saccharin, sucralose, aspartame—on the gut microbiome.[90] They gave mice the artificial sweeteners or natural sugars (glucose and sucrose) in their drinking water for eleven weeks and compared their gut bacteria to mice who consumed only plain water. They found that saccharin had the largest effect on the microbiota, with a 1.2-fold decrease in beneficial *Lactobacillus reuteri*. Recall that *L. reuteri* is an important gut bacterium that affects immunity, resists development of breast and colon tumors, and influences the gut-brain axis to produce the social hormone oxytocin.

An attraction of artificial sweeteners is that most do not contain any carbohydrates, so they rank very low on the glycemic index. Surprisingly, however, when mice were given artificial sweeteners versus natural sugar or just plain drinking water and then tested for their ability to metabolize glucose, scientists found that mice drinking the artificial sweetener had more impaired glucose tolerance compared to those drinking sugar water or plain water. This would not make sense if you only considered the chemical makeup of the sweeteners. But the possibility of their interacting with the microbiome has been investigated. When broad-spectrum antibiotics (ciprofloxacin, metronidazole, or vancomycin) were given to the mice in order to wipe out gut bacteria, all the mice had similar responses to the glucose tolerance test, revealing that the interaction of the artificial sweeteners with the microbiome was responsible for the observed glucose intolerance.

The Israeli group also studied 381 nondiabetic healthy people in their forties and found that long-term consumption of noncaloric artificial sweeteners correlated with changes in their gut microbiome.[91] They also had a bigger waist-to-hip ratio (a measure of obesity), higher fasting levels of blood glucose, and elevated levels of hemoglobin A1c, a blood marker that reflects long-term high blood sugar. Importantly, the researchers found that there seemed to be individual differences in the way people respond to artificial sweeteners, which may also be due to variations in their microbiome.

Another lab study by scientists from Case Western Reserve University, Ohio State University, the National Institutes of Health, and the University of Aberdeen in Scotland showed an artificial sweetener could cause dysbiosis. They studied mice that are prone to a Crohn's disease-like inflammation of the gut and fed them sucralose maltodextrin for six weeks. When their gut bacteria were examined after the feeding, they found an overgrowth of E. coli.[92]

These studies show how synthetic foods can impact the microbiome. In the case of artificial sweeteners, the potential consequences may influence how the gut bacteria control blood sugar metabolism and weight gain. This is important because, after all, the entire reason for using artificial sweeteners is to avoid these problems.

Putting It All Together

Everything you put in your mouth that goes down the hatch—fruits, vegetables, carbs, meats, junk food, soda, artificial sweeteners—feeds your human cells and then becomes food for your gut microbiome. Your bacteria can metabolize food components that the human body can't digest, and this can create beneficial bioactives that protect your health. So, the next time you shop at the market, look at a menu, plan a meal, grab a snack, or reach for a beverage, ask yourself, *What's good for my bacteria?* Treat your bacteria well, and they will return the favor by defending your health.

The best way to eat for your bacteria is by putting more dietary fiber in your diet and less animal protein and fat. Plant-based foods are excellent sources of fiber and bioactives that feed and stimulate the healthy microbiome. Your gut bacteria then create metabolites that reduce inflammation, help regulate blood sugar and cholesterol, and improve immunity. The benefits will not only help you but also your progeny.

Eating to help your microbiome allows you to venture beyond fruits, vegetables, and nuts. Eating traditional fermented foods and cheeses that contain useful bacteria add diversity to the bacteria in your gut. Beneficial gut bacteria also thrive on cocoa, and eating or drinking it decreases bad bacteria. Remember that certain fruit juices (pomegranate, cranberry, Concord grape) increase the gut bacteria called *Akkermansia*, which may help optimize your immune system to clean house of cancer. Healthy gut bacteria enjoy a glass of red wine as well as tea in many forms, from black to oolong to green.

If you have taken antibiotics for any reason, they will definitely disrupt your microbiome. You will want to take steps with your diet to rebuild your gut's ecosystem. Artificial chemicals are often found in processed foods, and they may have negative consequences for our bacteria and therefore our health, possibly for generations to come. So remember:

when it comes to eating a healthy diet, it's not just about you. Take care of your microbiome, too.

KEY FOODS AFFECTING THE MICROBIOME

Prebiotic		Probiotic
Apricots	Lentils	Camembert cheese
Arugula	Lion's mane mushroom	Gouda cheese
Asparagus	Mango	Kimchi
Bamboo shoots	Navy beans	Pao Cai
Black beans	Olive oil (EVOO)	Parmigiano Reggiano
Black tea	Oolong tea	Sauerkraut
Bok choy	Peaches	Sourdough bread
Broccoli	Peas	Yogurt
Cabbage	Pomegranate juice	
Cauliflower	Pumpernickel bread	
Cherries	Red wine	
Chickpeas	Rutabaga	
Concord grape juice	Shiitake mushrooms	
Cranberry juice	Tomatoes	
Dark chocolate	Turnips	
Green tea	Walnuts	
Kale	White button mushrooms	
Kiwi	Whole grains	

CHAPTER 9

Direct Your Genetic Fate

Pollution, industrial toxins, ultraviolet radiation, and emotional stress all cause damage to our genetic code. When DNA is damaged, genes can malfunction. The consequences, such as aging, wrinkled skin, can be visible. Or, the effects can be insidious and invisible, causing cancer or damaging the brain, heart, lungs, and other organs. But foods and beverages can help you protect your own DNA against environmental assaults, as well as naturally occurring mutations.

When we read about diet and health, one term that is frequently encountered is *antioxidants*. These are touted as natural substances found in superfoods that can neutralize free radicals and provide a range of benefits from fighting cancer to anti-aging. This general wisdom is correct. Free radicals are highly reactive chemicals made from oxygen and nitrogen that are produced by the natural chemical reactions taking place in the body. Our body naturally attempts to reduce the levels of free radicals using antioxidants made by our cells. If free radicals overwhelm natural antioxidants, they can cause a condition in cells called oxidative stress. When free radicals run rampant, they act like chemical shrapnel and can injure our DNA.

Many foods contain bioactive chemicals with antioxidant properties. Often, these foods and their antioxidants are hailed for their ability to neutralize free radicals, lower cellular stress, and protect DNA. Of course, you also see marketing of dietary supplements and functional foods with antioxidant properties almost everywhere you look. Selling antioxidant products has become a big business—it is projected to become a $278 billion market by 2024.[1]

But let's look at the scientific and clinical evidence for foods that protect our DNA and how they actually work.

First, there's the popular vitamin with antioxidant properties: vitamin C. One of the most commonly taken dietary supplements, vitamin C is naturally found in many plant-based foods. The antioxidant effects of vitamin C have been proven in many lab studies, but as always, clinical evidence is king.[2]

Researchers from the Hong Kong Institute of Vocational Education (Shatin) conducted a small but eye-opening clinical study to examine the DNA protecting effects of drinking orange juice.[3] Oranges are known for their high vitamin C content. The researchers recruited six subjects and took a blood sample before having them each drink 1.75 cups of pasteurized orange juice, and then took a second blood sample two hours later. On a separate occasion, the researchers repeated the experiment with the same subjects, but this time gave them a placebo beverage made of water, sugar, and a vitamin C tablet instead of orange juice. After both tests, researchers used a special test called the comet assay to analyze the ability of the blood to protect DNA before and after the subjects drank the beverage. In the comet assay, white blood cells, or leukocytes, are exposed to hydrogen peroxide, the same chemical used in hair lightening bleach. The peroxide creates massive free radical damage and shreds the DNA in the white blood cells. If drinking orange juice had a protective effect, there would be less damage in the DNA when cells are exposed to bleach.

The study found indeed that drinking orange juice improved the blood's ability to protect DNA. The DNA damage in people after drinking orange juice was reduced by 19 percent compared to when they drank the vitamin-enriched sugar water. This DNA protective effect was seen as quickly as two hours after having the juice. The improved DNA-protecting effect of the orange juice beyond the vitamin C content suggests that the benefits come from more than just vitamin C. Oranges contain many bioactives, including naringenin and hesperidin, which are also antioxidants. This would support the prevailing wisdom that the combined antioxidant benefits gained from consuming whole foods can be more powerful than swallowing a supplement. And when it comes to oranges, you actually derive more benefit if you eat the whole fruit, rather than just drink the juice. Oranges contain dietary fiber, which as we saw in chapter 8, is good for your microbiome. While fresh-squeezed orange juice is a good option, be cautious about processed fruit juices. Many are simply sugar-sweetened beverages containing very little actual fruit.

Eating foods containing antioxidants is only one part of protecting your genetic code. Here's the problem: neutralizing free radicals with antioxidants is like the military shooting missiles out of the sky. It can be successful if there are only a few missiles, but put enough missiles in the air, and some will get through and cause destruction on the ground. The analogy applies to health as well. If there are only low levels of free radicals in the body, antioxidants can easily shoot them down. But if the burden is high, as you might find in someone regularly exposed to environmental toxins, or in a smoker, or in a person with a chronic inflammatory condition, antioxidants in food (or supplements) will offer useful, but only partial, protection.

The good news is that antioxidants aren't the only mechanism for preventing damage to our genes. Foods can trigger health defenses that are naturally hardwired into our DNA. Some foods can speed up the repair of broken DNA, after the damage has taken place. What we eat can also switch certain genes on or off through so-called epigenetic changes. In addition to diet, exercise, sleep, and environmental exposures can also have good (and bad) epigenetic effects. But foods that have a positive epigenetic influence can unleash beneficial genes or turn off harmful ones to prevent and fight disease. Foods can also influence DNA by protecting telomeres. Recall that telomeres are protective caps that cover the ends of DNA strands. Protecting telomeres slows down the ravages of aging that wear them down. You can activate these DNA safe-guards by consuming familiar and tasty foods that are easy to include in your everyday diet. So, what we eat can protect us against DNA damage and support our DNA's natural ability to help us resist disease.

Before we discuss the many foods and beverages that can protect your DNA, let's take a look at the diseases that are associated with DNA damage.

Diseases with DNA Damage

DNA damage is found in many serious diseases, including every type of cancer. Skin cancer is perhaps the most common, caused by solar (ultra-violet) radiation that damages the DNA in every bit of exposed skin (think: sunburn at the beach). This is a process called "field canceriza-tion." Other cancers are linked with occupational, environmental, and dietary exposures in which DNA becomes repeatedly damaged in spe-cific organs. These include cancers of the lung, bladder, esophagus, stom-ach, and colon, where insults from the air and the diet can alter your DNA. Precancerous lesions such as colon polyps, carcinoma-in-situ of the breast, cervical intraepithelial neoplasia, and actinic keratosis, a pre-cursor to skin cancer, are filled with cells that contain damaged DNA in need of repair.

Infections by disease-causing bacteria and viruses can cause DNA mutations from which tumors can arise, as in cervical cancer, liver (hepa-tocellular) cancer, and in cancer of the mouth and upper airway. Some people carry inherited mutations in which the body has weakened DNA repair mechanisms. For those individuals, cancer is a very likely fate. Some of the conditions that carry this risk have tongue-twister names like Li-Fraumeni syndrome (no relation to the author of this book), ataxia telangiectasia, and Lynch syndrome. If you have one of these con-ditions, your DNA is not protecting you the way it should, and it needs all the help it can get. Foods that help defend DNA are invaluable in these conditions.

DNA damage can be a side effect of traditional cancer treatments such as chemotherapy and radiation therapy. While killing cancer cells, the indiscriminant treatments actually cause collateral damage to the DNA of normal healthy cells, too. This can lead to secondary cancers in patients who were successfully treated and survived their first cancer. Common medical imaging procedures, from X-rays to CAT scans to MRIs and PET scans all deliver radiation that traumatizes normal DNA.

Autoimmune diseases cause DNA damage, not only in the organs that are affected by an overactive immune system but even in the white blood cells circulating in their bloodstream. This has been seen in people with lupus, rheumatoid arthritis, celiac disease, and inflammatory bowel diseases, like Crohn's disease and ulcerative colitis, among others.[4]

Epigenetic changes can be harmful as well as helpful, and these take place over a person's lifetime. The changes in how the DNA is expressed can be passed down across generations. These alterations are being discovered to play a role in a remarkable range of diseases, including schizophrenia, autism spectrum disorders, Alzheimer's disease, Parkinson's disease, major depression, atherosclerosis, and autoimmune diseases.[5] Clearly, there is a huge range of health threats where DNA protection could prove useful. A mindful diet containing foods with DNA protecting properties could boost your health defenses.

Foods That Influence DNA Repair

Most nutrition textbooks describe the importance of micronutrients as the building blocks for normal DNA. These include vitamins A, B, C, D, and E, found in spinach, carrots, red peppers, lentils, navy beans, and mushrooms, as well as eggs, cod liver oil, sardines, and mackerel. Minerals like magnesium, found in almonds, oatmeal, bananas, and tofu, and zinc, found in oysters, crab, and lobster, are all needed for the upkeep of DNA repair mechanisms. But increasingly it's becoming clear that the benefits of whole foods are bigger than any one singled-out component, whether it's a vitamin, mineral, or even a bioactive. This is one reason why I pay special attention to the data coming from clinical and laboratory studies of whole foods and beverages, and from epidemiological studies in real world populations.

Berry Juices

While orange juice may be a go-to morning beverage, other tempting options can provide DNA protective effects. Mixed berry juices are found everywhere, from grocery stores to juice bars and smoothie stands. Red and dark-colored berries contain many bioactives, including anthocyanin and other polyphenols with antioxidant effects.

A research study conducted at the University of Kaiserslautern in Germany recruited eighteen healthy male volunteers[6] and gave them a mixed berry juice made of red grape, blackberry, sour cherry, blackcurrant, and chokeberry (also known as aronia) juices. The subjects drank the juice every day for three weeks, consuming a daily total of three cups, divided into equal parts over the course of the day. After completing the first three weeks, they were asked to refrain from eating berries for another three weeks. The researchers drew blood at the beginning and throughout the study. A comet assay showed that drinking the berry juice significantly increased DNA protection by 66 percent, which was seen one week after starting the juice, compared to levels before starting the juice. When the juice intake was stopped, the protective effects wore off, and the level of DNA damage in the blood steadily increased back to previous levels. To see if the effects were due to berry bioactives, the researcher removed the polyphenols from the juice, then repeated the study. This time, when the volunteers consumed this drink, their blood did not show the DNA protective effects, nailing down that the effect was due to the bioactives.

Kiwifruit

Bright green slices of kiwifruit make your breakfast plate look attractive, and its strawberry-like flavor is mouthwatering. As we saw in chapter 8, kiwifruit has a beneficial impact on the microbiome. Kiwi also contains high levels of vitamin C, chlorogenic acid, and quinic acid that each have antioxidant effects.[7] Researchers at the Rowett Research Institute in Scotland examined kiwifruit's ability to reduce DNA damage.[8] They recruited fourteen healthy volunteers and gave them one, two, or three kiwifruits to eat each day. The participants ate a different dose of fruit during each of three periods of time, and their blood was drawn for a comet assay at the beginning and end of each period. The results showed that eating kiwifruit, regardless of the number of fruits, could reduce DNA damage by approximately 60 percent. When the researchers looked more closely at the DNA, they found that eating three fruits per day actually increased DNA *repair* activity by 66 percent. So, eating kiwifruit not only neutralizes free radicals, but it also increases the repair rate of any DNA that has been damaged to get it back into shape.

Carrots

You may want to reach for carrot juice or carrot soup for more than their great taste. True to their name, carrots are rich in the bioactives called carotenoids, red and yellow pigments found throughout the plant-based food world. Carotenoids are powerhouses when it comes to antioxidant activity.

Researchers at the Quadram Institute Bioscience in the United Kingdom wanted to examine the DNA protection effects of eating carrots.[9] They recruited sixty-four male volunteers and fed them the equivalent of 2.5 cups of carrots (about five medium carrots) per day for three weeks, on top of their regular diet. The carrots were frozen Sainsbury brand and cooked for ten minutes in boiling water, drained, and then minced in a food processor. The researchers took blood at the beginning of the study, after three weeks, and then six weeks after that. After three weeks of eating carrots, subjects' blood exhibited an increase in DNA repair activity, but not a lowering of DNA damage rates. This means that carrots don't prevent DNA damage but instead repair damage that already exists. Interestingly, dietary supplements containing carotenoids decrease DNA damage, which is consistent with their well-known antioxidant effects. This is a great example of how whole foods can benefit your health in different ways than supplements.

Broccoli

It's true, eating broccoli *is* good for you, and one of its benefits is DNA protection.[10] Researchers from the University of Milan in Italy and the University of Copenhagen in Denmark recruited twenty-seven young male university students who smoked more than ten cigarettes per day.[11] Cigarette smoke contains a cloud of chemicals called reactive oxygen species that are guaranteed to cause DNA damage. So, smokers are a perfect group to study to determine if broccoli can provide any protection. The researchers steamed broccoli (Marathon cultivar) for fifteen minutes and fed each subject with 1.3 cups of the cooked vegetable per day for ten days. Blood samples were drawn at the beginning and end of the study, and tested for their ability to reduce DNA damage with the comet assay. The broccoli intervention led to a 23 percent decrease in DNA breakage in the blood of cigarette smokers. After the broccoli-eating period had ended, the blood tests were repeated. Not surprisingly, the blood of the smokers showed a return to the same levels of increased DNA damage that was seen prior to eating any broccoli.

Lycopene-Rich Foods: Tomato, Watermelon, Guava, Pink Grapefruit

The next time you go to the beach, consider drinking a shot of tomato, watermelon, pink grapefruit, or guava juice before heading out. It will protect you against sun damage. The red-orange color of these fruits comes from lycopene, which, among other benefits you've seen in earlier chapters, protects DNA from the ionizing radiation damage from the sun.[12]

Scientists from the National Institute of Public Health–National Institute of Hygiene in Poland wanted to study lycopene's effects. They recruited healthy, nonsmoking thirty-year-old women from Warsaw and collected their white blood cells. They then exposed the white blood cells to X-rays, analyzing the damaging effects of the radiation using the comet assay. The radiation damaged the DNA and killed most of the cells. However, if the cells were exposed to lycopene one hour *before* or just immediately before radiation exposure, the DNA damage was significantly reduced, and more cells survived. This showed a protective effect, especially at low levels of lycopene. However, when the lycopene was added to the cells *after* radiation exposure, there was no protective benefit at all, and the DNA damage significantly increased.

This finding shows that lycopene cannot repair DNA after radiation damage, but it can have a protective effect before exposure to the radiation. As a consequence of these results, also think about having a shot of tomato or watermelon juice before going to the dentist, who may take an X-ray of your teeth, or before getting on an airplane, where a dose of radiation during the flight will be unavoidable.

Lycopene is also protective against DNA damage caused by infection. The bacterium *Helicobacter pylori* infects the stomach and wreaks cellular havoc, causing gastritis, stomach ulcers, and even stomach cancer. More than 4 billion people worldwide are infected by *H. pylori*, making it a global health issue.[13] The bacterium does its damage by creating reactive oxygen species. In the stomach, these cause oxidative stress and DNA damage.

A study by scientists from Yonsei University in Korea and Tokyo Medical and Dental University in Japan found that the damage from

H. pylori can happen fast. As soon as fifteen minutes after the stomach cells are infected, free radicals are created. After exposure, their production continues for at least an hour, with an increasing amount of DNA destruction in the stomach cells.[14] But, when the cells were pretreated with lycopene one hour before *H. pylori* infection, the amount of damaging reactive oxygen species was reduced by more than 60 percent. Lycopene decreased the cell DNA damage by almost 40 percent, and the cells were rescued. This protective benefit by lycopene on stomach cells is parallel to its effect on white blood cells in the women in Warsaw.

Seafood

In addition to their antiangiogenic benefits, polyunsaturated fats (omega-3 PUFAs) from seafood can protect your DNA. There are many sources of marine omega-3 PUFAs, and you might be surprised to learn that while salmon is one source, it's not actually at the top of the list. The next time you are at the fish market or restaurant, consider these top sources of marine omega-3 PUFAs, which you read about earlier in chapter 6, for their DNA-repairing advantages: hake (a white-fleshed fish in the cod family), sea cucumber (a delicacy in Asia, related to the starfish), manila clams and cockles, tuna (watch out for high mercury levels), yellowtail, and bottarga (the dried roe of gray mullet that is considered a delicacy in the Mediterranean).

Health-producing omega-3 PUFAs have antioxidant effects that can counter the devastation of DNA caused by free radicals.[15] But they can also improve DNA repair in cells, which left unchecked might otherwise go on to become cancerous.[16] Researchers at Harvard Medical School and from the National Cancer Institute examined 1,125 cases of patients with colorectal cancer.[17] (These patients had been part of two large studies called the Nurses' Health Study and the Health Professionals Follow-up Study.) The researchers looked at the cancer specimens for signs of DNA instability. When a cancer's DNA is stable, its cells are less erratic and more predictable in their behavior. When cancer DNA is unstable, things can get wild, and even more dangerous. Cancers with stable DNA are called MSS (microsatellite stable), while those with high DNA instability are called MSI-H (microsatellite instability-high). As we said in chapter 4, cells are hardwired to be able to repair DNA by replacing damaged parts.

The researchers found that a high intake of marine omega-3 PUFAs was associated with a 46 percent reduced risk of the more aggressive MSI-H colon cancers compared to those with low intake of omega-3 PUFAs. High daily intake was equivalent to the amount of healthy fat you would find in 3.5 ounces of fish, a serving size roughly the size of a deck of cards. These data show that eating foods rich in omega-3 PUFAs not only reduces DNA damage through their antioxidant effects, but also can help improve the body's ability to repair DNA.

Pacific Oysters

If you are an oyster lover, you will love this research finding: oysters protect your DNA. Among the more than one hundred different varieties of briny bivalves, the Pacific oyster is a relatively small, sweet oyster that is widely cultivated and eaten around the world. They don't produce pearls, but they do offer antioxidant benefits. Oyster meat has high amounts of the amino acid taurine, which protects DNA against free radical damage. It also contains the amino acid cysteine and bioactive peptides that create a powerful antioxidant called *glutathione*.[18]

While oysters at the raw bar are a delicacy, oysters are also baked, used in stews, and made into sauce. The sauce is especially potent because oysters are boiled down, essentially creating an extract containing concentrated bioactives. Classic oyster sauce is a thick, dark sauce that was invented in Guangdong, China in the 1800s. It is commonly used in stir-fry recipes to add a rich umami flavoring to brassica vegetables, like broccoli and bok choy in Chinese and Southeast Asian cooking.

Researchers at the National Center for Scientific Research in France and Fox Chase Cancer Center in Philadelphia studied the antioxidant effect of oyster extracts in humans.[19] They recruited seven healthy men and gave them extracts from Pacific oysters prepared by heating fresh oysters for one hour at 176°F, then drying the extract into a powder. The powder was taken in the form of a supplement pill three times per day for eight days. The researchers drew blood throughout the study, inflicting and then measuring DNA damage in the blood to see the effects of the oyster extract. Remarkably, eating the oyster extract led to a whopping 90 percent reduction of DNA damage. The oyster extract also raised blood levels of the protective antioxidant glutathione by 50 percent.

The next time you enjoy a platter of oysters, you'll want to ask if they are Pacific oysters. And you can now relish adding oyster sauce as a flavor booster and DNA protector when you make a stir-fry.

Foods with Epigenetic Effects

Beyond protecting or repairing DNA, foods can influence DNA function through a process called epigenetic change. Remember, epigenetic influences are those that come from outside exposures, like diet or environment. These influences either unleash DNA that would otherwise be silent and not functioning, or block DNA that would otherwise be active. While some epigenetic changes caused by toxic exposures, for example, are harmful to your health, research has shown certain foods can cause beneficial epigenetic changes that tip the scales toward better health.

A quick recap of different epigenetic changes: Methylation is where a chemical methyl sits on top the DNA strand and silences a gene, so it cannot function to make its protein. Demethylation allows proteins that were once blocked to be made. Histone modifications uncoil or recoil DNA to make it more or less available, which can be beneficial for health, depending on the genes being influenced. By understanding the epigenetic effects, you can select foods with the ability to turn off a harmful gene or to activate a useful gene, so greater quantities of beneficial proteins are made. When beneficial DNA is activated and harmful DNA is silenced, you are boosting your health.[20]

Soy

In addition to its antiangiogenic cancer-starving effects, soy can suppress breast cancer by epigenetically activating the power of a tumor suppressor gene.[21] The job of these genes is to prevent tumor growth. When the genes are blocked, it becomes easier for breast cancer cells to grow, even though there are still other health defenses that cancer must overcome to become deadly. But the epigenetic effects of soy are particularly important because of the confusion surrounding soy and breast cancer.

Researchers at the University of Missouri and Iowa State University studied the effect of giving soy bioactives (isoflavones) to women to activate these tumor suppressor genes.[22] They recruited thirty-four healthy women in a prospective, randomized, double-blind clinical trial. The women were given either a high dose or a low dose of soy bioactives to consume twice a day for ten days. The daily low dose was equivalent to eating 1.2 cups of edamame beans, while the high dose was the equivalent of 4 cups. Blood levels of one soy isoflavone, genistein, were higher when the women consumed the high dose of soy.

The researchers specifically looked at a tumor suppressor gene called retinoic acid receptor B2 (RARB2). Tumor suppressor genes serve as guardians of the genome to prevent cancer development. In the case of RARB2, this protective gene is often found to be deactivated, or neutralized, in breast cancer. Recall that methylation blocks the function of a specific section of DNA.[23] The researchers found that even after consuming the low dose of soy isoflavone, the RARB2 tumor suppressor gene was turned on. This means that eating soy causes more tumor suppression and greater protection against cancer growth. Subjects who consumed the soy isoflavones also had increased levels of a second tumor suppressor gene, Cyclin D2 (CCND2).[24]

These findings have practical implications for women who are

BRCA (pronounced "brack-uh") mutation carriers, since carrying this gene is associated with a higher risk for developing breast cancer, ovarian cancer, and pancreatic cancer. Thanks to convenient DNA testing using saliva, more and more women are getting to know their BRCA status. Because BRCA is a tumor suppressor gene, when you have a mutation it means you have less protection against cancer. One study of patients with BRCA mutations showed that they also had other tumor suppressors blocked, including RARB2 and CCND2.[25] Soy helps to activate these cancer-fighting genes through epigenetic change, partly explaining why soy may help counteract the danger of having a BRCA mutation. Eating soy can spark an epigenetic change in your DNA with protective effects against breast cancer.

Cruciferous Vegetables

You've already seen the value of broccoli, but the entire family it belongs to, cruciferous vegetables, also cause beneficial epigenetic changes in your DNA. Broccoli, bok choy, kale, and cabbage all contain the bioactive sulforaphane. Scientists at the Institute of Food Research in Norwich (UK) showed, for example, that when colon cancer cells are exposed to sulforaphane, there is a profound change in the activity of genes in the cells. Sulforaphanes caused sixty-three genes in the cancer to be reduced in their activity by half.[26] Other studies have shown that sulforaphanes in cruciferous vegetables cause an epigenetic increase in the activity of tumor suppressor genes, similar to soy, which activate a hardwired defense against cancer.[27]

Coffee

Coffee beans contain polyphenols that trigger beneficial DNA functions. Similar to soy, coffee polyphenols epigenetically turn on the tumor suppressor gene RARB2. Scientists at the University of South Carolina have documented these effects in the lab, where they exposed human breast cancer cells to two bioactives found in coffee: chlorogenic and caffeic acid.[28] Both of these polyphenols changed the cancer cells so that the tumor suppressors in their DNA were unleashed, thwarting the ability for cancers to grow.

Tea

Similar to coffee, the major bioactive in green tea, called epigallocat-echin gallate (EGCG), causes epigenetic changes that amplify the influence of tumor suppressor genes, thus dampening the ability for cancer to form. Combined with its antiangiogenic and microbiomic effects, it's no wonder tea has clinical evidence for anticancer benefits.[29] Green tea also causes cells to experience epigenetic changes that increase production of a natural antioxidant enzyme called glutathione-S-transferase (GSTP1), which further protects DNA by neutralizing free radicals.[30]

Turmeric

If you've ever eaten at an Indian, Indonesian, or Thai restaurant, you have most likely had turmeric, a spice commonly used in Southeast Asian cuisine. This spice is also used in mustard to give it its characteristic golden color. Turmeric is a tropical plant whose underground stems are harvested, boiled, dried in an oven, and powdered to make an orange colored spice that has been used in cooking and Ayurvedic medicine for thousands of years. The main bioactive in turmeric is curcumin. Curcumin causes many beneficial epigenetic effects that increase the activity of tumor suppressor genes in our body known to counter the growth of colon cancer and leukemia.[31]

Curcumin's epigenetic effects also protect the health of your blood vessels.[32] In lab rats with hypertension, scientists at the China Academy of Sciences found that eating curcumin reduced injury to the coronary blood vessels feeding the heart by allowing their genes to produce a protein called tissue inhibitor of metalloproteinases (TIMP). This protein reduces inflammation. Because inflammation damages the blood vessel wall which leads to the narrowing of blood vessels by cholesterol plaques, curcumin's epigenetic action protects the heart from inflammation that could ultimately lead to a heart attack from blocked arteries.

Curcumin also benefits the brain. Scientists at Pusan National University in Korea showed that when brain cancer (glioma) cells are exposed to curcumin, it triggers an epigenetic effect that causes the cancer cells to commit suicide and die.[33] The same group in Korea exposed healthy neural stem cells from the brain to curcumin to see what would happen. In that case, the curcumin stimulated the stem cells to grow into mature normal neurons. This means that the epigenetic powers contained in a single spice, curcumin, can do triple duty: protect against cancer, reduce blood vessel inflammation, and help grow neurons.

Herbs

Many popular herbs used in Mediterranean cuisine contain a bioactive called rosmarinic acid, so named because of its original discovery in rosemary. Rosmarinic acid is also found in basil, marjoram, sage, thyme, and peppermint. Scientists at Poznan University in Poland examined its epigenetic effects and found that rosmarinic acid prevents the blocking of tumor suppressor genes in human breast cancer cells.[34]

Foods That Protect Telomeres

Your telomeres play an important role in protecting your DNA by shielding the ends of your chromosomes from damage. Telomeres naturally shorten with age like a fuse burning down, so any action that can help them stay longer will help protect your DNA and combat aging. Let's look at the foods and beverages that have been shown to counteract telomere shortening.

Coffee

Coffee has been enjoyed as a beverage for more than six hundred years. And if you are like me, it's part of a customary morning ritual to start your engine for the day—mostly due to its caffeine. But it turns out coffee has other benefits and bioactives beyond the morning jolt. It lowers your risk of dying.

In a massive study of 521,330 men and women in the European Prospective Investigation into Cancer and Nutrition, consumption of both caffeinated and decaffeinated coffee was associated with reduced mortality, specifically 12 percent lower in men and 7 percent in women—from any cause.[35] The greatest benefit was in lowering the risk of dying from a digestive-related disease, which makes sense, since the gut is exposed to the highest concentration of coffee bioactives.

Caffeine may give you the kick you want, but it may not play a significant role in the DNA protection provided by drinking coffee. In lab studies, caffeine actually shortens telomeres.[36] Yet, coffee drinking has just the opposite effect. In a study called the National Health and Nutrition Examination Survey (NHANES), researchers documented coffee and caffeine consumption in 5,826 adults and showed that drinking more coffee was associated with *longer* telomeres.[37] For each cup of coffee that subjects consumed each day, their telomeres were 33.8 base pairs longer. This means that drinking one cup of coffee every day effectively slows aging. Coffee contains many more bioactives than caffeine, and the multiple bioactives likely work together to offer a telomere-protecting effect. (Recall, too, that coffee also has benefits on the angiogenesis defenses.)

A third large study, the Nurses' Health Study, backed up the beneficial coffee findings. Researchers examined 4,780 women for their coffee consumption levels using a food frequency questionnaire and then measured their telomeres through blood samples.[38] Compared to non–coffee drinkers, women who drank three or more cups of coffee per day had longer telomeres.

In the old days, coffee was viewed as a possible risk for heart disease, since caffeine can speed up heart rate. Theoretically that made sense, but in fact, the opposite was seen when actual population studies of coffee drinkers were conducted. Researchers at the University of York in the United Kingdom conducted a meta-analysis of human studies examining coffee consumption and mortality after a heart attack in a total of 3,271 people. (A meta-analysis allows researchers to examine multiple studies and use statistical methods to combine their results and synthesize all of the findings to arrive at a common truth using the available evidence.) When applied to coffee, the analysis found that light coffee drinkers (one to two cups per day) had a 21 percent *reduced* risk of death from heart attack, while heavy coffee drinkers (two or more cups per day) had a 31 percent reduced risk of death. The many coffee bioactives likely act on the heart leading to this associated lower risk. The net benefit of coffee for health based on all the clinical evidence is a good example of why it's important to look at (and consume) the whole food and not come to sweeping conclusions on the basis of only one of its components like, in the case of coffee, its caffeine.

Tea

Given the mounting health attributes of tea, an obvious question is whether drinking tea benefits your telomeres. Researchers at the Chinese University of Hong Kong studied a group of 976 men and 1,030 women, age sixty-five and older.[39] The average age of participants was seventy-two, which is important for a telomere study because telomeres shorten with age. Each individual in the study reported how much and how often they consumed foods across thirteen categories common in China, including tea. Researchers drew blood and measured telomere length in the white blood cells. The results were striking: tea drinking was associated with increased telomere length, but only in elderly men, not women. When the amount of tea consumed by men was analyzed, those who drank three or more cups of tea per day had longer telomeres compared to those who drank less than a third of a cup of tea. The difference in telomere length was equivalent to a calculated difference of five years of additional life between high- and low-level tea drinkers. No other food group was associated with any telomere lengthening in this elderly population. The study did not specifically ask which type of tea, but green tea and oolong tea are the most commonly consumed teas in China.

Why did women not enjoy the same telomere-lengthening benefits of the tea? The only other statistically significant finding from this study was a negative effect seen in women (but not men) associated with the use of cooking oil and shorter telomeres. The researchers noted that women who do most of the cooking in Chinese culture may be standing over the fumes of oil heated to extremely high temperature in a wok, which could generate chemical byproducts that damage telomeres, thus potentially erasing any protective benefit of tea.

Nuts and Seeds

Nuts and seeds are popular snacks today, and all evidence points to their health benefits. They are a good source of dietary fiber (for the microbiome), and contain potent bioactives, like gallic acid and ellagic acid. At least two large studies have shown that eating nuts and seeds is associated with reduced mortality.[40] The Physicians' Health Study involved 22,742 male doctors and showed an association between eating five or more servings of nuts per week and a 26 percent lower risk of mortality, compared to people who rarely ate nuts or ate no nuts at all. The PREDIMED study showed an even higher level of benefit. In that study, which evaluated 7,447 healthy people in Spain who were at risk for cardiovascular disease, those who ate three servings of nuts per week had a 39 percent reduced risk of mortality compared to people who didn't eat any nuts.

Given these associations seen between nut consumption and mortality, researchers at Brigham Young University in Utah studied whether nut consumption influences telomere length. The researchers surveyed 5,582 men and women between twenty and eighty-four years old who were part of the National Health and Nutrition Examination Survey (NHANES) program led by the U.S. National Center for Health Statistics, asking them how much and how often they ate nuts and seeds.[41] In this study, "nuts and seeds" included almonds, almond butter and paste, Brazil nuts, cashews and cashew butter, chestnuts, flaxseeds, hazelnuts, macadamia nuts, peanuts and peanut butter, pecans, pine nuts, pistachios, pumpkin seeds, squash seeds, sesame seeds and tahini, sunflower seeds, and walnuts. The researchers then examined the participants' blood to determine telomere length and look for dietary correlations.

Their analysis showed that the more nuts and seeds consumed, the longer the telomeres. For every ten grams of nuts or seeds consumed per day, telomeres were 8.5 units longer over the course of a year. Ten grams is roughly one tablespoon of nuts, which is equivalent to: nine cashews; or seven walnuts; or six almonds; or four teaspoons of flaxseeds, pumpkin seeds, or sunflower seeds; or two teaspoons of sesame seeds. These amounts can easily be consumed in one day in a number of different forms, from individual nuts to baked into a bar or added to a salad.

What advantage does this offer in terms of aging? Normally, telomeres shrink by 15.4 base pairs per year. Since the NHANES findings showed that eating nuts or seeds increased telomere length by 8.5 units per ten grams consumed, the researchers calculated that for every half a handful of nuts or seeds eaten per day, there would be approximately a 1.5-year slowing of cellular aging.

Mediterranean Diet

Beyond its great flavors and fresh ingredients—and all the angiogenesis, stem cell, and microbiome influencing benefits—the Mediterranean diet is associated with healthy aging and improved telomere length. One study led by Harvard researchers examined 4,676 healthy middle-aged women from the Nurses' Health Study to investigate the association between dietary patterns and telomeres.[42] The women completed a food frequency questionnaire, which researchers then analyzed to see how closely the foods they ate resembled the Mediterranean diet. The scoring system used for this analysis was based on a higher consumption of vegetables (excluding potatoes), fruits, nuts, whole grains, legumes, fish, and monounsaturated fats; moderate alcohol intake; and lower consumption of red and processed meats. Researchers drew blood and measured telomere length in the white blood cells of the participants. Women whose dietary patterns were most similar to the Mediterranean diet had significantly longer telomeres. By contrast, women who ate a more typical Western diet, high in saturated fats and meat, had just the opposite effect. In fact, those whose diets *least* resembled the Mediterranean diet had shorter than average telomeres.

The Mediterranean diet is made up of foods and beverages that are known to be high in antioxidant, DNA repairing, and anti-inflammatory activity, which slows telomere shortening.[43] What was important from this study, however, is the finding that no single individual food documented in the diets was by itself a magic bullet for increased telomere length. The overall dietary pattern was the most important factor.

Vegetable-Rich Asian Diets

As a dietary pattern, there's no question that a plant-based diet is more beneficial to your health than a diet heavy in animal proteins. Besides the Mediterranean diet, the Asian diet is another pattern that is typically rich with plant-based foods—and known to be healthy. The first study to comprehensively collect data and analyze this diet was the China-Cornell-Oxford Project, which was elegantly described by nutrition and health pioneer T. Colin Campbell in his landmark book *The China Study*. This study detailed the links between nutrition, heart disease, cancer, and diabetes in Asia, and is widely considered one of the most comprehensive nutrition studies ever undertaken.

More recently, scientists have investigated the connection between the Asian diet and telomere length. Researchers from Sichuan University,

No. 4 West China Teaching Hospital, Sun Yat-sen University, and People's Hospital of Ganzi Tibetan Autonomous Prefecture in China studied 553 adults (272 women and 281 men) from Southwest China, who were in the age range of twenty-five to sixty-five years old.[44] Participants completed a dietary survey asking about the specific foods they ate during the previous year. The survey results revealed four real world dietary patterns among the subjects: (1) a vegetable-rich pattern that primarily consisted of fruits, vegetables, whole grains, nuts, eggs, dairy, and tea; (2) a "macho" pattern (researchers' term), heavy in animal protein and alcohol; (3) a traditional pattern that featured rice, red meat, and pickled vegetables; and (4) a high-energy-density pattern, which was high in sugar-sweetened beverages, wheat flour, and deep-fried foods. The researchers then drew blood, measured telomere length in white blood cells, and correlated the four dietary patterns with telomere length.

Only the vegetable-rich dietary pattern was associated with longer telomere length, and interestingly, only in women. This study found no correlation between any of the four dietary patterns and telomere length in men. The reason for the gender differences on telomere length and diet is not understood, reminding us that there is no universal one-size-fits-all diet for health, and that much more research is needed in this area before concrete dietary recommendations can be made for telomere lengthening.

Overall Diet and Lifestyle Change

A holistic and inclusive approach to diet and lifestyle was explored in an important study called Gene Expression Modulation by Intervention with Nutrition and Lifestyle (GEMINAL) led by Dean Ornish at the Preventive Medical Research Institute in Sausalito and Nobel Laureate Elizabeth Blackburn at the University of California, San Francisco. GEMINAL researchers studied twenty-four men who were diagnosed with low-risk prostate cancer and volunteered to undergo a comprehensive diet and lifestyle intervention for three months.[45] The intervention included a three-day residential retreat, followed by weekly lifestyle counseling, a weekly telephone check-in with a nurse, yoga six days a week, exercise (walking thirty minutes per day six days a week), and a one-hour weekly support group session. The dietary component of the intervention was similar in composition to the Mediterranean diet, and the subjects also received omega-3 PUFAs (fish oil), vitamins C and E, and selenium supplements.

Researchers drew blood at the start and end of the three-month intervention, analyzing white blood cells for activity of telomerase, an enzyme that helps lengthen telomeres. The results showed a striking 30 percent increase in telomerase activity following the diet and lifestyle intervention. Increasing telomerase activity extends a cell's longevity and ability to function normally.[46] The higher the levels of telomerase, the longer the telomeres were, which is a good thing for health.

Five years later, the GEMINAL researchers followed up with ten participants and compared their blood cells and telomeres to twenty-five other men with low-grade prostate cancer who opted for no intervention.[47] The researchers found that telomeres were significantly longer in the group that underwent the diet and lifestyle intervention compared to their original baseline. In the group that did not undergo the intervention, telomere length actually shortened. Sticking with the program proved to be beneficial. Those in the intervention group who were more adherent to the diet and lifestyle had longer telomeres than those who were lax.

Foods That Harm Our DNA Health Defense Mechanisms

Some foods are not so good for your DNA, and even contribute to its damage. While this book focuses on inclusiveness with diet, I feel it's important to tell you about the foods and dietary patterns that can potentially harm our DNA.

FATTY FOODS

The next time you reach for a strip of crispy bacon or carve into that beautifully marbled rib eye steak, think first about your DNA. Fatty foods can change your health through epigenetic effects. Researchers studied the epigenetic impact of saturated fat in human volunteers at the Uppsala University Hospital in Sweden.[48] They recruited thirty-one healthy men and women between eighteen and twenty-seven years old and of normal weight, and fed them high-calorie muffins for seven weeks. There were two kinds of muffins: one made with high (excessive) amounts of saturated fat (refined palm oil), and the other kind was with polyunsaturated fat (sunflower oil). The goal of the study was to compare weight gain caused by overeating too much of each kind of fat. The number of muffins each participant was asked to eat was tailored to cause a 3 percent increase in weight.

The researchers found that saturated and polyunsaturated fat had different effects. The participants who ate saturated fats increased their visceral fat as well as fat in their liver. Their blood triglyceride levels rose by 14 percent. In contrast, those who ate muffins made with unsaturated fats increased their lean body mass[49] and decreased their blood triglyceride levels by 8 percent.

The researchers were particularly interested in what epigenetic changes accompanied these fat-associated effects. So they biopsied the participants' abdominal fat at the beginning and end of the study in order to analyze the genomic changes in fat cells. The genes of both groups showed epigenetic changes. In fact, 1,442 genes were silenced through methylation by eating fat. Eating muffins made with the unhealthy saturated fats actually changed twenty-eight proteins produced by fat cells, whereas the PUFA muffins did not significantly alter gene expression. While the exact consequences of the individual methylated genes are not yet precisely known, this study clearly demonstrates that overeating fatty foods not only causes weight gain, but it also changes the function of your DNA.

In the lab, high-fat diets have been shown to cause undesirable epigenetic changes that shut down the liver's ability to regenerate. Since the liver is key to detoxifying the blood, this can lead to a buildup of toxins and contribute to a pro-inflammatory state in the body.[50]

PROCESSED MEAT

Everyone knows that eating processed meat is not part of a healthy diet, but it's even more telling that several large-scale studies have shown that eating processed meat actually shrinks your telomeres. The Multi-Ethnic Study of Atherosclerosis (MESA) is a study of six thousand men and women representing different ethnicities from six communities across the United States (Baltimore; Chicago; Forsyth County, North Carolina; New York City; Los Angeles; and St. Paul, Minnesota).[51] Among this group, researchers studied 840 white, African American, and Hispanic subjects who recorded their daily intake and frequency of eating twelve different categories of food over the previous year: whole grains, refined grains, fruit, vegetables, non-fried seafood, nuts and seeds, dairy, red meat, processed meat (including ham, hot dogs, lunch meats, sausage, organ meats, and ham hocks), fried foods (including potatoes, fish, and chicken), non-diet soda, and coffee. The researchers sampled their blood, measured telomere length in white blood cells, and correlated telomere length with their reported diet.

The findings of MESA were revealing. Only one food was associated with shorter telomeres: processed meat. In fact, for each additional serving of processed meat consumed each day, the telomeres became 0.07 units smaller. Since normal aging shortens telomeres by 15.4 units per year, this means that eating 220 servings of processed meat or having lunch meats four to five days a week is equivalent to accelerating your aging by one year for every year you eat this way.

The Strong Heart Family Study, a major study funded by the National Heart, Lung, and Blood Institute, also found a connection between processed meats and shorter telomeres. This study explores genetic and other factors contributing to cardiovascular disease in thirteen Native American tribes. Researchers asked 2,864 Native Americans to report their consumption of processed and unprocessed meat over the past year, then took blood and measured telomere length. Consistent with trend of the MESA study, the analysis showed that every serving of processed meat was associated with shortening of telomeres by 0.021 units.[52] The reason that eating processed meat causes shorter telomeres is not clear. Meat processing can generate chemicals called advanced glycation end products (AGEs). These AGEs are known to provoke inflammation, which can cause oxidative stress in cells and damage DNA. There may also be other chemicals found in the meat that can influence telomeres.

One surprise that came from the Strong Heart Family Study was the finding that eating *unprocessed* red meat one to two times per day was actually associated with *longer* telomeres. A possible explanation for this unexpected result is that certain bioactives found in red meat, such as vitamin B, heme-iron, and carnosine, can reduce telomere shortening.[53] Still, eating red meat has multiple downsides. Beyond unhealthy saturated fats, which are associated with increased risk of cancer and cardiovascular disease, red meat also contains L-carnitine, which your gut bacteria metabolize to generate a harmful chemical called trimethylamine-N-oxide (TMAO). TMAO has been implicated in the development of obesity, diabetes, gastrointestinal cancers, and heart disease.[54] A study by scientists at the Cleveland Clinic in Ohio showed that dietary L-carnitine accelerates the development of blood vessel–blocking atherosclerosis in mice.[55]

The method of cooking red meats, such as grilling, also can generate carcinogenic chemicals like heterocyclic amines, which are found in the char of barbecued meats. The crispy bits might be tasty, but they can be deadly. So, when it comes to eating meat, consider these risks, and steer clear of the char.

SUGAR-SWEETENED BEVERAGES

Soda and soft drinks are often regarded as the products of modern industry, but in fact, flavoring water with natural herbs and fruits originated in ancient times. Carbonating the beverage to create fizz was invented in 1767, when a chemist named Joseph Priestley infused water with carbon dioxide, setting the stage for today's carbonated beverages. The addition of loads of sugar and fruit juices to sweeten soda became popular in the twentieth century. As we saw in chapter 8, artificial sweeteners can alter the microbiome, but what are the effects of sugar-sweetened beverages on DNA? As we discussed in chapter 4, research suggests that toddlers who consume soda have shorter telomeres, but there is other work in this area.

Researchers from the University of California, San Francisco; the University of California, Berkeley; and Stanford University evaluated the impact of sugar on DNA in 5,309 adults whose health stats are part of the National Health and Nutrition Examination Survey (NHANES), managed by the National Center for Health Statistics. Data about food and health parameters collected over time include the amount consumed of sugar-sweetened soda, noncarbonated sweetened drinks (fruit juices, energy and sports drinks, sweetened water), diet soda, and 100 percent fruit juice.[56] In addition to dietary information, the participants contributed blood samples from which telomere length can be measured.

The NHANES study published in 2014 showed that the average daily intake of sweetened beverages in the United States was seventeen fluid ounces (the equivalent of one and a half cans of soda). The researchers then crunched the available data and found that each can of soda consumed in a day shortened telomeres by 0.01 units, accelerating the effects of aging. In those drinking a twenty-ounce bottle of soda daily, the telomere shortening was equivalent to that of 4.6 years of faster aging each year. The researchers noted this degree of accelerated telomere shortening was similar to that caused by smoking cigarettes, also 4.6 years.

The good news is that telomere shortening appears to be reversible. The positive benefit of moderate physical activity led to a nearly equivalent gain of telomere length (4.4 years) on a similar scale as the loss of telomere length in the sweetened soda and drinks NHANES study.[57] This is an example of how everything we do has an additive (or net) effect. Making more good choices will push you toward longer telomeres, while poor choices will chip away at whatever benefits you've gained.

Another study conducted by researchers at the University of California, San Francisco and the University of California, Berkeley examined the effects of soda drinking in 65 pregnant women ages eighteen to forty-five. The researchers asked women to report their beverage consumption and then drew blood for telomere measurements at the beginning of the study and then at three months and at nine months after delivery of the baby. The results showed that when the women reduced their consumption of sugar-sweetened beverages, their telomeres lengthened.[58]

Putting It All Together

Living the good life is full of dangers to your DNA. You can't avoid all of the damage, because aging eventually and inevitably takes its toll. But you can consciously use your dietary choices as countermeasures to protect, repair, and course-correct your DNA to defend your health. There are easy everyday decisions about food that can be made. Foods with bioactives that are antioxidants can neutralize harmful oxidizing chemicals in the bloodstream. But remember, that only protects DNA from damage. Some foods can actually help repair DNA by activating cellular machinery to mend the problems.

Foods with epigenetic effects can influence DNA to your advantage by unleashing genes that protect your health, like tumor suppressor genes that prevent the growth of cancer cells. Putting your DNA to work like this could literally save your life.

Finally, foods that protect and lengthen telomeres can protect your DNA and help fight the effects of aging. Although telomeres do shrink over the course of our lives and expose our DNA to damage, food and dietary patterns can slow this shrinking, and in some cases, even lengthen telomeres. Your DNA is not just a blueprint of your genetic code, it is a superhighway of information that needs to be protected, repaired, and in some cases rerouted to fight the assaults of our environment and the ravages of aging, as a way to defend our health.

KEY FOODS AFFECTING DNA

Antioxidation	Increases DNA Repair	Influences Epigenetics	Telomere Lengthening
Bottarga	Bottarga	Basil	Almond butter
Broccoli	Carrots	Bok choy	Almonds
Cockles (clam)	Cockles (clam)	Broccoli	Brazil nuts
Guava	Hake	Cabbage	Cashew butter
Hake	Kiwifruit	Coffee	Cashews
Kiwifruit	Manila clam	Green tea	Chestnuts
Manila clam	Sea cucumber	Kale	Coffee
Mixed berry juice	Tuna	Marjoram	Flax seeds
Orange juice	Yellowtail (fish)	Peppermint	Green tea
Oranges		Rosemary	Hazelnuts
Oyster sauce		Sage	Macadamia nuts
Pacific oysters		Soy	Peanut butter
Papaya		Thyme	Peanuts
Pink grapefruit		Turmeric	Pecans
Sea cucumber			Pine nuts
Tomato			Pistachios
Tuna			Pumpkin seeds
Watermelon			Sesame seeds
Yellowtail (fish)			Squash seeds
			Sunflower seeds
			Tahini
			Walnuts

CHAPTER 10

Activate Your Immune Command Center

Every grandmother, it seems, has offered her wisdom on choosing the right food to help fight sickness. When it comes to your immunity, some dietary traditions are now being looked at through the new lens of health defense. The science of modern immunology is revealing which foods affect immunity and telling us how they work.

Take chicken soup, one of the oldest home remedies known. We now know that soup made with chicken meat and bones indeed contains natural bioactives that, in the lab, can modify the inflammatory reaction of our immune systems. Less inflammation in the body translates to less misery from the symptoms of colds and the flu.[1] Or consider the nostrum "feed a cold, starve a fever." Actually, cycles of fasting can help the body rid itself of older, worn-out immune cells that are past their prime and cause it to regenerate from stem cells fresh new ones that are ready for battle to beat an infection.[2]

New discoveries reveal that specific foods can help fine-tune your immune system, keep it in prime shape, and help you thwart disease. There's a simple way to understand the impact of diet on the immune system. What we eat and drink can turn up or turn down the two arms of immunity—the innate and acquired immune system—to defend our health. In this chapter, we'll identify the evidence supporting specific foods that can boost your body's ability to resist disease through the immune system.

Let's first take a look at some major diseases where the immune system plays a role in making you sick. This will help you think about the different situations where diet can be used to your advantage.

Diseases Related to Immunity

The immune system is so inextricably linked to health that every disease is somehow tied to it. Two big principles connect immunity with health. First are conditions in which the immune system is weakened and unable to prevent invaders from taking root. Second are conditions in which the immune system is overly ramped up, and its exuberance causes inflammation and the unintended destruction of our own healthy tissues.

Weakened Immune Conditions

Let's first look at diseases that result from weakened immunity. A broken-down immune system can open the door to life-threatening infections, but infection is only one danger. Cancer can also take root because an ineffective immune system cannot detect cancer cells. This weakness can be addressed using the cancer treatments called immunotherapies, new medications that help the immune system locate and destroy cancer cells. These medicines have led to breakthroughs for the treatment of malignant melanoma; cancers of the lung, kidney, bladder, head and neck, and cervix; and some blood cancers like large B-cell lymphoma and acute lymphoblastic leukemia.

These FDA-approved therapies can help your body's immune system find and destroy cancer. But cancer can be spotted naturally and wiped out with an intact and optimally working immune system. Some cancers like multiple myeloma and leukemia are diseases of immune cells, taking down their ability to defend health.

The irony is that traditional cancer treatments based on high-dose chemotherapy and radiation actually weaken the immune system. They destroy fast-growing cells, which is an effective way to target cancer. But immune cells and other healthy cells are also decimated during the treatment, impeding the body's own ability to defend against the cancer.

Infection by certain viruses can also destroy the body's ability to mount an adequate immune response. As I described in chapter 5, acquired immune deficiency syndrome (AIDS) is the classic example of impaired immunity, resulting from infection by the human immunodeficiency virus (HIV). The human papillomavirus (HPV) lowers the immune system's ability to detect and destroy infected cells, which later increases the risk for cervical cancer, penile cancer, and cancer of the mouth and upper airway.[3] A vaccine against HPV trains the immune system to destroy the cancer-causing virus. Hepatitis B and Hepatitis C are other infections that compromise the body's ability to mount an attack with its immune system to eliminate infected cells.[4] These types of hepatitis can also lead to liver cancer.

Some diseases actually cripple the immune system. Although type 1 and type 2 diabetes are different types of disease, both make an individual more vulnerable to infection. Obesity also makes individuals more susceptible to infection and impairs the immune response by creating a chronic low-grade state of inflammation in the body.[5] In these conditions, consuming foods that enhance immunity would be beneficial.

Before we continue, here's an important caveat: not all immune deficiencies can be addressed using your diet. For foods to have an effect, you need to start with an intact immune system that has all its parts. With certain inherited diseases, however, where the immune cells are defective and unable to function properly, dietary factors are unlikely to help. Some of these conditions with life-threatening immune defects have tongue-twister names like ataxia telangiectasia, Chédiak-Higashi syndrome, and severe combined immunodeficiency disorder.

Overactive Immune Conditions

The flip side of weakened immunity is an overactive immune system. The result of this are autoimmune diseases, where the immune system is active in the wrong place at the wrong time, causing chronic inflammation and damaging organs. A classic example of autoimmune disease is type 1 diabetes, in which the body makes so-called autoantibodies against the insulin-producing beta-islet cells in the pancreas. When these cells are destroyed, insulin is not made adequately, and the body cannot process blood glucose properly. In rheumatoid arthritis, autoantibodies destroy joints and can cause severe disability and crippling pain.

Lupus erythematosus, commonly known simply as lupus, is actually a collection of autoimmune diseases in which antibodies launch vicious attacks on different organs, including the heart, lung, kidney, skin, joints, brain, and spinal cord.

Scleroderma is an insidious disease in which organs are replaced by hard scar tissue after they are assaulted by the immune system.

Although the exact cause of multiple sclerosis (MS) is still uncertain, the damage in this condition occurs from autoantibodies that destroy the insulating layer of nerve cells in the spinal cord and brain, leading to a gradual destruction that proves fatal over time.

The thyroid gland can also be an autoimmune target. In Hashimoto's thyroiditis, antibodies attack the thyroid, crippling its ability to make thyroid hormone. Graves' disease also involves antibodies attacking the thyroid, but in a twist, the body produces antibodies that mimic the hormone that signals the production of thyroid hormone. The effect is that the thyroid releases enormous, inappropriate amounts of thyroid hormone, with a host of side effects.[6] People with celiac disease suffer from autoantibodies stimulated by gluten in the diet, which trigger painful gut inflammation and destruction of the cells lining the small intestine.[7]

Overactive immunity leads to chronic inflammation. Asthma sufferers have a trigger-happy immune system that causes severe inflammation in their lungs when they are exposed to various environmental factors. The skin and joints are inflamed in people with psoriasis. In the conditions known as inflammatory bowel disease (Crohn's disease and ulcerative colitis), massive inflammation takes place in the gut, causing intestinal bleeding, bloating, and abdominal pain. In ulcerative colitis, the nonstop inflammation can lead to the development of colon cancer.

Foods That Stimulate the Immune System

As we consider foods that can help your immune defense, we will first look at foods that boost immune function. These foods may be of importance to you if you have a condition where you could benefit from a more active immune system. An important note: there are many claims on the internet about foods that supposedly enhance immunity, but many are not supported by evidence. In this chapter, I am going to describe the research that has been done on specific foods in humans demonstrating an immune benefit.

Mushrooms

The white button mushroom, one of the most common of all edible mushrooms, is eaten raw in salads or cooked with a wide variety of ingredients across world cuisines. White button mushrooms are a good source of bioactives, including beta-glucan, an immune-stimulating dietary fiber. Researchers at the University of Western Sydney in Australia studied twenty healthy volunteers who were assigned to eat either a normal diet or a normal diet plus white button mushrooms.[8] The mushroom-eating participants ate one hundred grams of blanched mushrooms per day, roughly equivalent to 1.3 cups of mushrooms for one week. As a test of whether the mushrooms affected immune function, the researchers measured the levels of two antibodies (IgA and IgG) in the subjects' saliva. More antibodies are produced in the saliva after immune activation. The researchers found a steady increase in IgA levels in the participants, with a 55 percent increase after one week of mushroom consumption and a continued rise to 58 percent above baseline levels up to two weeks after finishing the mushrooms. Eating the mushrooms activated the gut, which stimulated the immune system to produce the antibodies. The antibodies then circulated to the mucous membranes where they were secreted in saliva.

A number of other studies in the lab using extracts from other culinary mushrooms like shiitake, maitake, enoki, chanterelle, and oyster mushrooms showed that they, too, can activate immune defenses.[9] In addition to their culinary value, some of the most popular edible mushrooms have immune-boosting benefits.

Aged Garlic

Garlic is renowned as both an ingredient and a health remedy. Ancient Greeks used garlic to strengthen athletes and soldiers, and as a component of healing tonics. Fresh garlic has a strong, pungent smell valued for cooking, but when it is aged, garlic becomes almost odorless. Aged garlic is found as a dietary supplement and retains potent bioactives, such as apigenin, that can influence the immune system.

Researchers at the University of Florida in Gainesville studied the effect of aged garlic on the immune systems of 120 healthy men and women in their mid-twenties and early thirties during the cold and flu season.[10] Two groups received either an aged garlic extract or a placebo for ninety days, and had their blood drawn for analysis of immune response. The subjects were instructed to keep a daily illness diary to log any symptoms of being sick, such as runny nose, head congestion, sore throat, cough, fever, or body aches, and to record if they became ill enough to miss school or work.

At the end of the study, the group who consumed aged garlic extract had significantly more immune T cells and natural killer (NK) cells circulating in their bloodstream than the group taking the placebo. Remarkably, the T cells resulting from the aged garlic were supercharged and could replicate themselves eight times faster than in people taking the placebo. The NK cells, too, were enhanced by garlic. They were 30 percent more activated than similar cells in people on the placebo.

The illness diaries showed that people taking the garlic extract reported 20 percent fewer cold and flu symptoms, 60 percent fewer incidents of feeling sick enough to cancel regular activities, and 58 percent fewer missed days of work. This study showed a nice correlation between aged garlic, enhanced immune cell activity, and less illness.

Another study by researchers at the Kyoto Prefecture University of Medicine in Japan recruited patients who had inoperable cancer.[11] When they were given aged garlic for six months, the activity of their circulating NK cells increased. This opens the door to research on whether aged garlic could help augment the cancer fighting immune responses in patients receiving immunotherapy.

These studies offer clinical evidence that aged garlic can strengthen our immune defense against everyday infections and potentially even cancer.

Broccoli Sprouts

Delicious for salads, broccoli sprouts are three-to-four-day-old plant tendrils that have a mild, nutty taste. Remember that broccoli contains sulforaphanes, which are potent bioactives. Sulforaphanes activate the immune system, and, remarkably, broccoli sprouts contain up to one hundred times more sulforaphane than regular full-grown broccoli.[12] You can really taste the broccoli flavor when you chew them thoroughly. The chewing is important because it ruptures the plant cell walls to release an enzyme called myrosinase. This enzyme is important because it converts the sulforaphane, which is naturally inactive in the plant, to its active form in your mouth. Activated sulforaphane can affect the cells in your body.

Researchers at the University of North Carolina at Chapel Hill, Stanford University, and the University Children's Hospital Basel in Switzerland studied the impact of eating broccoli sprouts on the immune system by conducting a clinical trial involving the flu vaccine.[13] They wanted to know if the sprouts could help the body boost its response after vaccination. The scientists enrolled twenty-nine healthy volunteers in their late twenties and gave them either two cups of broccoli sprouts blended into a shake or a placebo shake to drink each day for four days. The volunteers received a nasal spray flu vaccine on the second day after starting to drink the shake. The vaccine delivered a live but weakened flu virus into the mucous membrane in the nose.

The results showed that volunteers who drank the broccoli sprout shake had twenty-two times more NK T cells in their blood compared to those who drank the placebo shake. Their NK cells also had more killing power. The proof in the pudding was that broccoli sprout shake drinkers also had less flu virus remaining in the cells of their nose, showing that their body cleared the invaders more effectively. Eating broccoli sprouts can boost your immune defenses against the flu virus.

Extra Virgin Olive Oil

Extra virgin olive oil is a critical component of the Mediterranean diet, and the bioactives it contains, such as hydroxytyrosol, oleocanthal, and oleic acid, can enhance your immune system.

Researchers at Tufts University, the University of Massachusetts, and the Institute for Food Science and Technology and Nutrition in Spain designed a clinical study to see if replacing the oil (butter and corn oil) found in the typical American diet with extra virgin olive oil would improve a person's immune response. The researchers selected forty-one overweight or obese volunteers from the Boston area, all over the age of sixty-five.[14] The subjects ate a typical American diet: high in saturated fat and refined and processed grains, and low in dietary fiber. The researchers gave all the subjects a bottle of oil and spread. One group received extra virgin olive oil from Spain in liquid and spreadable form.[15] The other group received a mix of corn and soybean oil and a butter spread. For three months, the participants continued to eat a typical American diet, but used only their assigned oil and spread. Both groups consumed on average about three tablespoons of oil per day. Blood analysis showed that the immune T cells in the olive oil group increased their ability to become activated and expand in number by 53 percent. The same immune cells in the group eating corn-soy oil and butter had no change.

Olive oil also helps reduce the body's reaction to allergens. The bioactive hydroxytyrosol found in extra virgin olive oil helps immune cells make interleukin-10, which calms inflammation.[16] These combined effects show that substituting extra virgin olive oil for other cooking oils used in a typical American diet can have both immune-boosting and anti-inflammatory health benefits.

Importantly, not all olive oils contain the same amount of hydroxy-tyrosol. A study from the Instituto de la Grasa in Spain compared the polyphenols found in four types of Spanish extra virgin olive oils made from olive monovarietals (Arbequina, Hojiblanca, Manzanilla, Picual).[17] The highest levels of hydroxytyrosol were present in the oil made from Picual olives.

Ellagic Acid

Many popular foods contain ellagic acid, a potent bioactive with health-defense-activating properties. Chestnuts, blackberries, black raspberries, walnuts, and pomegranate have among the highest levels. As noted in chapter 6, ellagic acid has antiangiogenic effects that can starve tumors and prevent them from growing. But when it comes to immunity, ellagic acid can assist immune cells by improving their ability to detect and destroy cancer cells.

Scientists at the University of Rome Tor Vergata in Italy discovered this immune effect in bladder cancer.[18] In the lab, ellagic acid slowed the growth of bladder cancer cells, preventing them from making proteins that stimulate tumor blood vessels. They had expected this reaction based on ellagic acid's angiopreventive effect. What they found in addition, however, was a surprise with important implications. Ellagic acid also reduced the cancer cells' production of the immune-cloaking protein PD-L1 by 60 percent. PD-L1 helps disguise the cancer cells so they escape detection by the body's immune cells, effectively making cancer invisible. When the cancer cell can't make as much PD-L1, the cancer cells are more easily seen by the immune system, which can then call in the immune troops to destroy them.

When ellagic acid was injected into bladder cancer growing in mice, the tumor growth was suppressed by as much as 61 percent. These results suggest that ellagic acid has the ability to suppress cancer by aiding two of the body's health defense systems: angiogenesis and immunity. Ellagic acid is the first dietary bioactive that has been shown to have the ability to target the cloaking protein PD-L1. This is the target of immunotherapies that help the immune system wipe out cancer. While the ellagic studies were conducted in the lab, it suggests that some foods may have immunotherapeutic properties that could complement cancer treatment, or potentially assist the body in its own ability to conduct surveillance to prevent cancer.

Fruit Juices with Immune Boosting Power

Cranberry Juice

For years, drinking cranberry juice has been touted as a way to prevent bladder infections. Researchers at Sapporo Medical University in Japan proved these benefits in a clinical study of women who suffered from recurrent urinary tract infections (UTIs). The women drank one-half cup of cranberry juice every night before going to sleep for twenty-four weeks. In women older than fifty, drinking cranberry juice reduced the recurrence of infection by 40 percent compared to women who drank a placebo beverage.[19]

The popular explanation for this effect is that cranberry juice changes the acidity of the urine, preventing bacteria from gaining a foothold for infection. But it turns out there's much more to the story. Researchers at the University of Florida in Gainesville designed a study to investigate how cranberry juice influences the immune system.[20] They recruited forty-five healthy volunteers and gave them either cranberry juice or a placebo beverage that looked exactly like the cranberry juice in color, matched in calories but containing no cranberries or cranberry bioactives.[21] The study took place during the spring flu season between March and May. Each subject drank a fifteen-ounce bottle (about two cups) of their assigned beverage every day for ten weeks. Just like in the aged garlic study, everyone kept an illness diary to record any symptoms of colds or the flu during the study.

Blood analysis showed that drinking real cranberry juice had a beneficial effect on gamma delta T cells, a special type of immune T cell. These cells are found in the lining of the gut and other mucous membranes of the body, including the urinary tract. Gamma delta T cells are first responders to bacteria and viruses that try to gain a foothold by invading these mucous membranes. Compared to cells from the subjects who drank the placebo, the gamma delta T cells in the blood of cranberry juice drinkers were three times more potent in their ability to divide and expand, which enhances immune defense.

The immune cells from subjects who drank cranberry juice also produced a whopping 148 percent increase in interferon-gamma, which is a chemical signal that amps up the immune response against infection, after drinking the juice. The placebo group actually produced 25 percent less of this immune signal, which rendered them more susceptible to infection.

All of these changes correlated with the reports in the illness diaries, as the group consuming cranberry juice had 16 percent fewer reports of cold and flu symptoms. The benefits of drinking cranberry juice are clearly more than an urban legend. Cranberries activate the immune system not just in the bladder, but throughout the body.

Concord Grape Juice

In addition to the DNA-protective properties we discussed in the last chapter, Concord grape juice has immune-boosting benefits, too. This purple-colored grape juice contains bioactives, such as anthocyanins, procyanidins, and hydroxycinnamic acid, that influence T cells. Other grape bioactives found in the juice, such as vitamin C and melatonin, can also activate the immune system.[22]

The same groups at the University of Florida in Gainesville that studied cranberry juice also conducted a randomized, placebo-controlled clinical study of Concord grape juice and its effects on the immune system.[23] Seventy-eight healthy men and women ages fifty to seventy-five were given twelve ounces (1.5 cups) of either 100 percent Concord grape juice or a closely matched placebo beverage to drink every day for nine weeks. Blood analysis showed that subjects drinking the Concord grape juice had 27 percent more protective gamma delta T cells than before they started drinking the Concord grape juice. There was no change to T cell numbers in the group who drank the placebo.

An important health consideration to keep in mind with any beverage, even naturally sweetened ones, as in the case of Concord grape juice, is the impact it can have on your blood sugar. Fruit juices can contain a lot of sugar, which can raise insulin levels and put stress on your metabolism. People with diabetes and others who need to watch their blood sugar levels should be cautious about adding fruit juice to their diets and check with their doctor. Cancer patients also need to be wary of high-sugar beverages because of the growing evidence that sugar does indeed fuel cancer cells and help them grow.

Blueberries

Blueberries have been shown to have remarkable immune influencing power through their bioactives. Researchers at Louisiana State University studied the immune effects of blueberries by conducting a randomized placebo controlled clinical trial in twenty-seven people in their late fifties who had metabolic syndrome.[24] This condition presages the development of cardiovascular disease. The participants drank either a blueberry smoothie or a placebo smoothie twice each day, at breakfast and at dinner, for six weeks. The blueberry smoothies were twelve ounces in size (1.5 cups) and made with freeze-dried blueberry powder and yogurt or milk. The amount of blueberry powder in each smoothie was the equivalent of two cups of fresh blueberries.[25] The placebo was made with the same ingredients but minus the blueberries.

Blood tests before and after the study showed that people who drank the blueberry smoothie had an 88 percent increase in immune cells called myeloid dendritic cells in their blood. These cells help to initiate immune responses against infection. Subjects who drank the placebo smoothie had no change in their myeloid dendritic cells or any other immune cell.

At the end of the study, the inflammatory markers of people drinking blueberry smoothies also went down, suggesting that blueberries calm excessive inflammation even while they boost immune function.

Researchers at Appalachian State University in North Carolina, the University of Montana, and Vanderbilt University in Tennessee collaborated on a study aimed at defining the impact of blueberries on the body after intense exercise.[26] It is known that intense workouts trigger a brief rise in immune cells, which then taper off immediately after the workout. The researchers recruited twenty-five physically fit volunteers in their early thirties and evaluated their baseline oxygen intake, heart rate, and respiration. Half of the group was given prepackaged bags of blueberries (equivalent to 1.7 cups per serving) to eat each day for six weeks. They followed strict dietary guidelines so everyone had a similar baseline diet. The other half of the group ate the instructed diet, but no blueberries.

At the end of six weeks of eating blueberries, the participants did a 2.5-hour treadmill run. First, researchers drew their blood before the run.

Then, an hour before exercise, the blueberry eaters ate a larger than usual amount of blueberries (375 grams, or 2.7 cups worth of fresh blueberries). Immediately after the participants' run, researchers took another blood sample. One hour later, blood was drawn one final time to see what happened to their immune cells and what the effect of eating blueberries was. The blood samples were analyzed for different immune cells, including T cells, B cells, and natural killer (NK) cells.

The results were eye opening. Blueberry eaters had almost double the number of NK cells *before* exercise compared to those who did not eat blueberries. Normally, NK cells would be expected to rapidly decline after intense exercise. But in the group that consumed blueberries, the NK cells remained elevated for at least one hour after exercise ceased.

The ability of blueberries to increase NK cell numbers is significant. NK cells are critical to immune responses that eliminate virus-infected cells or tumor cells, and they can help the immune system develop memory against foreign invaders. These studies are especially interesting because they reveal a dose of blueberries needed for this immune effect: in this case, 1.7 cups of berries per day.

Chile Peppers

Chile peppers belong to the genus *Capsicum*, which is the namesake of the formidable bioactive that carries the heat, capsaicin. The bright red, yellow, and green colors of chile peppers also alert you to the presence of bioactives like zeaxanthin, lutein, and beta-carotene, which each have their own biological activities. Capsaicin activates the immune system and has been shown to increase the numbers of circulating white blood cells and antibody-producing B cells.[27]

Scientists at the University of Connecticut studied the effect of capsaicin on the immune responses specific to cancer.[28] In the lab, mice with fibrosarcomas, a type of aggressive tumor, received capsaicin injections. Their tumors either stopped growing or, in some cases, shrank completely and disappeared. When the scientists examined under the microscope what was left of the cancers, they saw the capsaicin-treated tumors had forty-two times more dying cells than tumors that had not been treated with capsaicin. They found the response was consistent with immune killing of cancer.

The scientists studied how capsaicin engages the immune system in mice with growing colon cancer. They found capsaicin activates the immune dendritic cells, which actually have specific receptors for capsaicin.[29] Similar to a key fitting into a lock, the capsaicin turned on the immune cells. Again, when the mice were treated with capsaicin, tumor growth dramatically slowed. The capsaicin stimulated the immune system of the mice to produce cytotoxic T lymphocytes that would kill cancer cells.

While these experiments delivered capsaicin as an injection into the tumor, they demonstrate that a chile pepper bioactive has the power to activate and weaponize the immune system against cancer cells. To appreciate the potency of capsaicin used in these mouse experiments, the scientists used only two hundred micrograms of capsaicin for each treatment. This is the equivalent amount of capsaicin found in one-fifth of a habanero pepper.

Pacific Oysters

As I showed you in chapter 9, the Pacific oyster has DNA protecting properties. This oyster is one of the most cultivated oysters worldwide, and its creamy, briny taste makes it a popular choice for seafood connoisseurs. While oysters are renowned for having transformative properties as an aphrodisiac, more attention should be paid to their effect on boosting immunity. This activity comes from proteins found in the oyster.

Scientists at the Shandong University in China purchased Pacific oysters from a local fish market and extracted the immune-stimulating peptides.[30] For fourteen days, they fed this oyster extract to mice with growing sarcoma cancer cells and compared the effect of the oyster extract to that of a chemotherapy drug cyclophosphamide and to no treatment at all. The results showed that mice eating the oyster extract had a remarkable 48 percent reduced tumor growth compared to untreated mice. Although the mice treated with chemotherapy did experience the greatest tumor shrinkage, the chemotherapy also damaged the spleen and the thymus. Since these are both immune organs, this effect leads to an undesireable hit to the immune defense system. By contrast, the immune organs in the mice who consumed the oyster extract actually increased in size, suggesting that the oyster extract exerted its anticancer effects by improving immune function. Mice who received the oyster extract also had twice the number of cancer-fighting NK cells compared to untreated mice, and 38 percent more than those who received chemotherapy.

What is fascinating is that oysters contain multiple immune stimulators, even beyond its peptides. A group of scientists at Central Taiwan University of Science and Technology showed that an immune-stimulating polysaccharide is present in Pacific oysters. An extract containing these oyster polysaccharides can stimulate T cells as well as NK cells.[31] When these oyster polysaccharides were fed to lab mice growing melanoma, tumor growth was reduced by a remarkable 86 percent compared to untreated mice.[32]

Oysters also have anti-inflammatory benefits, as revealed by scientists at National Taiwan University. They prepared a solution by poaching oysters for four hours and then mixing the oyster meat with alcohol to extract its bioactives, including proteins and beta-glucans.[33] The scientists then fed the extract to mice who had gut inflammation because they are severely allergic to ovalbumin, the protein found in egg whites. This allergy caused severe diarrhea and severe inflammatory damage in the intestines. When these allergic mice ate the oyster extract, however, their reactions to ovalbumin were considerably milder. Their diarrhea improved by 30 percent, and there was 37 percent less inflammation in their intestines. Under the microscope, their intestinal cells looked almost normal despite exposure to the allergen.

Shellfish lovers take note: the briny oyster now has immune defense activation, anti-inflammation, and DNA protection to add to its résumé. These benefits should grow its reputation beyond being an aphrodisiac.

Licorice

Licorice—the root, not the candy—is traditionally used as a flavoring and for herbal medicine to treat stomach and respiratory ailments. It has now been discovered to boost immunity. Among many bioactives in licorice are isoliquitrin, glabridin, and 18-beta-glycyrrhetinic acid, a natural sweetener that is fifty times as sweet as sugar yet remarkably does not increase blood sugar. In fact, glycyrrhetinic acid actually reduces blood glucose by making cells more sensitive to the effects of insulin.

Scientists at Montana State University studying licorice showed that glycyrrhizin can improve immunity defenses against viral infection.[34] They fed glycyrrhizin to mice that were infected with rotavirus, a highly contagious pathogen that invades the intestines and causes diarrhea. In humans, rotavirus causes more than 30 percent of childhood deaths from infectious diarrhea worldwide.[35]

Their results showed that feeding mice glycyrrhizin sped up their body's ability to get rid of the virus by 50 percent. This was accomplished by increasing the activity of genes in the intestines that recruit immune T cells to fight infections. The number of T cells guarding the intestinal lining and in the lymph nodes was increased. Interestingly, the B cells in the intestines also increased. Recall from chapter 5 that B cells make antibodies to fight infections, and they memorize what bacteria and viruses look like so they can respond to future infection.

A note of caution about glycyrrhetinic acid: high levels can interfere with the body's regulation of sodium. This means that high licorice consumption can lead to salt retention and high blood pressure.[36] It can also alter blood levels of potassium, which can affect the heart, and it can also interact with certain medications.[37] Because of the potential side effects, extra caution should be taken when using licorice supplements. Consume it in moderation, and keep an eye on your blood pressure.

Licorice also contains bioactive polysaccharides. These can prompt the body to produce a protein signal called interleukin-7, which tells the body to generate more immune T cells. This can prompt an anticancer response in the body. Scientists at the Tianjin University of Traditional Chinese Medicine in China boiled dried licorice root and created an extract containing the polysaccharides. They tested for antitumor effects by feeding the licorice extract to mice with colon cancer every day for two weeks.[38] Mice with tumors normally lose weight, just like humans with cancer. Remarkably, however, the mice fed licorice extract actually gained weight, while at the same time, their tumors shrank by 20 percent. The immune organs of the mice—the spleen and thymus—both increased in size and weight, showing there was an enhancement of immune activity.

Bloodwork revealed the licorice-fed mice had increased numbers of both helper T cells and cytotoxic T cells. During the study, these mice kept to their normal activity, behavior, and appearance. By contrast, the mice that did not receive licorice became emaciated, just like cancer patients do, and their fur becme dull in appearance.

When the scientists compared the antitumor effects of licorice to chemotherapy treatment in the mice, they found that feeding licorice extract could achieve 61 percent of the antitumor effect as chemotherapy, but without side effects. This type of research sheds a scientific light on benefits associated with traditional remedies such as licorice root, which can support immune health.

Foods That Calm Inflammation and Autoimmunity

Sometimes, calming an overactive immune system can be as important as boosting it. Autoimmune diseases are seemingly intractable diseases that doctors treat with high-dose steroids to suppress immunity. But the problem with steroids is that they have side effects that cause unintended consequences, like weakening of bones, thinning of the skin, formation of cataracts, interfering with wound healing, and even causing psychosis. Steroids, while often effective, are an imperfect solution at best. Eating foods that tame the immune system is an important step for people suffering from an autoimmune condition. A dietary approach can help protect organs from being destroyed by friendly fire from your own immune system, as well as from the medicines used to treat autoimmune diseases.

Some foods can relieve suffering from autoimmune conditions by reducing inflammation. Many bioactives are able to achieve this by calming inflammatory immune cells. Other foods have a prebiotic effect and feed healthy gut bacteria, which, as we learned in chapter 8, can help the microbiome produce its own anti-inflammatory metabolites like *butyrate*. These metabolites can slow down overly active immune cells. When inflammation is quelled, the normal balance of immunity in the body can be more easily regained to achieve homeostasis. An effective dietary solution may even allow autoimmune sufferers to avoid the need for medications.

Anyone who has experienced or has taken care of someone with the painful and crippling symptoms of conditions like rheumatoid arthritis, lupus, scleroderma, multiple sclerosis, or inflammatory bowel diseases will attest to the importance of finding relief from the symptoms. And once over the hump, the goal of preventing future flares is often a major concern for both the person with an autoimmune disease and their doctor. Staying in remission makes life a whole lot better, and a dietary strategy to maintain remission is a major win.

One way to avoid flares is to avoid dietary patterns that are known to provoke inflammation.[39] Researchers at the Institute Gustav Roussy in France showed in a study of 67,581 women that eating a diet high in protein from meat or fish is pro-inflammatory and associated with increased risk for inflammatory bowel disease.[40] A high intake of sugar and soft drinks in people who also have low vegetable intake has been associated with a higher risk of ulcerative colitis, another inflammatory bowel disease.[41] Because some dietary patterns are known to incite inflammation, avoiding those foods is important if you are trying to calm your immune system.

In the next section, I will share evidence for some important foods and dietary patterns that can help calm an overactive immune system and help keep immunity in balance as part of an overall health defense strategy.

Foods Containing Vitamin C for Lupus

Lupus is not one disease, but a collection of severe autoimmune diseases in which autoantibodies attack the joints, kidney, heart, lungs, skin, and other organs. About 5 million people worldwide suffer from lupus. The treatments rely on medication with escalating potency to suppress the immune system, but they often come with the risk of severe side effects.

Foods containing vitamin C can help turn down the autoimmune response in the body. Researchers from the Miyagi Cancer Center Research Institute in Japan led a study of diet and lupus over a four-year period. They studied 196 women from twenty-one hospitals in Miyagi Prefecture in northeastern Japan who had inactive or mild lupus. Their mean age was forty. The women were assessed for organ damage from lupus and current lupus activity, and they filled in a food questionnaire.

When all dietary parameters were analyzed, the researchers found that consuming the greatest amount of foods with high levels of vitamin C was associated with a 74 percent decreased risk of active lupus compared to women with low vitamin C intake.[42] The amount of vitamin C showing the most beneficial effect was 154 milligrams per day, which is equivalent to the amount found in one and a half large oranges, 1.5 cups of sliced strawberries, two cups of raw broccoli, or eight cups of uncooked cherry tomatoes (which could be reduced to make a nice sauce). Other good sources of vitamin C include fruit juices from camu camu (a Brazilian fruit), acerola (West Indian cherry), guava, and grapefruit. The Miyagi study was the first to show an association between dietary vitamin C, at easily achievable levels, on lupus activity.

Vitamin C affects the immune system in multiple ways, including by increasing the body's production of immune Treg cells.[43] Remember from chapter 5 that Treg cells have a unique job. They turn down the immune response to restore immune balance in the body.[44] For an autoimmune disease like lupus, upping Treg levels could prove helpful for preventing flares by keeping the immune system calm, which may explain the beneficial effect of vitamin C.

Green Tea

Once again, green tea appears as a health booster—this time for autoimmune disease. The main bioactive that you have become familiar with, epigallocatechin-3-gallate (EGCG), turns down the activity of the immune system by lowering the number of pro-inflammatory T cells. At the same time, EGCG increases the production of Treg cells, which brings the activity of the immune system back down to normal levels.[45] Don't forget that EGCG is also antiangiogenic and DNA protective, showing how Mother Nature can roll together multiple benefits in a single bioactive.

Scientists at the Jean Mayer USDA Human Nutrition Research Center on Aging at Tufts University studied EGCG's effects in mice that develop an autoimmune brain disease similar to human multiple sclerosis (MS). In mice, this is called experimental autoimmune encephalitis. What happens in the brains of these mice is their nerves are stripped of insulation, just like what is seen in human MS. The result is nerve loss, brain inflammation, and scar formation. When the mice were given EGCG orally, however, their symptoms were much less severe. The immune cells produced fewer inflammatory proteins after the mice consumed EGCG.

When their brains were examined, there was less overall inflammation and nerve damage was reduced.[46] Thus, green tea was able to tip the scales of an overactive immune system back toward a more balanced state and reduce immune destruction in the brain.[47]

Researchers at the University of Shizuoka, Kansai Medical University, the National Institute for Longevity Sciences, and the University of Tokyo collaborated to investigate the benefits of green tea on a different autoimmune disease: lupus.[48] They used a different mouse model, in which mice spontaneously develop similar autoantibodies as seen in lupus. The effects of these autoantibodies include severe kidney damage, which is one of the feared complications of lupus in patients. The scientists mixed green tea powder into the diet of one group of mice for three months. A second group ate a regular mouse chow diet.[49] Blood tests showed that mice that ate the green tea extract had significantly lower levels of the autoantibodies, compared to the mice that ate regular chow. In fact, in the green tea-eating mice, the immune deposits from the disease were decreased by more than 80 percent compared to mice eating regular chow. When the scientists examined the kidneys, the green tea mice had four times less damage from their autoimmune disease compared to the other group. Because of less kidney damage, the mice fed green tea extract survived twice as long as their regular-diet-eating counterparts.

Scientists at the National Defense Medical Center in Taiwan found a similar protective effect.[50] When EGCG was given to lupus-prone mice for five months, there was much less kidney damage. What they discovered, in addition, was that green tea increased Treg cells. These cells tamed the immune reaction and reduced the disease severity.[51]

This benefit has been observed in human studies. Researchers at Ahvaz Jundishapur University of Medical Sciences in Iran conducted a randomized, double-blind, placebo-controlled clinical trial on sixty-eight women between the ages of fifteen and fifty-five who were suffering from lupus.[52] For three months, one group of subjects received green tea extract in a daily capsule containing an amount of EGCG equivalent to 4.7 cups of green tea. The other group received a placebo. The researchers monitored lupus disease activity with routine medical and laboratory tests. Participants provided blood and urine samples, and they filled out food and lifestyle surveys.

At the end of the three months, the researchers found that the women taking the green tea extract experienced a reduction in lupus disease activity by twofold. By contrast, participants who received the placebo experienced no significant change in their condition. Blood levels of anti-DNA antibody, a marker for lupus, were lower in the green tea group. When the quality of life surveys were analyzed, those who received the green tea extract had a 30 percent improvement in their physical function and general health compared to women who received the placebo.

Collectively, these studies paint a convincing portrait of the power of green tea for calming an overactive immune system and for preventing the symptoms and organ damage of lupus.

Dietary Patterns That Calm Autoimmune Disease

Raw Vegan Living Diet

Raw diets involve eating foods in their natural and unprocessed state, meaning that they are not cooked or heated above 104°F. Although some aboriginal cultures eat uncooked foods, the modern concept of raw foodism originated as part of the late nineteenth and early twentieth century Lebensreform (back-to-nature) movement in Germany that rebelled against the "perils" of civilization. Although technically a raw diet can be omnivorous, the health culture version of a raw diet is vegetarian or vegan. Proponents of the raw diet claim that uncooked foods contain more natural nutrients and antioxidants and fewer toxins than cooked. Critics point out that a raw food diet carries a higher risk of foodborne illness and may not provide an adequate nutritional balance for your body and that some beliefs about raw diets are based on fallacies about the harms of cooking. Genetic studies have, in fact, shown that the human body has evolved to adapt to eating a cooked diet.[53]

Some raw diets are further called living diets because they emphasize sprouted plants, which are considered to have beneficial enzymes produced during sprouting. Living diets can include fermented foods that contain high levels of beneficial bacteria like *Lactobacillus*. Together, raw, living, and vegan diets are believed to have lower inflammatory potential and a less immune-provocative state. A plant-based living raw diet may thus be able to calm autoimmune diseases such as rheumatoid arthritis.

Researchers at Turku University Central Hospital in Finland studied the impact of a raw living diet on forty-three individuals, mostly women in their late forties and fifties, who had chronic and active rheumatoid arthritis.[54] All the patients had swollen joints and elevated inflammatory markers in their blood. The researchers randomized the patients into two groups and gave them either an uncooked living vegan diet or allowed them to eat their usual omnivorous diet for one month. The intervention diet was composed of plant-based ingredients that were soaked, sprouted, fermented, blended, or dehydrated. The ingredients included almond butter, apples, avocados, bananas, beetroots, blueberries, carrots, cashew nuts, cauliflower, fermented foods (cucumber, sauerkraut, oats), figs, garlic, millet, red cabbage, seaweed, sesame seeds, sprouts (mung bean, lentil, wheat), strawberries, sunflower seeds, tamari sauce, germinated wheat, and zucchini. All animal products were excluded. The researchers conducted interviews and urine tests to ensure compliance with the diet. They took blood and stool samples and scored the improvement of symptoms as "Hi" or "Lo."

The results showed that 28 percent of patients eating the living vegan diet were in the Hi improvement group, while none of the other group consuming the control omnivorous diet received a Hi score. The makeup of the fecal microbiome changed significantly in the living diet group, but not in the omnivorous group. These findings suggest that a living diet may improve the symptoms of rheumatoid arthritis by triggering changes in the microbiome that reduced inflammation.

High-Vegetable/Low-Protein Diet

An immune-dampening diet could help patients with MS avoid a flare-up of symptoms or relapse of disease. Researchers at the Don Carlo Gnocchi Foundation in Italy explored twelve months of a plant-based diet as an intervention for MS.[55] They recruited twenty volunteers who had a history of relapsing-remitting MS, a frustrating sequence of rebounding flares of the disease. The participants were chosen because their self-reported dietary pattern over the past twelve months fell into one of two distinct groups. One group had consumed a diet that was high in vegetables but low in protein. Their diet consisted primarily of fresh fruits and vegetables, legumes, nuts, whole grains, and extra virgin olive oil. They had very low intake of fish, poultry, eggs, and dairy products; ate little sugar or salt; and consumed no alcohol, red meat, or saturated animal fats of any kind. The other group reported eating a typical Western diet consisting of regular red meat, processed meats, refined grains, sugar-sweetened foods, and saturated fats. During the study, a professional nutritionist interviewed each participant every four months to make sure they were still eating the same kind of diet.

At the beginning and end of the study, the participants received an assessment of their MS symptoms. The results showed the participants who ate the high-vegetable/low-protein diet had a threefold reduction in relapse of MS and reported less disability compared to people consuming a Western diet. In fact, those who ate the Western diet reported an *increase* in disability over twelve months. Blood analysis demonstrated that participants eating the vegan diet had fewer activated immune T cells in their blood, and lower levels of cells called monocytes, which are associated with inflammation. This was consistent with protection against MS relapses and symptoms.

The researchers took stool samples because they were looking for a link between the participants' diet, microbiome, and immune responses. They found one: participants on the plant-based diet had 35 percent higher levels of a gut bacteria called *Lachnospiraceae*, which produces the anti-inflammatory short-chain fatty acids we saw in chapter 8. *Lachnospiraceae* also helps Treg cells to mature. Tregs dampen down the immune response in MS, which can suppress the disease.[56] Although this study involved only a small number of patients, the differences in improvement seen between the two dietary patterns and T cell activities is encouraging, and may sway those affected by MS to shift their dietary pattern to be plant-based.

Autoimmune Protocol Diet

Another dietary pattern, called the autoimmune protocol diet, borrows heavily from the Paleo diet. It has been explored as a strategy for providing relief from inflammatory bowel disease (IBD). People with IBD suffer from severe gastrointestinal symptoms like abdominal cramping, bloating, diarrhea, rectal bleeding, loss of appetite, and unintended weight loss. While sophisticated medicines called biological therapies can be helpful, they are not always able to put the disease into remission—and they are accompanied by side effects.

Let's first look at the Paleolithic (Paleo) diet. Paleo is an elimination protocol based on the idea that foods consumed by humans during the Paleolithic period did not cause inflammation in the body compared to modern processed foods. While there is, in truth, sparse evidence of what people truly ate during Paleolithic times, the Paleo diet has been evaluated in small studies to determine its impact on gut inflammation, and anti-inflammatory effects have been speculated to be useful for an overactive immune system.

A group of researchers led by the Scripps Research Institute in California set out to determine if a stricter version of the Paleo diet, called the autoimmune protocol diet, would benefit patients with IBD. In this protocol, all foods that are thought to irritate the gut and cause intestinal "leakiness" are eliminated. These foods, according to the principles behind the autoimmune protocol, include all grains, nuts, seeds, dairy products, nightshade family vegetables (tomato, potatoes, and peppers), all vegetable oils, and all sweeteners. (Remember, many of these foods have been discussed throughout this book and I have shown you the compelling evidence for their delivering health benefits through various health defense systems.) The autoimmune protocol does allow for most vegetables, omega-3 PUFA–rich seafood, animal protein (including liver), extra virgin olive oil, fermented foods, and some fruits. To start the protocol, there is an elimination phase in which all the "offending" foods are removed. This is then followed by a month of strict maintenance of the diet until all IBD symptoms disappear and overall well-being improves. Then, the foods that were eliminated are slowly reintroduced, one at a time, to restore diversity to the diet until IBD symptoms start again. The offending foods are removed and you keep your diet to what is tolerated.

In the Scripps clinical study, fifteen patients with active inflammatory bowel disease (either Crohn's disease or ulcerative colitis) were placed on an eleven-week autoimmune protocol diet.[57] Although this was a small study, starting on the autoimmune protocol led to a very clear improvement in the severity of IBD. For participants with Crohn's disease, the protocol led to a 51 percent improvement in their score on the Harvey-Bradshaw index, which is used to assess severity. In participants with ulcerative colitis, the protocol significantly reduced rectal bleeding after six weeks, and their partial Mayo score, a scoring system for disease severity, improved by 83 percent. By week six, 73 percent of the patients had experienced remission, remaining in remission for the entire eleven weeks of the study.

The researchers also found evidence for decreased intestinal inflammation in people on the autoimmune protocol. A protein called calprotectin, which reflects inflammation, dropped by 76 percent over the course of the study.[58] By visual inspection of the gut using endoscopy, the researchers saw improvements in the gut lining of patients at the end of the eleventh week of the study.

An important factor to keep in mind when evaluating the results of the Scripps study is that diet was not the only intervention for the disease. Half of the patients were also on medical treatments for IBD, including biological therapies as infliximab, adalimumab, and vedolizumab. More study needs to be done testing the diet alone, but the autoimmune protocol appears to be helpful in conjunction with medical therapy, although it is not a replacement for it. The Scripps study also did not examine the benefits of reintroducing foods to the diet, which is important in real-life situations where a more diverse diet is desirable. Because the autoimmune protocol is an elimination diet, it is not easy for people to adhere to it for a sustained period of time. While I don't believe long-term elimination diets are ideal for healthy eating, it is definitely useful to identify foods that provoke symptoms and to avoid them. This alone can bring relief for sufferers of active IBD.

Putting It All Together

Eating to help your immune system defend health is like listening to music on your headphones. It's easy to do, if you pay attention to the volume. Sometimes you need to turn it up, and other times you need to lower the volume to more tolerable levels. There are times you need to boost the immune system to protect you against infection, such as during flu season. As under stressful situations, we need to fortify our immunity. A strong immune defense can protect you against a myriad of diseases that come from outside the body, like infections, but it can also defend us against internally developed diseases, like cancer or autoimmune conditions. And if you have cancer, you definitely need to do everything possible to protect your immune system and give your immune defenses the best shot at finding and wiping out cancer cells. This is especially a concern if you receive high-dose chemotherapy and/or radiation, both of which deliver a smackdown to immune defenses. An immune-boosting diet during cancer therapy may help your medical treatments be even more successful.

The take-home message is this: protect your immune system with everything you've got. If you are receiving one of the new cancer immunotherapies, which rely on your immune system to wipe out cancer cells, it's critical for your immune system to be in prime shape. Your doctor can't do that for you, but you can eat right at home.

Remember, too, that your gut microbiome communicates with your immune system through the jellyroll-like layer of the intestines called the gut-associated lymphoid tissue (GALT). When your gut bacteria are healthy, they help your immune system keep you healthy. So, all the foods in chapter 8 that keep your microbiome healthy also help support your immune defenses. This is why it's important to not isolate the health defenses by paying attention to only one of them—they work in concert. All five of the health defense systems I've discussed in this book interact with one another in ways that collaborate to support your health.

On the other hand, autoimmune diseases are serious conditions in which your immune system is overly aggressive and can cause serious, even life-threatening damage to your organs. Certain foods and dietary patterns can calm the immune system, reduce symptoms and prevent autoimmune flares. These diseases teach us that when it comes to immunity, you want to aim for the Goldilocks zone, where the system is not too active or too inactive, but just right. For autoimmune diseases, this may require a continuous fine-tuning of your diet to keep inflammation quelled.

As you've seen, the ancient wisdom about eating to strengthen your immunity has entered the scientific age. Using the information in this book, it is easier than ever to put our knowledge about immune-influencing foods into everyday practice.

KEY FOODS AFFECTING THE IMMUNE SYSTEM

Immune Boosting		Immune Calming
Aged garlic	Enoki mushroom	Acerola (vit C)
Black raspberries	Licorice root	Broccoli (vit C)
Blackberries	Maitake mushroom	Camu camu (vit C)
Blueberries	Olive oil (EVOO)	Cherry tomatoes (vit C)
Broccoli sprouts	Oyster mushrooms	Grapefruit (vit C)
Chanterelle mushrooms	Pacific oysters	Green tea
Chestnuts	Pomegranate	Guava (vit C)
Chile peppers	Shiitake mushrooms	Oranges (vit C)
Concord grape juice	Walnuts	Strawberries (vit C)
Cranberry juice	White button mushroom	

PART III

PLAN, CHOOSE, AND ACT

Putting Food to Work

It's not how good you are now, it's how good you're going
to be that matters.

—*Atul Gawande*

Right now is the time to improve the way you approach food and choose what to eat. Every day, multiple times a day, you are making important choices that can tip the odds in your favor for living longer and better without a dreaded chronic illness. In part 3, I will show you how to put your new knowledge about health defenses and the many foods that influence them into practice.

I have created a 5 × 5 × 5 framework that makes it super easy to incorporate foods that offer health benefits into your daily life. My approach is not a one-size-fits-all diet, nor is it a weight-loss plan. It is a simple way that helps you make healthy choices consciously and consistently, no matter what you do or where you live.

The best part is that the approach you are about to learn is not based on elimination, restriction, or deprivation, but rather is based on the foods you like best—your own personal preferences. How great is it if the foods that are healthy for you are the very ones you love. That's exactly what is possible based on the research I've shared in parts 1 and 2.

In the chapters ahead, you will learn how to rethink your kitchen, discover some exceptional foods, put the 5 × 5 × 5 framework into practice, and receive some easy, delicious recipes to get your new healthier life started. Finally, I'll provide you with a unique peek into the cutting edge of the "food as medicine" movement: food doses that have been shown to thwart illnesses. You *can* eat to beat disease, and I'm about to show you how.

CHAPTER 11

The 5 × 5 × 5 Framework: Eating to Beat Disease

You've made it! You first learned about the health defense systems that help your body resist disease, and then about the foods and beverages that boost those defenses. Now, you are ready to take action to make your own body healthier and armed to fight disease. This chapter is about applying this new knowledge. I'm about to give you a lifelong eating plan that is based on fortifying the five defense systems you've learned about: angiogenesis, regeneration, microbiome, DNA protection, and immunity.

This is not a weight-loss plan, a fitness diet, or a mental clarity plan. It is not a meal-by-meal, or a day-by-day plan that instructs you how to strictly live your life. It's much better. This plan is about freedom, because I'm not going to tell you every last thing you have to eat (or not eat) every single day. Instead, I'm going to give you a new enjoyable way to integrate health-defense-boosting foods into your lifestyle that will make you look better, feel better, and live longer.

I call it the 5 × 5 × 5 framework. Simply put, it is a way to eat to beat disease. It will help you use your body's own ability to heal itself to save your own life. The 5 × 5 × 5 framework is a strategy I've developed to support the five health defense systems by working a minimum of five health-supporting foods you already like to eat into meals and snacks and incorporating them up to 5 times each day into the opportunities where you eat or snack: breakfast, lunch, dinner, and a couple of moments where you snack or eat dessert.

Because the 5 × 5 × 5 is a framework, not a prescription, it is adaptable to whatever diet plan you're currently following, whether it's Paleo, Whole30, Ornish, low-carb, plant-based, gluten-free, allergen-free, or ketogenic—and it's easy to adopt if you don't follow a plan at all. The 5 × 5 × 5 framework doesn't exclude anyone, because it is a larger concept into which you can easily integrate other protocols. Anyone can do it.

The framework is also personal and unique to you, because you create it based on your own food preferences—what you enjoy. And, if you like strict guidelines and are a diet program aficionado looking for calorie counting and a week-by-week plan, the 5 × 5 × 5 framework will also work for you.

The 5 × 5 × 5 framework is flexible and requires little effort to implement, which makes it easy to stick to. And it's not restrictive. It's all about *adding* beneficial foods into your diet, not about excluding foods. This plan encourages you to add to the food choices you are already making, rather than cutting foods out. The plan works if you enjoy batch prepping and prepare many meals at once. The plan also works if you prepare new meals each day, or if you love leftovers.

Everything in the 5 × 5 × 5 framework is backed by the science you've read about in this book, and it is universally appealing because it provides lots of options. This makes it work well for beginners, health enthusiasts, nutritionists, and wellness coaches alike.

The 5 × 5 × 5 framework is not a grueling seven-, ten-, or thirty-day program to sweat through. Instead, this plan is designed to be easy to adhere to and integrate into your everyday life for the long term. It is fluid and flexible, and it takes into account that each day is different, every person is different, and situations change all the time.

I'm going to show you how the framework can be adapted so you can practice healthy eating in diverse environments and different situations. For most people, it's just not realistic to force a single diet plan into every situation you are in. My philosophy is that your diet should be able to adapt to changes in the foods you can find, social situations, and your budget. The 5 × 5 × 5 framework works because it's not about perfection; it's about choices. Daily choices do matter, and even more importantly, they add up!

How to Use the 5 × 5 × 5 Framework

- First, use my lists of foods on page 260, and from those identify your favorites from the two hundred plus items that benefit at least one of the five health defense systems. This helps you create your personalized preferred food list.
- Then, choose five foods to eat each day. Make sure each supports at least one of the defense systems, and be sure you are covering all five systems across these five food choices.
- Finally, eat all five foods in a day as part of one or all of five meals, snacks, or other "occasions" that you eat. Most people have five encounters with food each day (breakfast, lunch, snack, dinner, dessert) and you may find it easiest to incorporate your chosen foods across these five occasions. But you can eat them all together in groups. You can eat however frequently or infrequently you want, depending on personal preference. Just make sure you get all five foods in each day.

Later, in chapter 14, I'll provide a sample meal guide for how to apply the framework every day and share some delicious easy-to-make recipes that will show you how health-promoting ingredients can easily fit into your week. I'll also provide more specific details about how to eat this way. But first, let me tell you about a few guiding principles that I used to craft this framework.

Life's Not Always Perfect

Positive choices with food strengthen your health defenses, but every now and then, you will be in a situation where good choices are not easy or even possible. This is why making good choices regularly can help balance out the effects of the not-so-healthy choices that we all occasionally make. This is also why it's so important to know your overall health risk, which you can find out in the Risk Assessment in appendix B. The Risk Assessment will allow you to develop a sense for how much urgency or wiggle room you have. If you're in the green zone, you can allow yourself a little more leeway. But if you're in the yellow or red zone and are in a situation where you're unable to make healthy choices, it's worth getting back as quickly as you can to being able to control your choices within your 5 × 5 × 5 framework.

In my own life, when I know I'll be in situations where my food choices are limited to less-than-healthy ones, I'll load up with healthier choices either before or later that same day or the next day. The more healthy food you eat, the less room you have in your stomach—and in your life—for unhealthy food. Let the good displace the bad.

Eat What You Enjoy

The 5 × 5 × 5 framework gives you the freedom to choose what you eat and when you eat it. The starting point is selecting your favorite foods from a list of foods known to boost your defense systems. These foods become part of your personalized framework for health—you get to choose them. Everyone prefers eating foods they like. My intent was to create a framework that is neither a prescription telling you what you *must* eat nor a proscription telling you what you have to *remove* from your diet.

People on highly restrictive plans tend to fall off the wagon and revert to their old (often unhealthy) habits when they have to give up too many of the foods that they love. And if you are like me, you get bored having to eat the same things over and over. The 5 × 5 × 5 framework is designed to avoid this problem by starting with your personal favorites, and you can vary your food. It's easier to stick with healthy habits when you're eating what you already enjoy.

Make It Personal

My philosophy says there is no one-size-fits-all approach to health that is right for everyone. We doctors know that in the future, our work with patients will become increasingly personalized. We are shifting from a cookie-cutter approach to embracing unique recommendations for each individual, based on the specific needs of their bodies (and cells, and even genetics) and desires. The goal will be to combine the best treatments with lifestyle modifications, based on each patient's individual makeup and situation.

But you don't have to wait for the future to start benefiting from a personalized approach to health. You can create your own solutions using the 5 × 5 × 5 framework by eating a personalized diet every day, taking into account your own likes and dislikes, food allergies and sensitivities, health risks and worries, life circumstances, budget, and whatever else matters to you. If you have medical reasons not to eat certain foods, that's personal, too. Choose the healthy foods that you like and avoid the ones you dislike.

Make It Sustainable

A sensible plan is one you can adhere to and is meant for you. Trying to fit into a plan designed for someone else is like trying to squeeze into a pair of shoes that are a size too small. You won't feel good, and you won't be able to stand it for long. For longevity and disease prevention, dietary diversity is beneficial. The health payoff does not come from any single item on the menu. It's the mix of foods that go into your body over time that tip the odds in your favor against disease. The 5 × 5 × 5 framework is sustainable because it's personal, based on your likes, and adaptable to life's circumstances—so you can stick with it.

Be Adaptable

Everyone's situation changes over time, from day to day, and even throughout a single day. When you are at your workplace, for example, your access to food is different from when you are home over the weekend. The choices you have at a restaurant vary greatly from what you have available in your own kitchen. When you are invited to someone's home, what they've graciously decided to feed their guests might be very different than what you would normally choose to eat on your own. If you are on the road or on vacation, your destination may have entirely new food options than what you have at home. The 5 × 5 × 5 framework is designed to be flexible and adaptable to any situation as life changes.

As with many areas of life, being able to adapt and be resilient is a key to success. I like to think of eating to beat disease like mixed martial arts (MMA). In MMA, two fighters enter a cage to compete in five-minute rounds of combat. They are not restricted to just one style of fighting, like boxing. Instead, they can use multiple fighting styles (aikido, boxing, judo, jujitsu, kung fu, wrestling) in facing their opponent. The goal of scoring and winning trumps rigid adherence to any one style or philosophy. The martial arts master Bruce Lee, who is considered one of the pioneers of MMA, once explained that the effectiveness of his fighting style was to have no style at all. He incorporated techniques from various martial arts to his practice in order to be fluid and adaptable. Lee even used techniques from fencing to beat his opponent.

This kind of flexibility is just as important for long-term health when it comes to food. Here's what I mean: First, you need to have a heightened situational awareness (how your emotions, hunger, and stress levels affect your food choices), the right convictions based on scientific evidence, and the willingness to act. Next, you need to use every tool at your disposal. Not everyone can always find organic, non-GMO, sustainably farmed, locally grown, grass-fed and wild-caught food all of the time. People are on the go, moving through their lives, often at a breakneck pace, and many times they have limited access to, or time for, the foods they might otherwise like to eat in a more ideal situation.

The 5 × 5 × 5 framework works in these circumstances. By taking a fluid approach to food selection, the 5 × 5 × 5 framework allows you to maintain a healthy diet using whichever healthy foods, beverages, and ingredients you can get your hands on to activate your defense systems against disease. Be aware of the healthy choices in your surroundings, anticipate situations where you might encounter difficulty in gaining access to good quality, healthy food, and improvise with whatever you have. Once you've practiced being flexible, eating to beat disease will become a natural and relaxed everyday reflex.

Putting the 5 × 5 × 5 Framework into Action

The 5 × 5 × 5 framework puts all the information you've learned in this book into a simple action plan that will enhance your health, satisfy your taste buds, and protect you against diseases.

Here's how it works. Each of the three 5s stands for an action that you can take for your health:

5 health defense systems
5 health-defending foods to select each day
5 opportunities to eat them each day

Let's define them.

The First 5 in 5 × 5 × 5: The Health Defense Systems

There are five health defense systems in your body: angiogenesis, regeneration, microbiome, DNA protection, and immunity. These systems maintain your health in a state of perfect balance. When mild disruptions occur in your health, the systems adjust themselves to take care of the problem and continue functioning behind the scenes, so you don't even notice—that's what you want your health to be like your entire life.

If you do something for each system each day, you'll fortify your overall resistance against disease and develop a lifelong habit of covering your bases. To support and fortify all five of your defenses, you will use the second 5.

The Second 5 in 5 × 5 × 5: Health-Defending Foods

The second 5 is about *your* choice of at least five *favorite* foods to include in your diet each day. You don't need permission to eat what you like, because I'm going to help you create your own list of your favorite foods. This will be drawn from a database of foods and beverages with proven scientific association with one or more of the five health defense systems. Some foods you love will influence one system, while others influence more than one defense, and a few even boost all five defenses. (I will share this list with you in chapter 13.)

What is amazing is that when you choose five different foods to hit each of the five health defense systems each and every day, this adds up to eating thirty-five health-promoting foods per week—or 1,820 healthy food choices in a year! These are deposits you make in the bank for your health and they go a long way to counteract the less healthy food choices which we all occasionally make. Let's do the math: let's say you make a stunning one hundred poor food choices a year (fried foods, grilled red meat, etc.). If you follow the 5 × 5 × 5 framework, 95 percent of your food choices will still be healthy ones. Again, let the good choices outweigh the bad.

To be clear, these aren't the only five foods you will eat each day, but rather five foods that you are deliberately choosing to add alongside any other foods you eat in a day. Also, they probably won't be the same five foods every day. You can have repeats from day to day if you like, but the point is to eat *at least* five of them each day. Of course, this does not limit your healthy choices. You can have as many healthy ingredients as you like. The more you stack one healthy food upon another, the more you feed your fortress, and build up your bank of health.

The Third 5 in 5 × 5 × 5: Opportunities to Eat the Health Defense Foods

This last 5 refers to *when* we eat: meals and snacks. The fact is, most of us eat on five occasions each day: breakfast, lunch, and dinner, and perhaps a snack and dessert. This means you get five shots every day to eat the five healthy foods you've chosen. The great news is that the five occasions are just options. You can choose to eat all five of your daily selections in one meal or spread them out over a few meals. This allows you the flexibility to adapt healthy eating into changing circumstances, including when you are on the go and may have to skip a meal.

I am highlighting five meals to underscore the message of abundance. I do not advise that you skip or eat more meals. You can still use the 5 × 5 × 5 Framework if you prefer to eat more or fewer meals. You can also use the 5 × 5 × 5 Framework if you prefer to graze throughout the day. Most people find it easiest to incorporate their five foods by eating them during the five encounters with food each day, but you can do whatever works for you.

Once you get started, you'll find it is very easy to do, since it's flexible, customizable, realistic, and habit-forming. Most importantly, it's rooted in your preferences.

Let's get started.

STEP 1: Create Your Personalized Preferred Food List

For the 5 × 5 × 5 framework you first create your own personalized preferred food list (PFL) based on foods you actually enjoy. You create your list from the master list of all of the foods that follow. You've read about all of them in this book. Now, get a pen, review the list, and check the box next to *each* food or beverage that you know you enjoy consuming. Be honest. Take your time, because some of the items might not be immediately identifiable. Google an item you're unfamiliar with for an image. Do you recognize it? Have you eaten it before? Even if you are not a health food devotee, with the 5 × 5 × 5 framework you'll soon become an expert at picking out foods that support your health defenses. For any listed food that you really dislike, are allergic to, or just plain can't stomach, ignore it (do not check its box).

Preferred Foods List

Fruits

- ☐ Acerola
- ☐ Apples (Granny Smith)
- ☐ Apples (Red Delicious)
- ☐ Apples (Reinnette)
- ☐ Apricot
- ☐ Bitter melon
- ☐ Black chokeberry
- ☐ Black plums
- ☐ Black raspberries
- ☐ Black raspberries (dried)
- ☐ Blackberries
- ☐ Blackberries (dried)
- ☐ Blueberries
- ☐ Blueberries (dried)
- ☐ Camu camu
- ☐ Cherries
- ☐ Cherries (dried)
- ☐ Cranberries
- ☐ Cranberries (dried)
- ☐ Goji berries
- ☐ Grapefruit
- ☐ Grapes
- ☐ Guava
- ☐ Kiwifruit
- ☐ Lychee
- ☐ Mangoes
- ☐ Nectarines
- ☐ Oranges
- ☐ Papaya
- ☐ Peaches

- Persimmon
- Pink grapefruit
- Plums
- Pomegranates
- Raspberries
- Strawberries
- Sultana raisins
- Watermelon

Vegetables

- Aged garlic
- Arugula
- Asparagus
- Bamboo shoots
- Belgian endive
- Bok choy
- Broccoli
- Broccoli rabe
- Broccoli sprouts
- Cabbage
- Capers
- Carrots
- Cauliflower
- Celery
- Cherry tomatoes
- Chicory
- Chile peppers
- Chinese celery
- Collard greens
- Eggplant
- Escarole
- Fiddleheads
- Frisee
- Green beans
- Kale
- Kimchi
- Mustard greens
- Onions
- Pao cai
- Puntarelle
- Purple potatoes
- Radicchio
- Red-leaf lettuce
- Red black-skin tomatoes
- Romanesco
- Rutabaga
- San Marzano tomatoes
- Sauerkraut
- Spinach
- Squash blossoms
- Swiss chard
- Tangerine tomatoes
- Tardivo di Treviso
- Tomatoes
- Turnips
- Wasabi
- Watercress

Legumes/Fungi

- Black beans
- Chanterelle mushrooms
- Chickpeas
- Enoki mushrooms
- Lentils
- Lion's mane mushrooms
- Maitake mushrooms
- Morel mushrooms
- Navy beans
- Oyster mushrooms
- Peas
- Porcini mushrooms
- Shiitake mushrooms
- Soy
- Truffles
- White button mushrooms

Nuts, Seeds, Whole Grains, Bread

- Almond butter
- Almonds
- Barley
- Brazil nuts
- Cashew butter
- Cashews
- Chestnuts
- Chia seeds
- Flax seeds
- Hazelnuts
- Macadamia nuts
- Peanut butter
- Peanuts
- Pecans
- Pine nuts
- Pistachios
- Pumpernickel bread
- Pumpkin seeds
- Rice bran
- Sesame seeds
- Sourdough bread
- Squash seeds
- Sunflower seeds
- Tahini
- Walnuts
- Whole grains

Seafood

- Anchovies
- Arctic char
- Bigeye tuna
- Black bass
- Bluefin tuna
- Bluefish
- Bottarga
- Caviar (sturgeon)
- Cockles (clam)
- Eastern oysters
- Fish roe (salmon)
- Gray mullet
- Hake
- Halibut
- John Dory (fish)
- Mackerel
- Manila clam
- Mediterranean sea bass
- Oyster sauce
- Pacific oysters
- Pompano
- Rainbow trout
- Razor clams
- Red mullet
- Redfish
- Salmon
- Sardine
- Sea bream
- Sea cucumber
- Spiny lobster
- Squid ink
- Swordfish
- Tuna
- Yellowtail (fish)

Meat

- Chicken (dark meat)

Dairy

- Camembert cheese
- Cheddar cheese
- Edam cheese
- Emmenthal cheese
- Gouda cheese
- Jarlsberg cheese
- Muenster cheese
- Parmigiano-Reggiano
- Stilton cheese
- Yogurt

Spices/Herbs

- Basil
- Cinnamon
- Ginseng
- Licorice root
- Marjoram
- Oregano
- Peppermint
- Rosemary
- Saffron
- Sage
- Thyme
- Turmeric

Oil

- Olive oil (EVOO)

Sweets

- Dark chocolate

Beverages

- Beer
- Black tea
- Chamomile tea
- Cloudy apple cider
- Coffee
- Concord grape juice
- Cranberry juice
- Green tea
- Jasmine tea
- Mixed berry juice
- Oolong tea
- Orange juice
- Pomegranate juice
- Red wine (Cabernet, Cabernet Franc, Petit Verdot)
- Sencha green tea

Now, stand back and take a look at your handiwork. Congratulations, you've just selected the foods that you enjoy from the Master List. Each one has evidence for activating at least one of your health defense systems. Now, let's incorporate this information in the next step.

STEP 2: Snap It

Now that you have identified your preferred foods, it's time to highlight how your preferences help each health defense. Go to appendix A and make a copy of the 5 × 5 × 5 Daily Worksheet. The worksheet has several pages listing foods under the heading of their defense systems: angiogenesis, regeneration, microbiome, DNA protection, and immunity. Take the list from step 1 and transfer the marks you've checked from step 1 onto the worksheet under the defense system they activate. No worry if some of the foods you check appear multiple times on the worksheet. This is because there are foods that influence multiple defense systems. Check the food you prefer *each time* it appears on the worksheet.

Once you've transferred your preferred foods onto the worksheet, get out your cellphone and take a photo of each of the worksheet pages. This is now a record of your personal 5 × 5 × 5 preferred food list (PFL) you can carry with you and refer to wherever you go.

Now that your PFL is on your phone, it's easy to whip it out to select foods at a grocery store, restaurant, or even dinner party. At first, you may find yourself referencing the list a lot, but once you become familiar with your own preferences, identifying your healthy favorites will start to become second nature. The photos also make for a great year-round shopping list for those times when you are trying to decide what to buy at the market.

STEP 3: Choose Five Each Day

Now, you are ready to put the entire 5 × 5 × 5 framework in motion. For each day of the week, you'll go through your PFL and select five different foods, one from each defense category. It's okay if some foods influence more than one defense system. These five foods are the ones you will assign yourself to eat that day. This way, you'll be supporting each of the five defense systems daily.

Beyond these five foods, the foods you eat the rest of the day are your free choice (please choose healthy ones—and feel free to draw from the lists in this book). Write down or make a note of the five foods you've chosen for each day. To make it easy, you can do this in the notes application on your phone. Or, you can write down the food on a piece of paper, or in a datebook or journal. If it's in your mobile device, you will have the list with you throughout the day. If you are meal planning or shopping for the entire week, start making your daily list on Sunday and map out all the foods you want to incorporate into your meals over the entire week.

Many foods impact more than one defense system. That's a good thing. For example, mushrooms are both immune-boosting and enhance your microbiome. Oranges are antiangiogenic, help repair DNA, and calm your immune system. Here's the rule: if you choose a food that does more than one thing, it will count only as one of your five foods. You still need to find four more foods for that day that hit each of the defense systems. If one of your foods hits all the systems, you still need to pick four more to reach a total of five foods.

These actions are easy to stick to, and they don't call for a complete overhaul of your diet for the rest of your life. It's a practical way to add health-defending foods into your lifestyle. You may find after using the 5 x 5 x 5 framework that you feel so good, you want to add more foods each day. I encourage this. I also want to challenge you to new foods you didn't realize you like. Just add a check in the box and take a new photo.

Your PFL list should grow and change over time. Eventually you'll find yourself making multiple healthy food choices per meal, because you'll have the knowledge of which foods empower your health. Your friends, family, and colleagues will be asking you why you've chosen the foods on your plate—and you'll be able to tell them something they didn't know. Eating to beat disease will become instinctive and fun.

If you are interested in choosing foods based on their ability to fight a specific disease, I will show you how to think about these choices later in this chapter and in chapter 15. For quick reference on which foods impact each defense system, see appendix A. You'll find charts showing which defense systems influence diseases in part 1.

STEP 4: Eat the Five

Now, you are ready to execute. Go get the five foods you've chosen and eat them at the times you choose. Flexibility is important because your schedule and the ease of eating certain foods may change from day to day and from circumstance to circumstance. It's completely up to you. The key is to activate all five health defense systems every day. That's the 5 × 5 × 5 framework. Eventually, you'll naturally make so many good choices that almost all of the foods you eat on a given day defend your health.

STEP 5: Navigate Your Life

One question I get a lot is, Is this framework compatible with being paleo, pescatarian, ketogenic, vegetarian, vegan, gluten-free or dairy free, or another restriction? The answer is yes. If you follow a specific food philosophy, you can still use this framework because the food choices on the preferred list are so broad. You'll just need to be familiar with which foods you cannot have given the rule of your diet and eliminate those foods from your preference list.

Another question people have is, what if I fail and miss a day? The 5 × 5 × 5 framework is all about doing the best you can and taking the long view—remember, the goal is good health and lowered disease risk over your lifetime. A few days of straying from the framework are not going to break your health over the long haul. And there's no need to "cheat," because with the 5 × 5 × 5 framework, every choice is yours from the beginning.

The 5 × 5 × 5 Archetypes

Most of us have lives that fit into a few common scenarios that pose certain challenges to consistent, healthy eating. So, I've created a series of archetypes to show you how to use the 5 × 5 × 5 framework to navigate your life. See if one of these archetypes describes your life (you may not relate to any, and that's okay, too). These are just examples, and everyone is different, but I'll provide tips that have helped others (and me) stay solidly on the path of healthy eating. The tips are designed to be valuable to all, even if you don't identify with the situation—use them anyhow!

The "Busy Parent"

If you have children, you know exactly what I'm talking about. You may have children of mixed ages, maybe even have an infant. You feel like you're being pulled in multiple directions at all times by your children, your partner, your boss, your extended family, and the friends it's hard to find time for. You feel it's hard to excel in any one area of life because you're spread so thin. You may be getting little or interrupted sleep if you have little ones or a sick child. You may be bringing your children to and from school, or daycare, or from activity to activity. It's hard to find time for self-care at this stage in life, but you really want to have a healthy diet among your many priorities. If you don't have proper fuel, your health will suffer. Your children need you to model good behavior, and they deserve to have a healthy parent. So does your partner. Planning your meals can help you achieve better health during this busy time in your life.

Here's how the 5 × 5 × 5 framework can help when you need to plan ahead:

- Set aside some time on Sunday to look at your Preferred Food List. Take a look at the week ahead. Pick the five foods you want to get in every day.
- If you have a partner, have them make their own list separately, so you can compare or combine lists for shopping, planning, and cooking.
- Plan batch cooking with your chosen health-defending foods, so you have meals ready to go throughout the week and leftovers you can eat for lunch. This way, you are getting your five foods in during dinner and lunch with a minimal amount of mental energy spent thinking about healthy food each day. One day of cooking and prep can cover your five foods per day during the workweek. Some ideas for batch cooking include:
  - Make a pot of soup or a stew that can serve both as dinner and lunch the next day.
  - Roast vegetables and add to multiple meals over the course of the week.
  - Bulk cook grains like quinoa and brown rice to use throughout the week.
- In the meantime, keep some healthy snack items like nuts and fruit within easy reach.
- Use a grocery delivery service that can bring fresh produce and other ingredients to your door to save you time.
- Refer to your PFL every time you order food online.

The "Frequent Flyer"

You're a busy professional. Maybe you are growing a business, or perhaps your job requires you to travel often. You feel like you are always on the run, traveling from place to place. Let's face it, whenever you have to eat on the road, whether it's in an airport, on a flight, on a bus, in a car, or at a hotel, the food is usually not very good for you. In fact, it's often terrible. Eating out for every meal gets old. And because you are on the move, it gets hard to make healthy choices consistently.

You'll encounter situations where you have to use the mixed martial arts technique and adapt to the circumstances, using whatever is at your disposal. If you have to eat in an airport or during a flight, the first thing to do is open your camera app and check to see if there's anything on your preferred list on the limited menu, and order that. Remember, each meal or snack is a shot to build your defenses. Take the same approach if you are staying at a hotel and have to order room service, or eat at the restaurant.

Here's how to use the 5 × 5 × 5 framework when you need to be on the road:

- As you get ready to leave, look at your Preferred Food List and pick out the foods you are most likely to find where you are going. This will allow you to mentally adapt to your choices when you get to your destination.
- Choose nonperishable foods from our PFL that you can easily pack and take with you before you leave the house. Some examples of these are nuts, trail mix, homemade breakfast bars, and chocolate.
- When you dine at a restaurant, as soon as you open the menu, cross-reference what's being offered with your PFL, and order as many of your five daily selections as you can. Make special requests of the kitchen for ingredients to suit your 5 × 5 × 5 framework needs if you don't see anything that fits your needs.

- Sometimes you'll find great ingredients on your PFL in the appetizers but not the entrées. In which case, order two appetizers that contain healthy ingredients in place of a less healthy entrée.
- If you're going to be staying at a hotel for a few days and you're feeling ambitious, book a room with a refrigerator. You can go to a nearby market and stock your fridge with items from your preference list.
- Get coffee and tea at a local coffee shop, or bring your own tea packets, which are convenient for travel. (My personal favorite is a custom blend of angiogenesis teas developed by the Angiogenesis Foundation with Harney & Sons.)

The "Young Rock Star"

Everyone in their young adult years is a rock star. Here's the archetype. You are a twentysomething living with roommates or maybe on your own. You work hard and also play hard. You are enjoying your freedom and independence. Looking good and feeling good are important to you, so you go to the gym, you run half-marathons, and maybe you have a trainer. Being fit is your thing, but healthy eating tends to come in waves. Let's face it, when you go out at night, you may party a little too hard sometimes, and you definitely know that's not great for your health. But you are young, and your body is resilient, so you easily bounce back from a little overindulgence. From reading this book, you now know that the damage you do today will catch up to you later in life. Your health defenses are working their magic now, but the long-term toll on them could make you seriously suffer in the next phase of your life a decade or two from now. You don't want that to be you, but you also don't want to spend time worrying about the future.

Here's how to use the 5 × 5 × 5 framework to have your cake and eat it, too:

- Each morning, review your PFL and mark the five foods you will eat that day. Make it part of your daily personal challenge to find the foods, eat them, and check them off your daily list. If you get most of them in earlier in the day, it gives you more leeway to wander off the path later and explore new things you might encounter with friends.

- Download an app that lets you track your daily goals. Since you are no doubt a 100 percent kind of person, you should be able to eat at least those five foods every day.
- If you work out, eat most of your five either before or after you work out, so it becomes part of your health and fitness routine.
- If you drink coffee or tea every day, just think: you've just taken in one of your five, so now you only have to choose and eat four more for the day.
- Motivate yourself by making this competitive. Find a friend or coworker who is up for a friendly challenge and see who can keep up 100 percent with the 5 × 5 × 5 framework the longest without breaking the streak.
- Cook for yourself. Learn how to prepare meals. Having some of the basic equipment that I'll discuss in the next chapter will make cooking in healthy ways much easier. Cooking regularly gives you more control and flexibility than dining out every day for following the 5 × 5 × 5 framework.

The "Middle-Age Sage"

This is another classic archetype. After building your career and household, you've finally reached a point where you've (mostly) got a good handle on life. You are good at planning and have managed to master the balancing act of family, work, social life, and your personal interests. You have control over your decisions and resources at your disposal. By now, you know yourself and are comfortable with what you like and what you dislike.

When it comes to food, you know what you will eat and what you probably won't try. You've become a creature of habit, by choice. Even though you think of yourself as being younger than your chronological age, the reality is your friends are now starting to look old, and get sick with diseases you weren't thinking about ten years ago. You may even have lost a few friends or family members to a chronic disease. Like it or not, your own mortality is slowly creeping into your own mind.

Here's how to use the 5 × 5 × 5 framework, even if you are wise and set in your ways:

- Use your self-knowledge and experience to check the boxes of all the preferred foods on the list and identify the ones that you absolutely love the most. Put a circle around your favorites.
- Plan ahead for the weekend and select the five foods you want to eat each day in advance. Be ultra-focused and think exactly how you will hit your marks with the 5 × 5 × 5 framework, being sure to focus on the foods that bring you the most enjoyment.
- If you go out to eat, think about where you might dine to find foods on your PFL. You probably already know which restaurants are likely to use healthier ingredients found on your list. See how many foods on your list you can eat in a single meal.
- If you are not already an accomplished cook at home, cooking healthy foods could become your new hobby. Watch online cooking tutorials or take a cooking class to amplify your skills in the kitchen. By cooking your own meals, you're not only able to give yourself the gift of health, but you can also provide it for your family and friends. (I'll have many useful kitchen tips and tricks in the next chapter, so be sure to check it out.)

Person Facing Serious Disease

If you are battling a disease, you probably are experiencing a sense of urgency as you read this book. You want to beat the disease, and restore your health or the health of someone you care about to what it was. Even though the situation may feel overwhelming, you probably have family, friends, and doctors who are doing their best to provide help. You may not have the energy for meal planning or cooking. If you are the one who is sick, you may not even feel like eating at all right now. Keep in mind, though, that food is a weapon that can activate the body's natural health defense systems. When properly fired up, your health defense systems know how to bring your body back to a stable position of health.

Here's a practical way to use the 5 × 5 × 5 framework in your situation:

- Always discuss any changes to your diet with your doctor.
- Enlist the help of your family, friends, or support network to help go over the list of foods in the PFL. Let them read the list to you. You tell them which boxes to check. If they already know what foods you love, let them do it for you, and then check the list to make sure they got it right. Ask them to take a photo with their phone, as a reference for when they want to bring something for you to eat.
- Ask whoever is involved with helping you grocery shop, meal plan, and cook to take your PFL and create a weekly plan.
- Since you may not be eating as much, try to squeeze all five foods into a single meal or two.
- If you are in the hospital, ask to see the dietitian in charge and request their help in fulfilling your PFL. Few actually enjoy eating standard hospital food, so ask the dietitian if a meal can be created for you. If you need help getting your requests fulfilled, ask for the hospital's patient advocate to assist.
- No matter which disease you're facing, you should pay special attention to what you are eating, because your diet can help fortify your body's health defenses, and the right foods can work alongside with the medicines you may be taking.

Insider Tips for Incorporating the 5 × 5 × 5 Framework

To help you integrate the 5 × 5 × 5 framework into your life, here are some insider tips. These five tips have been very helpful in guiding the way I've approached my own diet.

Quit the Clean Plate Club

Regardless of how you were raised, the reflex to eat every morsel on your plate, regardless of how much is on it, is an unhealthy one. We have all experienced the terrible feeling of eating until we are full, and then being pressured to finish all the food that someone else heaped on our plate. Cleaning the plate is an outdated idea dating back to 1917, during World War 1 when food was scarce, that contributes to overeating and obesity.[1]

Be moderate in your portions at every meal. Eat until you are no longer hungry. The Japanese have a principle called *hara hachi bun me*, which means "eat until you are eight parts [out of ten] full" or "belly 80 percent full." This is a smart approach, because your body has had enough food before you feel full. The first bite of food tastes really great. When you start to feel fuller, you may notice the food isn't as tantalizing as that first bite, but maybe you keep eating out of habit or because you've been conditioned to clean your plate lest you let the food "go to waste."

I am hereby giving you permission to leave food on the plate. Slow down your eating and let the food in your stomach trigger the release of satiety hormones that tell your brain to switch off your appetite. It can take up to twenty minutes before this happens. If you wolf down your meal, everything on the plate will be down the hatch and in your body before your natural satiety responses kick in. The result: you will overeat.

When food starts to lose its appeal, pause and take note. Tune into your body while you're eating, so put away your phone or laptop and turn off the television while you eat. Don't put too much food on your plate. And walk away from each meal before you feel like you need to be carried away.

Skip a Few Meals Each Week

Most research studies on diet and longevity show that restricting your calories increases life span. A 15 percent restriction of calories over two years not only slows metabolic aging, but in one study it also led to a nineteen-pound weight loss.[2] Beyond its antiaging and weight loss benefits, caloric restriction is beneficial because it activates all five of your health defense systems. Trendy diets like 16:8, 5:2, Eat-Stop-Eat, and the Warrior Diet all restrict calories, but there are other easy ways to do it.

Here's one easy way: skip breakfast or lunch a few days each week. You may already be doing this if you live a busy and hectic life. This cuts down your meals by 15 percent. If you decide to skip a meal, however, make sure you are still getting the five foods that day. This is easy to do if you incorporate them into at least one of the meals you do eat or during a snack. When it comes to fasting, however, be aware that the long-term effects of extreme fasting and ketogenesis in healthy individuals are not yet known. Like anything related to diet, extreme measures usually lead to short-term gains but may have long-term consequences for your health. Keep it reasonable if you skip any meals.

Eat Mindfully

Each time you have something to eat, be deliberate: take a moment and think about what you are about to consume. Think about why: your intent is to help your body become healthier, not just to cram bulk or calories into your system. Foods contain bioactives. Have the intent to put them to work for your health. Listen to your body. Before the era of packaged foods, processed foods, fast foods, and online meal delivery, people ate what was instinctive and natural to them. Left to its own devices, the body is designed to be in tune with itself, and it will tell your brain what it needs. Now we know the signal may also be coming from your microbiome. Eat with the intent of taking good care of your gut bacteria.

Eat with People You Like

Eating is not only an act of survival, but it is an act of culture, tradition, and pleasure. The people who live to be centenarians in the so-called Blue Zones—Okinawa (Japan), Sardinia (Italy), Ikaria (Greece), Nicoya (Costa Rica), Loma Linda (California)—eat in very different, sometimes surprising ways that lead them toward health and longevity. But what they do share in common is community and strong social bonds. Enjoying your food is best done in the company of friends and family.

Avoid dining alone whenever possible. Humans are a social species, and eating for enjoyment usually involves others. Even hunter-gatherers ate with their own trusted social networks so they could share the precious food they collected. In many cultures, eating with a group allows the kitchen to prepare more offerings, so greater diversity of food becomes available to all. Eating together often means preparing the meal together. Cooking makes you appreciate the food you prepare and gives you a better connection with the ingredients you are putting into your body.

Try New Foods

Having new experiences is part of self-growth. This is part of the appeal of watching television cooking shows, food travelogues, and looking at a restaurant menu. As you master the 5 × 5 × 5 framework, you'll realize there are more foods that support health defenses than you ever thought. Many of those foods you'll like, and some perhaps you don't care for. But, there will certainly be some new foods that you've not yet experienced. I'm recommending that you update your PFL every six months for a couple of reasons. First, because research is going to be revealing new foods with evidence for beating disease, and you should look to see if you want to add them to your life. Second, because I'm encouraging you to explore foods you haven't tried yet because discovery is part of the joy of life, especially when it comes to good food. In chapter 14, I'm going to give you recipes and a sample week's meal plan, so you can get off to a great start.

But first, let's go to the kitchen.

CHAPTER 12

Rethinking the Kitchen

Now that you know how to create your personal 5 × 5 × 5 framework, you'll need the tools to execute it—starting in your kitchen. You may be one of those people who leads such a busy life that you dine out most of the time, and that's not the best path to health. Having the tools you need to prepare a healthy meal or snack at home makes do-it-yourself health easy.

The information in this chapter will help you get the most benefit from the foods you want to eat. To eat to beat disease, you need to choose the right foods, store them properly, and prepare them in the way that best serves up their health benefits. These are important not just for flavor and food safety. The right cooking process can help retain, or even amplify, the health-promoting properties of your ingredients. When you dine out, you don't have control over ingredients or preparation. When you cook at home, you have complete control.

You need the proper tools for prepping and cooking, as well as the right ingredients in your pantry. In this chapter, I'm going to take you through a rethink of your own kitchen and tell you exactly what you need to have on hand.

The kitchen has always been the center of my home. Growing up, when I came home from school, my mom always had something delicious cooking on the stovetop. My memories of the smell of childhood dinners brings me a sense of comfort to this day. Because I was always interested in what was being sliced, chopped, mixed, stir-fried, stewed, or steamed, my mom taught me about the ingredients and the methods of preparation she used. Eventually, I learned to cook my favorite dishes from her recipes.

Today's home kitchen is different from those of our grandparents' generation. Basic kitchen tools and implements used to be ubiquitous, often given as wedding gifts to help a couple start out in life or passed down from one generation to the next. Nowadays, although many people own kitchen-cluttering gadgets inspired by television cooking shows and infomercials, some home kitchens are missing the basics. You don't need to have lots of fancy equipment to create tasty, healthy meals, but there are some basic tools you should own.

Let's take a look at some of the things every healthy-minded kitchen should have—from the cabinets to the pantry. I'll also tell you about some of the best techniques every home cook should know for simple, healthy cooking.

Tools

Every kitchen must have some basic tools for preparing and cooking food in healthy ways. Some people prefer a no-frills minimalist kitchen, but here are the basic tools you should have, so you can whip up healthy meals at home.

- **Knives (eight-inch chef's knife, paring knife):** Stainless steel or ceramic knives will give you cutting performance and durability. Plus, they are easy to clean.
- **Metal tongs:** Tongs help you move hot ingredients around a pot or pan while they are cooking.
- **Metal colander:** For draining pasta, washing vegetables, and rinsing fruit.

- **High-quality pans (ceramic coated, stainless steel, or cast-iron skillet and sauté pan):** Pans should contain no plastic so they can go from the stovetop into the oven and be easily cleaned.

- **Stockpot with lid:** For making stock and soups.

- **Cast-iron Dutch oven or casserole dish with lid:** For simmering stews in the oven.

- **Glass or ceramic baking dishes:** For roasting vegetables, seafood, and poultry.

- **Baking sheets:** Stainless steel is best, but aluminum conducts heat more evenly for performance (bake on a sheet of parchment with aluminum pans).

- **Bamboo steamer:** Easy to clean, lightweight, and cooks food quickly without the need for oil.

- **Wok:** Get cast iron or carbon steel; never buy a nonstick wok. Look for one that has an all-metal handle (no plastic).

- **Rice cooker:** Makes cooking rice easy and a no-brainer. Just add water and push down the button, and it will let you know automatically when the rice is done. No need to watch the stove for perfect timing or worry about burning the rice and having it stick on the bottom of a pot.

- **Food mill:** Used to mash and sieve foods to remove seeds, skin, and large chunks. Get one that is stainless steel with multiple blades.

- **Toaster oven:** An alternative to the microwave for quickly heating food.

- **Cutting board:** Get a wooden one; wood is best for your knives and the most natural surface for cutting or chopping food.

- **Vegetable peeler**

- **Can opener**

- **Whisk:** Metal only.

- **Microplane grater:** For grating cheese and nuts, and zesting peel.

- **Pepper mill**
- **Wooden spoons**
- **Stainless steel ladle**
- **Blender:** For making smoothies and soups.
- **Glass liquid measuring cup**
- **Stainless steel dry measuring cups**
- **Metal measuring spoons**
- **Coffee mills:** Get two: one for coffee, one for spices.
- **French press coffeemaker:** Allows the coffee bioactives to be in the water, not trapped in a paper filter.
- **Automatic hot water dispenser:** Makes it convenient to make tea by just pushing a button to dispense heated water.
- **Wine opener or corkscrew**
- **Food storage containers**: Always glass, never plastic.

Equipment in the "nice to have" category will allow you to have a more sophisticated approach to preparing and storing healthy foods. These are by no means necessary but are great additions to your tool kit.

- **Immersion blender:** A handheld mixer that can puree foods in a container (great for blended soups).
- **Juicer:** An easy way to make all varieties of juice.
- **Mortar and pestle:** Perfect for crushing garlic and making pesto.
- **Mushroom brush:** Cleans mushrooms without having to wash them, which removes dirt from the forest floor if wild harvested or compost (often straw and horse and chicken manure) from farmed mushrooms.
- **Plancha:** A metal cooking surface to place on top of a flame or other heat source. This provides a uniform heating surface and prevents fats from dripping on the coals or flame, which could cause toxic fumes to flare up. It should be cast iron and can be used on stovetop or on a grill.

- **Pressure cooker:** For nutrient-preserving speed cooking.
- **Slow cooker:** An electric-powered heavy ceramic pot that makes it possible to cook a meal unattended during the day and have dinner ready when you come home.

Make Room for the New

When I help outfit a kitchen, the first thing I do is get rid of the old to make room for the new items that are useful for health. If you take a close look, you probably have equipment that's no longer needed, not working, and probably a few items you are better off without. Get rid of these if you have them:

- **Nonstick pans made with Teflon:** Avoid Teflon, because it is so easy to overheat on the stove. When the coating is overheated to high temperatures, it releases toxic fumes that can cause an illness called Teflon flu that kills birds exposed to it. In humans, the condition is called polymer fume fever, and it can seriously damage your lungs.[1]
- **Plastic storage containers:** Plastic will break down over time and contaminate food. Save leftovers, soups, and stews in glassware, not plastic.
- **Plastic utensils and tools:** Spatulas, spoons, colanders, measuring cups, etc.
- **Styrofoam and plastic cups:** Both contain chemicals that can leach out with hot liquids. Use ceramic mugs for your hot beverages. Whenever possible, take your own mug to be filled at the coffee shop.

Your Pantry

The word *pantry* comes from the French word for bread, which is *pain* (pronounced like *pen*). During the Middle Ages, the pantry was a room where bread and other foods were stored. In modern times, the pantry is often a closet or cabinet in the kitchen used to store dried goods, jars, and packaged foods that don't require refrigeration. When your pantry is properly stocked with the right ingredients, you'll be prepared to create healthy meals on a regular basis and you can focus on picking up the fresh items at the market. The pantry, however, often becomes a cluttered closet where unused and long-forgotten food items occupy shelf space, so I encourage you to regularly audit and clean out your pantry.

Are there foods in there that you received as a gift and never intend to eat? Old packaged foods that you bought for one recipe and never used again? Food items you picked up on a vacation that you threw in the closet and are now years old? If the answer to any of these is "maybe," it's time to check it out. Do a visual audit of your pantry now, and then again every six months. Clean out any old stuff that has expired, and throw away (or give away) what you have no intention of eating. By doing a regular purge of your pantry, you will prevent expired items from accumulating. And you will be reminded of the useful health-generating items you already have that you can use for cooking.

Here are the key items to get on the pantry shelves. Information on how long each can be stored is given at the end of this chapter.

Oils and Vinegars

- **Extra virgin olive oil:** Stock up on cold press olive oils made from one of the following monovarietals, which have the highest levels of polyphenols: Koroneiki (Greece), Moraiolo (Italy), or Picual (Spain). Store olive oil in a dark tinted jar or bottle to protect it from light, which can make the oil become rancid and degrade the health-producing bioactives.

- **Vinegars:** Real aged balsamic vinegar comes from Modena or Reggio Emilia in Italy, and it is expensive but worth it. If your local store doesn't have it, you can order it online. In addition to fantastic taste, it contains the bioactive melanodin, which prevents DNA damage.[2] Apple cider vinegar is another good pantry item that's been shown to reduce blood cholesterol levels.[3] Store in a cool, dark location. Some balsamic vinegars are aged one hundred years, so they will likely outlast your pantry.

Dried Goods

- **Dried Spices:** Basil, cardamom, cinnamon, clove, herbs de Provence, nutmeg, oregano, paprika, rosemary, thyme, turmeric, vanilla bean. Store sealed tightly in glass containers.
- **Black pepper:** Contains piperine that increases the absorption of other food bioactives, like curcumin in turmeric.[4] Get whole peppercorns and grind them fresh in a pepper mill when needed.
- **Beans:** Dried varieties (adzuki, black, chickpeas, fava, flageolet, Great Northern, kidney, lentils, navy, pinto). Beans begin to lose their natural moisture in one to two years. Their vitamins will degrade eventually and are gone after five years.[5]
- **Rice:** Brown (rice from California, India, or Pakistan is regarded as safer with less chance of having arsenic; avoid rice from Arkansas, Louisiana, or Texas[6]) or haiga (half-milled, leaving the beneficial germ). Because of natural oils present in brown rice, it lasts for only six to eight months in the pantry.
- **Flour:** Whole wheat, gluten-free, arrowroot, coconut, and amaranth. Store in an airtight container.
- **Pasta/noodles:** Whole wheat pasta, squid ink noodles, and buckwheat soba (buckwheat boosts immunity).[7]

- **Coffee:** Buy roasted beans and grind them when needed. Store in an airtight container and protect beans from light and heat, which degrade both flavor and bioactives. The jury is out on whether freezing beans is better for preserving flavor, and the effects of freezing on coffee bioactives are not known.[8]

- **Tea:** Green, oolong, black, and chamomile come in tea bags, sachets, or as loose leaf. Store in a dark container.

- **Nuts:** Almonds, cashews, macadamia, pecans, pine nuts, and walnuts. Due to their high oil content, most cannot be stored for very long. You can freeze nuts to make them last longer, but I recommend you simply buy only what you can eat over the course of a few weeks.

- **Dried fruits:** Apricots, blueberries, cherries, cranberries, mango, papaya, and raisins are great for mixing with nuts for snacking. Sulfites are often used as a preservative and can cause allergic reactions, but many organic brands are sulfite-free.

- **Dried mushrooms:** Dried morels, porcini, shiitake, and chanterelles can be soaked and reconstituted in warm water, adding flavor and intensity to any dish during cooking. Store in an airtight container.

- **Tinned seafood:** Spanish or Portugese tinned anchovy, sardines, mackerel, bonito tuna, clams, and baby squid in ink are delicacies. Tins can last several years, but discard if the tin is leaking or seriously dented.

- **Whole grains:** Whole wheat barley, buckwheat, couscous, farro, oats, and quinoa. Store in an airtight container.

- **Seeds:** Chia, pumpkin, sesame, and sunflower. They are rich in natural oils, and will go rancid quickly at room temperature, so they don't keep well. Buy only in small quantities.

- **Capers:** Jarred Sicilian capers from the island of Pantelleria, preserved in salt, are considered among the best. Refrigerate after opening.

Sauces and Pastes

- **Sriracha sauce:** A popular spicy sauce made from chile peppers, vinegar, and garlic, used for dipping, and named after Si Racha, a coastal town in eastern Thailand. The sauce should be refrigerated after opening.
- **Chile paste:** A spicy paste made with chile peppers, used for cooking and seasoning.
- **Canned tomatoes:** San Marzano tomatoes are best for high lycopene.
- **Tomato paste:** Sold in a can or in a tube. The best tube versions are made with San Marzano tomatoes, and the double-concentrated product has an intense flavor. Once opened, store in the refrigerator and use within three months.
- **Anchovy paste:** A paste made of anchovies, salt, and olive oil in a tube, for flavoring foods. Unopened tubes can last for years. Refrigerate after opening.
- **Miso paste:** Made with salty fermented soy, rice, and barley and packed with umami flavor. Refrigerate after opening.
- **Oyster sauce:** An umami sauce from Asia. Refrigerate after opening.
- **Soy sauce:** A fermented product, best kept in a cool, dark place. It's best to store it in the refrigerator after opening.

Natural Sweeteners

- **Honey:** Manuka honey from New Zealand stimulates the immune system and is good with tea and lemon for soothing a sore throat.[9]
- **Maple syrup:** Grade A amber contains more than twenty polyphenol bioactives.[10]
- **Maple sugar:** A natural sweetener made from maple syrup. It has been found to contain thirty bioactive polyphenols, some of which have antioxidant and anti-inflammatory properties.[11]

A Note on Bottled Water

Many people keep bottled water in their pantry for easy hydration, but I recommend you avoid regularly consuming water stored in plastic bottles. Studies have shown that even without BPA plastic, plastic particles called microplastics will shed into water that you drink. One study found as many as 2,400 pieces of microplastic in eight fluid ounces of bottled water.[12] As an alternative, keep a glass pitcher of chilled water in the refrigerator. You can add useful bioactives to it by dropping sliced citrus, stone fruit (such as peaches), berries, celery, or cucumber into the pitcher to create refreshing, lightly flavored water.

Basic Cooking Techniques

Healthy eating starts with fresh, high-quality ingredients. But once you have them, you need to know how to cook them. Many cooking techniques can be used to prepare healthy foods, but some are easier for a home cook than others. With the plethora of cooking shows on television, you've probably seen just about every culinary method that restaurants use, but let's focus on the ones that you can use at home.

The following are basic kitchen techniques that you should have in your repertoire. They will allow you to take your favorite preferred foods and prepare them in diverse ways to keep your meals interesting, fresh, and nonrepetitive. You are probably familiar with some of the techniques, but since we are putting together your plan, the tools, and the ingredients, let's review some of the best ways to prepare your meals. Note that none of them involve deep-frying or microwaving your food.

- **Steaming:** A very healthy cooking method that uses steam to heat and cook food in a metal or wooden vessel. A bamboo steamer can be set inside a cast-iron wok with water heated to boiling. You can do a variation by wrapping the food into parchment paper with some liquid or herbs and baking it. This is known as cooking en papillote. The liquid inside will create steam within the package, which seals in the cooking juices.

- **Blanching:** A technique that involves placing vegetables in boiling water for a very brief time (the time depends on the amount and type of vegetable), moving it to cold water to stop cooking, and then draining. This is an excellent technique for preparing vegetables for stir-frying, removing skins, and taking away some of the bitterness from vegetables.

- **Stir-frying:** A technique of rapidly cooking sliced foods in a small amount of hot oil (don't let it smoke) in a wok while being quickly stirred. This sears the outside of ingredients to seal in nutrients and flavors while swiftly cooking them all the way through. Be careful not to use too much oil or to overheat the oil to its smoking point. If you use olive oil for stir-frying, use light olive oil, not extra virgin, which will burn and impart an off-flavor to stir-fried foods.

- **Sautéing:** A technique using a pan heated with a little oil on the stovetop to cook foods, usually sliced into pieces, until finished.

- **Poaching:** Gently placing delicate foods, like fish, in simmering water (between 176 and 194°F) to cook slowly at a low temperature while extracting flavors and bioactives into the poaching liquid, which can be used for a sauce or broth.

- **Simmering:** A gentle way of cooking foods in liquids by first bringing to a boil and then reducing heat and continuing to cook just below the boiling point. Simmering tomatoes into a sauce will change their lycopene to a beneficial, more readily absorbable chemical form.

- **Braising:** Food is seared in a heavy-bottomed pan, then liquid (often a stock) and other ingredients are added to the pan, which is then covered tightly with a lid. The food is simmered until fully cooked and all the flavors meld together. The braising liquid becomes highly flavorful and can be used for a sauce.

- **Slow cooking:** Inspired by traditional stewing in the oven, this technique cooks food by simmering in liquid at low temperature for hours, usually in an electrical appliance, such as a Crock-Pot, which allows for unattended cooking. Slow cooking is a convenience for the cook who is not home or is otherwise busy most of the day, but still wants to prepare a substantive meal.

- **Pressure cooking:** A method of rapid cooking that uses steam to create high temperatures inside a tightly sealed container to reduce cooking time. Especially useful for cooking at high altitude, where the boiling point of water is lowered and it is hard to cook even pasta because the water will not get hot enough before it turns to steam. Be careful: special precautions are built into pressure cookers to prevent trapped steam from causing an explosion or serious burn injury.

- **A la plancha:** *Plancha* means griddle in Spanish. This is a way to cook vegetables, fish, or meat on an extremely hot flat metal or stone surface situated above but not in contact with an open flame. The plancha quickly sears the outside and keeps the nutrients and flavors locked in, similar to stir-frying in a wok but on a flat surface.

- **Grilling:** Everyone knows this primitive cooking technique that places food (usually on metal racks or a spit) above a flame or hot coals. Grilling with the heat source above the food is known as broiling and is usually done inside an oven. What you might not know is that grilling meats (but not vegetables) produces polycyclic aromatic hydrocarbons (PAH). These are carcinogens that form when oils from the meat drip into flame and smoke. The rising smoke deposits the carcinogens on the cooking meat. High grilling temperatures also convert amino acids and proteins[13] in meat into toxic heterocyclic amines (HCA). Marinating animal proteins ahead of time with olive oil, turmeric, soy, and fruits has been shown to reduce carcinogen formation during cooking.[14] If you cook vegetables on a grill, cook at medium heat. Make sure you clean the grates thoroughly beforehand, so you are not picking up carcinogenic polycyclic aromatic hydrocarbons that are in the char of the last piece of meat that was grilled. Grilling vegetables on a clean grill surface does not create carcinogens, so long as the veggies are not burned. Remember, burnt food tastes bad and is unsafe to consume.

- **Roasting:** Cooking by enveloping a food (like vegetables or a meat) with dry heat diffused in an oven. The tenderest results for roasting meats and vegetables are achieved using very low oven temperature (250–300°F) and checking for doneness using a thermometer. To add flavor and maintain as much moisture as possible in the food, you can use a marinade, baste the food frequently, or add a little olive oil.

- **Baking:** Using dry heat in an oven to cook a food, usually one that starts out as batter or dough.

- **Marinating:** A preparatory step, marinating is the coating, soaking, or immersing of a food in a seasoned liquid before cooking, whether it is roasting, sautéing, stir-frying, or even steaming. Marinating foods can help tenderize tough meats and offers some protection against the forming of carcinogens when meat is cooked on a grill. For fish and vegetables, marinating can be used as a way to add the health-defense-boosting spices, herbs, and oils.

- **Pickling:** An ancient technique of immersing and fermenting vegetables in brine or vinegar to extend the food's edible life span. The process changes the texture and taste, resulting in a distinct version of the food itself. Controlled use of salt, vinegar, and natural bacteria contribute to the pickling process. Pickling allows summer vegetables to be preserved and eaten during winter months. As you saw in chapter 8, many fermented foods like kimchi, sauerkraut, and pao cai are pickled vegetables rich in healthy bacteria, so the foods deliver probiotics.

Even More Health-Promoting Techniques

Here are a few more health-promoting cooking and preparation tips:

- **When cooking vegetables, make use of all the edible parts.** For broccoli, don't just cook the florets; prepare the stems, too. Same with mushrooms. Although we traditionally cook the tops and throw away the stems, use them! The stems of both broccoli and mushrooms contain higher levels of bioactives that support health defenses than their tops (floret and caps). Similarly, with carrots, buy whole fresh carrots, including their green tops, and cook the greens, which have potent antiangiogenic properties. And when you cook with tomatoes, keep the skin on, which contains high amounts of lycopene.
- **Avoid deep-frying, and never reuse oil you've cooked with once before.** Each time oil is heated, it breaks down. Upon reheating, its chemical structure becomes more destabilized, and the oil starts to become rancid and decompose into oxidizing products that can damage your DNA.
- **If oil is used, choose extra virgin olive oil.** But do not overheat olive oil (or any other oil) to its smoking point, which can generate toxic fumes as well as convert the oil into harmful trans-fats. If you are sautéing or stir-frying, use a cast-iron, stainless steel, or nonstick ceramic pan only.
- **Reheat food gradually in the oven or on the stovetop, instead of in the microwave.** Avoid microwaving starchy foods, because the high heat changes starch into a harmful polymer (advanced glycation end products) that can build up in your body and cause

damage to your organs.[15] If you bring your lunch to work, pack the food in a glass or metal, not plastic, container. Bring hot food in a Thermos container to avoid having to reheat it in the microwave if your workplace doesn't have a toaster oven or stove.

Keeping Food in the Refrigerator

One of the first things you do when you return from the market with fresh foods is put things away. Here's a list of fruits and vegetables that should be put in the fridge unless you are eating them right away, and how long they should remain fresh. Checking and cleaning out your refrigerator is important for a healthy diet. Knowing how long things will last will help you plan your shopping and how much you should buy at a time.

Store These in the Fridge

Food Item	Will Last For
Apples	3 weeks
Blackberries	2–3 days stored as a single layer on a paper towel
Blueberries	1 week
Bok choy	3 days
Broccoli (including Broccoli rabe)	1 week
Cabbage	1–2 weeks
Carrots	2 weeks
Celery	2 weeks
Chard	3 days
Cherries	3 days kept in an open bowl

Chile peppers (fresh)	2 weeks
Cranberries	4 weeks
Endive	5 days
Ginger (fresh)	3 weeks
Grapes	3 days
Green beans	1 week
Kale	3 days
Kiwifruit	4 days
Lemons	3 weeks
Lettuce	5 days
Mango	4 days
Mushrooms	1 week stored in a paper bag
Oranges	2 weeks
Peas (fresh)	4 days kept in their pods
Pomegranate (whole)	3 weeks
Radicchio	4 days
Raspberries	3 days stored as a single layer on a paper towel
Spinach	3 days
Stone fruit (apricot, nectarines, peaches, plums)	5 days
Strawberries	3 days
Watermelon	1 week uncut; 2 days cut
Zucchini	5 days

How to Keep Seafood

Eating fish regularly is important for your health. If you eat seafood regularly, you are already familiar with the logistics of buying and cooking fish. If you are a fish novice, I want to give you an overview to show you how easy it is. Buying freshly caught fish from a fishmonger is something that people who live near a coast can easily do. Fishermen go out

292

at night, and sell their fresh catch to the fishmonger the next morning. But for most people who live inland, the fish in the grocery store has been shipped in and is found in a display case on ice. Wherever you buy fish, the best plan is to bring it home, rinse it with cold water, pat it dry, and plan on eating it the same or the next day. Keep it in the refrigerator until you're ready to cook it. Fish that has been flash-frozen and vacuum-sealed on the fishing boat is a good alternative to fresh fish for inlanders. In fact, it may be even higher quality, since it was frozen minutes after being brought on board. If you buy frozen fish, store it in the freezer in its package until you intend to cook it.

Live shellfish such as clams and mussels need to be refrigerated immediately, as soon as you get them home. Place them in a bowl without any water (fresh water will kill them) and cover them with a damp towel to maintain humidity (never seal them in a plastic bag or they will die). Place the bowl in the refrigerator. Clams can be kept alive for up to one week this way, while mussels can last for up to three days. Fresh lobster, crab, or previously frozen squid are highly perishable and must be eaten the same day you buy them.

What to Keep on the Kitchen Counter or in the Pantry

Food Item	*Will Last For*
Anchovy paste	Several years; <1 year in fridge after opening
Beans (dried)	1–2 years
Black pepper	1–3 years
Black teas	2 years
Canned tomatoes	1 year
Capers (sealed)	1 year
Chile paste	1+ years
Coffee (ground)	3–5 months

Coffee (whole beans)	9 months
Dried fruits	6–12 months
Dried mushrooms	1+ years
Dried spices	1–3 years
Extra virgin olive oil	2 years
Flour	6 months
Garlic	2 months
Grapefruit	1 week
Green teas	1 year
Honey	2 years
Maple sugar	4 years
Maple syrup	4 years
Miso paste	1+ years; <1 year in fridge after opening
Nuts	6–9 months
Onions	2 months
Oyster sauce	1 year; 6 months after opening
Pasta/noodles	1–2 years
Pine nuts	2 months
Purple potatoes	3 weeks
Rice	6–8 months
Seeds	2–3 months
Shallots	1 month
Soy sauce	Indefinite; 2–3 years after opening
Sriracha sauce	1+ years
Tinned seafood	3+ years
Tomato paste	1+ years; 3 months in fridge after opening
Tomatoes (fresh)	3–4 days
Vinegar	5–10+ years
Whole grains	6 months

Your kitchen has been revamped, your tools acquired, and kitchen techniques sharpened. Now, let's take another look at food. Throughout part 2, you learned about the evidence supporting the health benefit of many foods and beverages. In chapter 11, you got to choose from an evidence-based list of foods to build your personal preference list and selected the foods you like to eat that defend your health. Next, let's have some fun with how we choose foods to cook and eat. I'm going to show you why some foods are truly exceptional and tell you about some foods that you may not yet have tried but would be well worth exploring for those who are open to some experimentation.

CHAPTER 13

Exceptional Foods

I want to tell you about another group of foods, the ones I find exceptional. Everyone has their own definition of exceptional, and your idea
might be shaped by what you've seen in the media. Television shows
follow chefs traveling to foreign lands eating so-called bizarre foods.
Culinary game shows feature unusual secret ingredients. Online wellness
gurus wax on about the latest fad food from the jungle. Food companies, wellness pundits, and restaurant chains push ingredients branded
as superfoods. The appeal of the exceptional is understandable, but we
should rely on science and evidence, not commercial messages to decide
which foods stand out. The goal is to choose substance over style.

In this chapter, I'm going to give you a rundown on some of the foods
that I consider exceptional, based on their culinary and health virtues.
Think of this as a deep-cut version of the *Eat to Beat Disease* playlist. I
encourage you to seek them out and give them a try. Not only can these
foods easily fit into your 5 × 5 × 5 framework, but they will also open
both your mind and your palate to exciting new flavors.

In my collection of exceptional foods, I'm presenting foods sorted
into four categories. The first is "Global Finds," which includes lesser-
known foods that you might not yet have encountered, much less tried.
These are delicacies in certain regional food cultures that could surprise
and delight you if you tasted them expertly prepared.

Next, we go to "Jaw-Droppers," foods whose benefits are surprising,
or even astonishing. Many of these foods are not usually associated with

health, but the science now says otherwise. The benefits will truly make your jaw drop, and you'll learn some cool facts that you can use to wow friends and colleagues at your next social gathering.

From there I'll introduce you to "Grand Slammers." These are the foods I've mentioned in this book that hit not just one or two but *all five* of the health defense systems. Eating these is equivalent to a home run for your health.

Finally, I'll give you some tips on how to find the greatest versions of already good-for-you foods, what I call "Market Standouts." This section takes you on a virtual tour of the market and tells you how to shop like an expert to get the best of the best.

Global Finds

Everywhere around the world, palates are becoming more sophisticated as cultures blend and new foods are introduced across borders. The result is that in North America, Europe, and Asia today, you can find many foods in your local grocery store that were once considered exotic, such as fish sauce, burrata, and black rice. You may encounter interesting foods yourself on a vacation or a work trip, perhaps by chance or because a friend, colleague, or local encouraged you to expand your horizons and try something new.

Even if you are not a jetsetter, online videos, cooking shows, pop-up restaurants, and even food trucks are giving us access to tastes that most people would never have encountered a generation ago. These foods offer you the chance to take culinary adventures. Here are some interesting foods from culinary traditions around the world that are exceptional not only because of their delicious taste but also because science supports their health benefits:

Squash blossoms. During the summer months, this blossom, sometimes called a zucchini flower, can be found in farmers markets. The entire flower is edible and has a slightly sweet taste. Used in salads or soups, added to pasta, or stuffed and baked, the flower contains a natural bioactive called spinasterol that protects DNA against mutations, aids immunity, and kills breast and ovarian cancer cells.[1]

Persimmons. A sweet fruit resembling a tomato, the persimmon originated in China but became popular in the Mediterranean and Turkey and is now found around the world. It is the national fruit of Japan. There are different varieties of persimmon, and one of them, called Hachiya, becomes so soft and sweet when ripe that you can eat it like a custard, using a spoon. Extracts from persimmon have been shown to kill colon cancer and prostate cancer cells.[2]

Fresh wasabi. The edible part of a Japanese relative of horseradish, real wasabi is a stem called a rhizome that grows underground and is harvested by hand in the spring or early fall. The stem is finely grated to create wasabi paste, a delicate and fragrantly spicy condiment that enhances the flavor of sushi. Wasabi extracts have been shown to kill breast, colon, and liver cancer cells.[3] (Note: the green mound typically served with sushi in restaurants is not real wasabi, but an imitation made with powdered horseradish colored with green food dye.)

Bitter melon. Thin-skinned, cucumber shaped, and either warty or spikey in appearance, the bitter melon is a prized gourd used in Chinese, Indian, Indonesian, and Caribbean cuisine, as well as for herbal healing. Its unique, bitter flavor mellows dramatically with cooking and somehow enhances the flavors of other ingredients in the dish. Bitter is often better when it comes to health benefits, and the bioactives of this melon that are responsible for its taste have been shown to kill colon cancer and breast cancer cells, lower cholesterol, and improve blood sugar levels in diabetes.[4] This is not a vegetable for you to solo cook as a novice at home. Your first taste of bitter melon is best experienced at a restaurant or at the home of a friend who knows how to prepare it.

Fiddleheads. The edible, green coiled tendrils of young ferns appear at the market for a few short weeks in early spring in some parts of the world. Named after the curved ornamental scroll at the head of a fiddle, they are, like other living foods, chock-full of bioactives that activate your health defense systems, including your stem cells and microbiome.[5] They can be sautéed with some extra virgin olive oil, or eaten raw sliced in a salad. Just make sure you wash the forest soil off before using them.

Truffles. These are another treat from the forest. If you want to treat yourself to something really special, try having some fresh truffle shaved on your pasta, rice, vegetables, fish, or poultry. These lumpy, bumpy, golf-ball-shaped delicacies (after which the chocolate version was named) are underground fungi foraged by pigs and dogs in France, Italy, and Spain during the fall and winter. Truffles release an unmistakable scent, which results from natural chemicals resembling human pheromones. They also contain an immune booster called anandamide that does double duty as a neurotransmitter. Remarkably, anandamide activates the same reward centers in the brain stimulated by cannabis that produce a sense of euphoria.[6] Other bioactives in truffles protect DNA and improve muscle function and energy metabolism.[7] As one of the most expensive foods on the planet, truffles are a rare treat worth a splurge if you get the chance.

Now a few global finds from the sea that light up your taste buds as well as your health defense systems:

Bottarga. Bottarga is the salty dried roe of a fish called the gray mullet found in the Mediterranean. The classic version from Sardinia is called bottarga di muggine and can be found in Italian specialty stores. It's a true delicacy grated like cheese over pasta or rice and it adds a rich briny seafood flavor to any dish. Like most fish eggs, bottarga is a source of omega-3 PUFAs. There's an added benefit: extracts from this delicacy have been shown in the lab to kill colon cancer cells.[8]

Squid ink. Most cephalopods (squid, cuttlefish, octopus) squirt a black ink to escape predators. This ink is collected by fishermen from a sac in the creature's body and is a flavorsome delicacy used to make rice and pasta dishes in the seaside cuisine of the Mediterranean. Some famous dishes featuring the ink include Spain's black rice (arroz negra), Venice's risotto di nero di seppia, and black spaghetti known as pasta al nero.[9] Lab research on the ink has shown it can have antioxidant, anti-angiogenic, stem cell–protecting, and immune-enhancing effects.[10] Squid ink can even protect the gut microbiome against the side effects of cancer chemotherapy.[11]

Razor clams. If you are a shellfish aficionado, you'll really love razor clams. These unusual clams are named for their resemblance to an old-fashioned barber's straight razor. About six to ten inches in length, they are sold live in fish markets around the world and can be simply steamed or cooked a la plancha with some olive oil, garlic, and white wine. You never need to deshell them by hand because when they are cooked, their shells pop wide open, brimming with juice and the easy-to-remove clam body. The meat of the razor clam is sweet and mouthwatering. In the lab, extracts from the meat obtained by soaking in hot water have been found to increase the production of antibodies from immune cells, while being capable of directly killing breast and liver cancer cells.[12]

Jaw-Droppers

Research on food and health sometimes leads to jaw-dropping discoveries. Some studies even reveal that foods once scorned as completely unhealthy or considered guilty pleasures actually may have health benefits and deserve another look. The beauty of science is that it allows us to open our minds to whatever the evidence shows us. Sometimes this gives us an entirely new perspective on foods. The following are not recommendations, but simply the surprising facts from research:

Beer. Overindulgence of any alcoholic beverages is harmful to your health defenses, and beer does deliver a load of calories you probably don't need.[13] But, beer contains bioactives that float into the liquid during its fermentation. One of them, xanthohumol, has anticancer effects, is antiangiogenic, and can retard the growth of fat cells (yes, actually).[14] An epidemiological study of 107,998 people showed that drinking beer is associated with a reduced risk for kidney cancer.[15] The nonalcoholic part of beer also stimulates stem cells that are good for the heart, as we saw in chapter 7.[16]

Cheese. Cheese does contain saturated fat and can be high in salt, which pose health dangers on their own. But studies of tens of thousands of people in Sweden have shown that eating *small amounts* of cheese (up to six slices per day) is associated with a reduced risk for heart attack.[17] A major study in Germany of 24,340 people found that eating the equivalent of two slices of hard cheese, like Gouda, Jarlsberg, Emmenthal, or Edam, each day was associated with a reduced risk of lung cancer and prostate cancer.[18] These benefits, as noted in chapter 6, are linked to the vitamin K2, which is found in hard cheeses. Other cheeses like Parmigiano-Reggiano, cheddar, and Camembert supply healthy gut bacteria for your microbiome.

Chocolate. As a sweet, chocolate is a confection that contains saturated fat and processed sugar, two ingredients that are not healthy. But dark chocolate contains high amounts of cocoa solids, the core ingredient that does deliver a number of health benefits. A greater percentage of cacao along with less sugar and little dairy is what makes dark chocolate a healthier confection. Consuming dark chocolate has been found to lower risk of heart disease and diabetes, protect your DNA, and improve gut bacteria.[19] As we saw in chapter 7, drinking hot chocolate made with high concentrations of cocoa can increase your stem cells and improve blood flow. It can even switch cells in your immune system from a proinflammatory to an anti-inflammatory state.[20]

Prosciutto and jamón. Processed meats are definitely not healthy food choices. While willpower and self-discipline are virtues, some people just can't stop themselves from eating bacon. If you must have ham to enjoy your quality of life, remember from chapter 6 that jamón Ibérico de bellota from Spain is made from pigs fed on acorns, and Italian prosciutto di Parma is made from pigs fed on the whey of Parmigiano-Reggiano cheese (beneficial to gut bacteria) and chestnuts. Both acorns and chestnuts contain omega-3 PUFAs. For your health, you should minimize your intake of all meats, especially processed meat (there are no human studies supporting the health benefit of eating any processed meat), but it is surprising that these two specialty hams do offer some healthy fat.

Spicy food. There was a time when spicy food was considered a health hazard, if only due to the potential for heartburn. But research led to a complete rethink about the heat-generating, health-promoting properties of capsaicin found in chile peppers, both fresh and dried. A massive study from China, where entire regions eat fiery cuisine, showed that eating spicy food at least once a day was associated with a reduced risk of death from any cause, including cancer, heart disease, stroke, diabetes, respiratory disease, and infections.[21] Your gut bacteria also like the heat. Research has shown that a chile-fed microbiome can ward off inflammation and obesity.[22]

Purple potato. These distinct potatoes with inky-colored skins and blue-purple interiors are now found in modern markets and on restaurant menus. The healthiest way to eat them is probably roasted or boiled, and sliced into a salad. But scientists in the lab have found that purple potatoes are antiangiogenic, and they can kill cancer stem cells. The anticancer effects are preserved whether the purple potato is boiled, baked, or cooked as potato chips.[23]

Tree nuts. Nuts (almonds, cashews, chestnuts, macadamias, pecans, pine nuts, pistachios, and walnuts) by themselves are not jaw-dropping— we know eating them is good for you. But what they can do to change your fate from cancer is jaw dropping. One major European study showed that consuming one and a half servings of tree nuts (twenty-two walnut halves) per day was associated with a 31 percent reduced risk of developing colon cancer.[24] Even more stunning was the study from thirteen major cancer centers, including Harvard University, Duke University, the University of California, San Francisco, and the University of Chicago, that showed eating just two servings of tree nuts per week was associated with a whopping 53 percent reduction in the risk of death in patients with stage 3 colon cancer who were being treated conventionally with chemotherapy.[25]

Grand Slammers

Throughout this book you've seen how more than two hundred specific foods can activate one or more of your health defense systems. If you have sharp eyes, you've noticed some foods appear more than once across the chapters because they influence more than one defense system. I've pulled them together into a list of all-star foods that hit all five of the health defense systems at once. Like a baseball player hitting a home run with the bases loaded, these foods cover all the bases—thus I call them the Grand Slammers.

I am often asked if there were just one food I would recommend for someone to eat, what would that one be? There's never just one solution when it comes to food. But, if I had to choose for myself (and I do every day), I would select from this list.

GRAND SLAMMERS

Fruits		Vegetables	Beverages
Apricots	Mangoes	Bamboo shoots	Black tea
Blueberries	Nectarines	Carrots	Chamomile tea
Cherries	Peaches	Eggplant	Coffee
Kiwifruit	Plums	Fiddleheads	Green tea
Lychee		Kale	

Nuts/Seeds	Seafood	Oils	Sweets
Flax seed	Squid ink	Olive oil (EVOO)	Dark chocolate
Pumpkin seeds			
Sesame seeds			
Sunflower seeds			
Walnuts			

Keep in mind there are many other health-defense-promoting foods and ingredients that can be eaten alongside these Grand Slammers, so I recommend not getting too focused on them and try combining different foods to mix things up and keep your diet interesting and diverse. The Grand Slammers, however, will be great foods to regularly include in your PFL as you plan your week. If you are focused on a specific disease, and want a refresher on which specific diseases the Grand Slammers have been shown to influence, see the chart on page 349 in chapter 15, or refer to chapters 6 through 10 to see how each defense system connects with specific diseases.

Note that this chart lists only foods that are mentioned throughout part 2. As the science progresses, additional research will expand this list, and I encourage you to sign up on my website (www.drwilliamli.com) to get the latest updates on new data and new foods joining the list.

Market Standouts

Shopping at the grocery store or market can seem repetitive, and it's easy to get stuck in a rut. Even though the aisles and stands are rich with choices, somehow you tend to always go for the old standbys. If this describes your experience, you may find that buying food is boring. You know there have to be other, better choices, but maybe aren't sure which ones to choose. The PFL you've created will give an array of colorful and delicious choices. But I'm going to take you on a virtual tour of the grocery store and market and point out the standouts that I look for myself when I shop. To have a little knowledge and focus on the best choices to take home can really expand your horizons. My philosophy is, when it comes to food, great is better than just good.

Produce. Always look for seasonal fresh foods, because they will represent the best quality of what is in the market. Everything in the produce aisle is plant-based, and there are so many choices that you can always find some new things to try. Among the vegetables, if you're tired of kale, try the many varieties of chicory. This is a big category of healthy greens, including Belgian endive, escarole, frisée, punterelle, radicchio, and tardivo di Treviso. These all have bioactives with cancer-fighting properties and can add interest and variety to your eating experience.[26] There are plenty of YouTube videos showing you how to cook with chicory, including sautéing, roasting, stewing, and other techniques with delicious recipes.

Tomatoes are a great source of health defense activating bioactives, but some are greater than others. For high lycopene levels, look for: San Marzano tomatoes, cherry tomatoes, red black-skin tomatoes, and Tangerine tomatoes.[27] If you are looking for other great sources of lycopene, consider watermelon and papaya. Some papayas even have higher levels of lycopene than tomatoes.[28]

When it comes to choosing fruit, the varieties of apples available during the fall can be dizzying. The ones with the highest levels of health-promoting polyphenols are Granny Smith, Red Delicious, and the Reinette. I specifically look for these when I choose great-tasting apples for health.

In the section with mushrooms, go for fresh, whole mushrooms with stems that are sitting in wooden baskets. Avoid the packaged pre-sliced mushroom tops because their bioactives break down faster than whole mushrooms. Chanterelles, morels, porcini (cepes), maitake, and shiitake (fresh or dried) are my standouts for taste, but don't forget that the common white button is a great healthy choice.

Seafood. Everyone knows that salmon is healthy, but if you want more variety than just salmon, or simply don't like its taste, try other seafood that are high in omega-3 PUFAs. I have researched multiple international databases for the levels of omega-3 PUFAs in seafood, and some of my favorite choices with the high levels are: Manila clams, yellowtail (also known as amberjack, not a type of tuna), sea bass, bluefin tuna, and cockles (a type of small clam). Also, don't forget about the benefits of oysters if you can get fresh ones, because of their DNA-protecting and immune-boosting properties.

When you are in the seafood section of the market, keep in mind that some of the most popular large fish, such as tuna and swordfish, can contain high levels of mercury. If you are an ardent sushi eater and love tuna, you might even want to get your mercury levels checked. Pregnant women should, in general, be very cautious about eating sushi for this reason.

Don't overlook tinned fish, which tend to be smaller mercury-free fish loaded with omega-3s. The highest-quality traditional tinned fish are made in Spain, Portugal, and France, but these are exported and can be found in many markets around the world. They are usually found along with canned goods in the middle of the store. The most common tinned fish containing the highest levels of omega-3 are salmon, mackerel, tuna, sardines, and anchovies.

SEAFOOD HIGH IN HEALTHY FATS

High level omega-3 PUFA (>0.5 g/100 g of seafood)		
Anchovies	Gray mullet	Redfish
Arctic char	Hake	Salmon
Bigeye tuna	Halibut	Sardine
Black bass	John Dory	Sea bream
Bluefin tuna	Mackerel	Sea cucumber
Bluefish	Manila clam	Spiny lobster
Bottarga	Mediterranean sea bass	Swordfish
Caviar (sturgeon)	Pacific oysters	Yellowtail
Cockles	Pompano	
Eastern oysters	Rainbow trout	
Fish roe (salmon)	Red mullet	

Olive oil. By now, you know that extra virgin olive oil is the best to use for low-heat cooking, as an accompaniment to food, and for salad dressing. But when most people buy olive oil, they choose the brand that's most familiar to them. But not all olive oils have the same levels of bioactives, and I look for the oils made from one of three monovarietals that are high in polyphenols: Koroneiki, Picual, and Moraiolo. The next time you stand in front of dozens of types of olive oil, pick up the bottle and inspect the label carefully to look for the type of olives used to make the oil.

*   *   *

The foods you've just read about are some of the exceptionals I believe are worth knowing about and trying. They not only support your health defenses but also can excite your taste buds. They can add a sense of adventure to your diet. When you try something new, and you discover you love its taste, add it to your PFL so it can be part of your personal food repertoire. Feel free, of course, to venture beyond the foods in this chapter—explore new foods to find ones that bring you joy.

At this point, you are solidly armed with knowledge of your health defense systems. You have chosen a list of your own preferred defense-boosting foods. You've learned about the repertoire of techniques and ingredients for your home kitchen. You have seen some surprising and exceptional foods. Now is the time to put it all together and start eating! In the next chapter, I will share recipes using the delicious foods in this book and a sample meal plan. My goal is to inspire you with options so you can make this simple, flexible way of eating a satisfying and tasty approach for the rest of your life.

CHAPTER 14

Sample Meal Guide and Recipes

Freedom to choose is a wonderful thing, but it can become overwhelming when you're doing something new. *New* doesn't have to mean *intimidating* or *confusing*. It is helpful to have a guide or a template to follow while you become familiar and comfortable in creating your own approach to healing eating using the 5 × 5 × 5 framework. This chapter provides guidance and inspiration, so you can practice implementing the framework into your life.

I've put together some delicious recipes that include many of the tastiest health-promoting foods I enjoy so that you can use them to start preparing some delicious eat to beat disease dishes.

Sample 5 × 5 × 5 Framework Meal Guide

The sample meal guide is not meant to be followed as gospel. Its purpose is to demonstrate a few versions of what the 5 × 5 × 5 framework can look like in real life. You will see how to create different options for eating, and can begin practicing using the sample guide.

You will only be effective in eating to beat disease if you have a plan you can follow. Your plan has to account for the realities of day-to-day life, which is why rigid diets are so difficult to sustain. For this reason, I deliberately designed the 5 × 5 × 5 framework to allow for the fact that, despite our best intentions, our days and weeks don't always go according to plan. Each day is at least a little different from the day before. Things crop up, and schedules get interrupted or have to change.

Remember this, even as you practice the sample plan and try the recipes: the only prime directive of the 5 × 5 × 5 framework is that you eat at least five health-defending foods per day and to make sure that your choices touch each of the five defense systems at least once. That's it. Beyond this one rule, you can adapt the framework to any situation, and practice the method any way you want. Of course, you should cut down on the foods that you know are unhealthy for you, but my emphasis is always focus on the good to displace the bad. It's a good general philosophy when it comes to life.

How to Read the Sample Meal Guide:

- Each column represents a hypothetical day of the week.
- At the top of each column is a list of the five selected foods for the day and its associated property: A = angiogenesis, R = regeneration, M = microbiome, I = immunity, D = DNA protection.
- When you look closely, you'll notice that some days, the five foods are spread out across all five meals, while other days, they are concentrated into two or three. This is to demonstrate how you can flexibly fit this framework into any day, anywhere you are, no matter what is going on.

SUNDAY	MONDAY	TUESDAY
Five Daily Foods	**Five Daily Foods**	**Five Daily Foods**
• Nectarines (A) • Dark chocolate (R) • Broccoli stems (M) • Salmon (D) • Tomatoes (I)	• Chicken thighs (A) • Green tea (R) • Sourdough bread (M) • Walnuts (D) • Orange (I)	• Capers (A) • Whole wheat (R) • Pomegranate juice (M) • Tomato (D) • Dark chocolate (I)
Breakfast Nectarine with yogurt	**Breakfast**	**Breakfast** Dark chocolate breakfast bar Pomegranate juice
Lunch Broccoli stem and oregano soup	**Lunch**	**Lunch**
Snack Homemade tomato salsa + toasted sourdough bread	**Snack** Orange + walnuts Green tea	**Snack**
Dinner Baked salmon	**Dinner** Chicken curry + sourdough bread	**Dinner** Fresh tomato sauce with whole wheat pasta topped with capers
Dessert Healthy chocolate mousse	**Dessert**	**Dessert**

WEDNESDAY	THURSDAY	FRIDAY	SATURDAY
Five Daily Foods	**Five Daily Foods**	**Five Daily Foods**	**Five Daily Foods**
• Halibut (A) • Soy (R) • Gouda (M) • Oolong tea (D) • Dark Chocolate (I)	• Tofu (A) • Chinese celery (R) • Shiitake mushrooms (M) • Mangoes (D) • Chile peppers (I)	• Walnuts (A) • Purple potatoes (R) • Sourdough bread (M) • Tomato (D) • Kale (I)	• Chicken (A) • Oysters (R) • Yogurt (M) • Kiwifruit (D) • Coffee (I)
Breakfast Oolong tea	**Breakfast**	**Breakfast**	**Breakfast** Yogurt with kiwifruit Coffee
Lunch Salad with Gouda cheese	**Lunch**	**Lunch** Summer vegetable stew (contains tomato and kale) Sourdough bread	**Lunch** Half platter of Pacific oysters
Snack Dark chocolate breakfast bar (leftovers)	**Snack**	**Snack**	**Snack**
Dinner Steamed halibut with ginger, soy sauce, sesame oil, and scallions	**Dinner** Stir-fry with tofu, shiitake mushroom, chiles, and Chinese celery	**Dinner** Walnut pesto, and purple potato gnocchi	**Dinner** Chicken with mint and fish sauce
Dessert	**Dessert** Mango	**Dessert**	**Dessert**

In the rest of this chapter, I share with you twenty-four recipes containing eat-to-beat-disease foods. I want to show you it's possible to use and combine ingredients in ways that are incredibly delicious. All of these recipes have been tested, and they can all be prepared in thirty minutes or less (some recipes require additional unsupervised cooking time to complete).

Like the foods in this book, these recipes draw upon techniques and flavors from different cultures and culinary traditions: Mediterranean and Asian are strong influences, because these regions favor plant-based, fresh, whole foods, prepared with simple cooking methods, using healthy oils low in saturated fat. From part 2 of this book, you'll recognize broccoli stems, dark chocolate, chestnuts, cooked tomato, walnuts, chicken thighs, and more. All of these recipes can be made easily with the kitchen tools described in chapter 12. These are the kinds of recipes that I enjoy cooking and sharing with family and friends.

That said, I want you to view the sample meal guide and the recipes only as a starting point, not a destination. The principle of the $5 \times 5 \times 5$ framework is that it is easily adaptable to your real life and encourages you to explore. Even though we have discussed more than two hundred foods in this book, there are many more foods that can promote good health. If you spot an ingredient that intrigues you at the grocery store or market, I encourage you to give it a try. If it's not already mentioned in this book, I suggest you look it up to see whether it affects a defense system and which health benefits it has.

Here is how you can look it up like a pro. Get online and go to PubMed. This is an amazing search engine that taps into a gigantic research database maintained by the United States National Library of Medicine at the National Institutes of Health. PubMed accesses over 28 million scientific studies. It is free to use and accessible to the public at https://www.ncbi.nlm.nih.gov/pubmed, where you can search through a treasure trove of data. PubMed contains brief abstracts of almost every credible publication, which will tell you about the basic premise, methods, and conclusions of the study, so you can quickly get a sense for what health benefits a food may have.

Here's how you can use it. Type into the search bar the name of the food you are interested in and another search term related to the defense systems, like "angiogenesis" or "regeneration" or "stem cell" or "microbiome" or "DNA" or "immune." PubMed will search its 28 million research articles and return any studies that contain those key words.

I'll help you keep up with the growing list of foods that I've analyzed by adding them to a regularly updated preferred foods checklist, which you can get at: www.drwilliamli.com/checklist.

You can also greatly expand on the recipes given here by going online and searching the ingredients in your preferred food list for recipes. Just go to your favorite search engine and enter the name of the food and "recipe" and you'll be presented with a number of recipes. Just be discriminating. Choose recipes that use healthy ingredients and cooking techniques.

Here are the recipes I'm sharing with you to get started.

Recipes List

Recipes

Dark Chocolate Breakfast Bar

A breakfast bar that stimulates your microbiome and stem cells is a good way to start the day—especially if it is made with dark chocolate.

Servings: 12 bars
Cooking Time: 15–20 minutes
Prep Time: 15 minutes, plus 2–3 hours cooling time

Ingredients:
½ cup cashews, roughly chopped (can be omitted if nut allergies)

2 cups old-fashioned or quick-cooking oats

¼ teaspoon sea salt

¼ cup organic dried apricots, chopped

¼ cup organic dried mango, chopped

¼ cup organic dried cranberries

¼ cup organic dried blueberries

½ cup mini dark chocolate chips (70% or greater cacao) or chopped dark chocolate

½ cup whole dates (approximately 6–7 large), pitted and roughly chopped

¼ cup maple syrup

½ teaspoon vanilla extract

Preparation:

Preheat the oven to 350°F.

In a large mixing bowl combine the cashews, oats, and salt. Add the apricots, mango, cranberries, blueberries, and chocolate and mix well. To the bowl of a food processor add the dates, maple syrup, and vanilla, and puree until smooth. If the mixture is too thick or chunky, add warm water one spoonful at a time to obtain a smooth consistency similar to applesauce. Pour the date-maple puree over the oat and fruit mixture and mix thoroughly until all ingredients are coated and sticky.

Add the mixture to a parchment-lined 8- or 9-inch square baking pan and press firmly with your fingers or the back of a spatula. It is important to press mixture *firmly* before baking. Place on the middle rack of the oven and bake for 15–20 minutes, until the edges just start to brown. Remove and cool completely on a cooling rack, and then place in the refrigerator to set, approximately 2–3 hours or overnight, before cutting into individual bars. Store covered in the refrigerator.

Ginger Orange Hot Chocolate

Drinking hot cocoa made with dark chocolate can increase your body's ability to regenerate itself by increasing stem cells circulating in your blood. The most important part is using dark chocolate. This recipe was prepared for me by my good friend and chocolatier extraordinaire Katrina Markoff, with whom I have collaborated on creating chocolates containing unique combinations of healthy ingredients.

Servings: Four 6-ounce servings
Cooking Time: 5 minutes
Prep Time: 5 minutes

Ingredients:

3 cups almond, coconut, oat, or cows' milk
3 ounces (½ cup) 72% dark chocolate
1 ounce (¼ cup) cocoa powder
¼ teaspoon dried ginger or ½ teaspoon freshly grated ginger
1 4-inch furl of orange peel
1 tablespoon coconut sugar (optional)
Whipped Coconut Cream (optional; recipe follows)

Preparation:

Add the milk, chocolate, cocoa, ginger, orange peel, and sugar, if using, to a small saucepan. Place on medium heat and stir until well dissolved and all the chocolate is melted. Remove the orange peel and serve.

Top with homemade Whipped Coconut Cream, if desired.

Whipped Coconut Cream

1 14-ounce can coconut cream or milk
2 tablespoons agave syrup
½ teaspoon vanilla extract
Pinch of sea salt

Chill the coconut cream/milk in the refrigerator overnight, being sure not to shake or tip the can so you achieve a strong separation of the cream and liquid. The next day, chill a large mixing bowl 10 minutes before whipping. Remove the coconut cream/milk from the fridge without tipping or shaking and remove the lid. Scrape out the thickened cream from the top and reserve the remaining liquid for use in smoothies or your drinking chocolate above. Place the hardened cream in the chilled mixing bowl. Beat for 45 seconds with an electric mixer until creamy. Then add the agave syrup, vanilla, and salt and mix until creamy, 1 minute more. Taste and adjust sweetness as needed.

Use immediately or refrigerate—it will become quite firm in the fridge the longer it's chilled. It will keep for up to 1 week.

Warm Carrot Top Salad

A cumin-scented warm salad made with antiangiogenic carrot tops and shiitake mushrooms, with the sweet tang of cherry tomatoes.

Servings: 4
Cooking Time: 15 minutes
Prep Time: 15 minutes

Ingredients:

1 bunch carrot tops, tender leaves chopped into 1–2-inch lengths; discard tough stems

2 tablespoons extra virgin olive oil, plus more for garnish

½ medium onion, diced

2 cloves garlic, minced

1 cup shiitake mushrooms caps and stems, thinly sliced

½ teaspoon sea salt, plus more for garnish

½ teaspoon crushed red pepper flakes (optional)

½ teaspoon ground cumin

1 cup cherry tomatoes, halved

Grated zest of one lemon

Freshly ground black pepper, to taste

Preparation:

Arrange the carrot tops in a large serving bowl or platter and set aside. Heat the olive oil in a sauté pan over medium-high heat. Add the onion and garlic and cook until translucent, fragrant, and lightly golden brown, about 2–3 minutes. Add the mushrooms and cook until soft, about 3–5 minutes longer. Add the sea salt, red pepper flakes, if using, and cumin. Add the tomatoes and sauté until softened. Pour the cooked vegetable mixture over the carrot tops and toss to combine and wilt leaves. Season with salt, pepper, lemon zest, and a drizzle of extra virgin olive oil. Serve immediately.

Classic Lemon Vinaigrette Dressing

Salads can be made with interesting combinations of greens, herbs, and cut vegetables. Whatever you choose, the right dressing can make all the difference between a great versus just a good salad. You can easily add many healthy additions from the preferred food list to any salad.

Servings: 4–6
Cooking Time: 0 minutes
Prep Time: 5 minutes

Ingredients:
I small clove garlic, minced
I salt-packed anchovy, rinsed
½ lemon, juiced
I teaspoon Dijon mustard
¼ cup extra virgin olive oil
Freshly cracked black pepper, to taste
Sea salt, to taste

Preparation:
Using a mortar and pestle (or a small bowl and back of a spoon), smash the garlic and anchovy together into a paste. Add the lemon juice and mustard, and mix. Pour in the olive oil, whisking to blend the ingredients. Grind in some fresh black pepper to taste. Add a pinch of salt. The dressing can be stored in a container if you bring your lunch to work and poured over the salad during the meal.

Roasted Mushrooms

A perfect way to enjoy a mélange of immune-boosting mushrooms that benefit your microbiome and help your angiogenesis defenses, too.

Servings: 4
Cooking Time: 30 minutes
Prep Time: 10 minutes

Ingredients:

2 pounds mushrooms (white button, shiitake, cremini, chanterelle, morel, maitake, and/or porcini), both caps and stems, cleaned and thickly sliced on the diagonal

¼ cup extra virgin olive oil

4 cloves garlic, minced

Freshly cracked black pepper, to taste

6–8 sprigs of thyme or rosemary

Sea salt, to taste

1 sprig Italian parsley, finely chopped

Preparation:

Preheat oven to 450°F. In a large mixing bowl, combine the mushrooms, olive oil, garlic, and black pepper and lightly stir together. On a large parchment-lined baking sheet or roasting pan, evenly spread the mushroom mixture, top with thyme sprigs, and place in the oven. Roast 25–30 minutes, until the mushrooms are golden brown. Allow to cool slightly, season with salt, sprinkle chopped parsley on top, and serve warm.

Note: Mushrooms should not be washed or soaked in water; to clean, wipe gently with a wet paper towel or kitchen towel. Do not add salt to mushrooms until done cooking.

Grilled Eggplant

Eggplant contains chlorogenic acid which activates your regenerative system and other health defenses. In this recipe, it's grilled first, then it's dressed with many health defense-boosting ingreidents that lend incredible flavor and bioactives that are absorbed into the flesh, creating a truly mouthwatering and healthy dish.

Servings: 4–6
Grilling Time: 5–6 minutes
Prep Time: 20 minutes, minimum 30 minutes rest time

Ingredients:

4 small or 2 medium eggplants
2 teaspoons fresh oregano, chopped, or 1 teaspoon dried oregano
Large bunch fresh mint leaves, chopped (can use parsley if preferred)
3–4 cloves garlic, finely chopped
Salt, to taste
Crushed red pepper flakes, to taste (optional)
¼ cup extra virgin olive oil
Good-quality balsamic vinegar, to taste
6–8 basil leaves
Chopped olives, to taste (optional)
Capers, to taste (optional)

Preparation:

Heat an outdoor or stovetop grill. Wash and dry the eggplant. Trim and discard the top and bottom ends. Slice the eggplant into ¼-inch slices lengthwise.

Grill the eggplant slices 2–3 minutes per side. When the eggplant is done cooking, place in a single layer in a large casserole dish. Top with the oregano, mint, garlic, salt, and red pepper flakes, if using. Drizzle with olive oil. Top with a very light drizzle of balsamic vinegar. Repeat with up to three layers of eggplant and seasonings.

Cover tightly with plastic wrap and allow the dish to sit at room temperature or in the refrigerator for at least 30 minutes for all flavors to permeate the eggplant. This recipe can also be prepared ahead and refrigerated overnight or stored in the refrigerator in a tightly sealed container for 7–10 days.

To serve: arrange the eggplant slices on a serving platter and top with basil leaves either left whole or julienned. Garnish with olives and/or capers, if desired.

This recipe makes a great appetizer or side dish or can be served over arugula as a salad. The eggplant also can be cut into bite-size pieces before serving and served on toasted bread as a bruschetta.

Broccoli Stem and Oregano Soup

This is a great way to incorporate antiangiogenic broccoli stems and florets into your diet. In this recipe, I've added broccoli sprouts to give it an extra immune system boost.

Serves: 6–8
Cooking Time: 20 minutes
Prep Time: 10 minutes

Ingredients:
1 head broccoli
2 tablespoons extra virgin olive oil
1 medium yellow onion, peeled and chopped
4 cloves garlic, finely chopped
2 teaspoons dried oregano
5 cups vegetable broth
2 cups spinach, rinsed
1 cup flat-leaf parsley, rinsed with the stems removed
Zest of ½ lemon
Kosher salt, to taste

Freshly ground black pepper, to taste

Broccoli sprouts (for garnish; optional)

Preparation:

Remove the broccoli florets from the stalk; set aside. Peel the bark from the broccoli stems and chop the stems into 1-inch cubes. Keep the florets and stems separate.

Heat the olive oil in a large pot over medium-high heat. Add the onions and garlic and cook until translucent and fragrant, about 5 minutes.

Add the chopped broccoli stems and oregano and sauté for 3–5 minutes before adding the vegetable broth. Bring to a boil and reduce to a simmer over medium heat; cook for 10 minutes until the broccoli is tender and set aside.

In a medium pot, bring 4 cups of water to a boil. Blanch the broccoli florets for 2–3 minutes before rapidly transferring to an ice bath to cool. Repeat this process with the spinach and parsley and dry on a kitchen or paper towel.

Add the broccoli stem broth mixture to a blender and begin blending on medium-high speed. Slowly add the drained broccoli, spinach, and parsley and blend on high speed until smooth and vibrant green. Season with salt and pepper to taste and garnish with lemon zest and broccoli sprouts.

Chestnut Soup

A delicious way to get ellagic acid from chestnuts, this soup is comfort food for autumn. You can serve this with sautéed mushrooms and crusty sourdough bread.

Servings: 4
Cooking Time: 30 minutes
Prep Time: 10 minutes

Ingredients:

2 tablespoons extra virgin olive oil, plus more for garnish
1 large shallot, chopped
2 ribs of celery with leafy tops, chopped
1 medium carrot, chopped
1 clove garlic, chopped
2 sprigs thyme, leaves picked
3 fresh or 1 dried bay leaf, left whole to be removed later
Sea salt, to taste
Black pepper, to taste
1½ cups cooked chestnuts
4 cups vegetable stock

Preparation:

Heat the extra virgin olive oil in a medium saucepan over medium-high heat. Add the shallot, celery, carrots, garlic, thyme, bay leaf, salt, and pepper and sauté until fragrant, about 5–7 minutes. Add the chestnuts and stir well to combine. Add the vegetable stock, bring to a boil, and then reduce heat and simmer over medium heat for 20 minutes. Remove the bay leaves. Using an immersion blender, process the soup until smooth and creamy. Season with salt and pepper to taste. Top bowls of soup with a light drizzle of good-quality extra virgin olive oil.

Mushroom Soup

This warm and comforting soup can be made with a variety of immune-boosting mushrooms that add savory umami flavors. Be creative and get a range of mushrooms to experiment with using this basic recipe.

Servings: 4

Cooking Time: 30 minutes

Prep Time: 10 minutes

Ingredients:

2 tablespoons extra virgin olive oil

1 large shallot, chopped

4 cloves garlic, minced

1 pound mushrooms (button, shiitake, chanterelle, cremini, and/or oyster), chopped

3–4 sprigs thyme, leaves picked

Sea salt, to taste

4 cups vegetable stock

Black pepper, to taste

¼ cup Italian parsley, chopped

Preparation:

In a medium saucepan, heat the olive oil over medium-high heat and sauté the shallot and garlic until fragrant, about 4–5 minutes. Add the mushrooms and thyme leaves, and season with a dash of sea salt. Sauté until golden brown, about 4–5 minutes. Set aside a few attractive mushroom pieces to garnish the soup when serving. Add the stock and simmer for an additional 15–20 minutes. Using an immersion blender or regular blender, process the soup until smooth in consistency. Season with salt and pepper to taste. Garnish with the reserved mushroom pieces and chopped parsley.

Pumpkin Soup

A classic autumn soup wherever pumpkins (called potimarron in Europe) can be found.

Servings: 4

Cooking Time: 45 minutes

Prep Time: 10 minutes

Ingredients:

2–3 small sugar pumpkins, or 2½ cups organic pumpkin puree (2 15-ounce cans)

2–3 tablespoons extra virgin olive oil

Sea salt, to taste

2 cloves garlic, chopped

1 medium white onion, chopped

¼ teaspoon black pepper

½ teaspoon cardamom

½ teaspoon cinnamon

½ teaspoon turmeric

¼ teaspoon nutmeg

2 cups vegetable stock

1 cup coconut milk

Pumpkin seeds, to taste

Preparation:

Line a baking sheet with parchment paper and preheat the oven to 350°F. Prepare the pumpkins by cutting them in half and removing the seeds and strings. Drizzle with extra virgin olive oil, season with sea salt, and place facedown on the baking sheet. Bake for 30–45 minutes until a knife can be easily inserted into the flesh of the pumpkins. Wait until they're cool enough to handle, and then peel. Set aside.

Heat the olive oil in a medium pot over medium-high heat. Sauté the garlic and onion, season with pepper and ¼ teaspoon salt, and cook until fragrant, about 2–3 minutes. Add the cardamom, cinnamon, turmeric, and nutmeg, and stir well to combine. Add the pumpkin flesh and mix well to coat and combine. Add the stock and coconut milk and simmer until hot and bubbling. Using an immersion blender, process the soup until smooth and creamy. Season with sea salt to taste. Sprinkle with pumpkin seeds.

Roasted Purple Potato Soup

Potato soup never tasted so good. The natural dye in purple potatoes kills cancer stem cells and is antiangiogenic. This soup can be served with a dollop of yogurt to help your microbiome.

Servings: 4
Cooking Time: 45 minutes
Prep Time: 10 minutes

Ingredients:
1 pound (4–6 medium) purple potatoes, peeled and cut into 1-inch pieces
3 tablespoons extra virgin olive oil, divided
Sea salt, to taste
Freshly ground black pepper
½ small red onion or 1 large shallot, diced
2 cloves garlic, minced
1 rib celery with leafy top, chopped
2 small stalks rosemary, left whole for removal later
4–6 cups vegetable broth
Finely chopped parsley or dill
Yogurt (for garnish; optional)

Preparation:
Heat oven to 400°F. Place the potatoes on a large baking sheet, either nonstick or lined with parchment or nonstick foil. Drizzle with 1 tablespoon of the extra virgin olive oil and season with salt and pepper. Roast until the potatoes start to caramelize and become tender, about 25–30 minutes.

In a medium stockpot, heat the remaining 2 tablespoons of olive oil over medium-high heat. Add the onion and sauté for 1–2 minutes. Add the garlic, celery, and rosemary, season with salt and pepper, and sauté until fragrant and tender, about 4–5 minutes. Add the roasted potatoes and enough broth to generously cover the potatoes. Bring to a boil, then reduce the heat to low and simmer for 8–10 minutes, or until potatoes are tender. Remove the stalks of rosemary and discard. Using an immersion blender, process the soup until smooth and creamy. Season with sea salt to taste. Top with chopped parsley or dill and freshly ground black pepper.

Spoon a generous dollop of yogurt, if using, on top of the soup.

Variation:

Roast chunks of purple carrots and/or purple cauliflower with potatoes.

Summer Vegetable Stew

During the bounty of summer, there's no better way to get the benefits of the many fresh vegetables and herbs available than making a stew. In this power-packed recipe, there are 18 ingredients that boost your health defenses.

Servings: 4–6
Cooking Time: 45 minutes
Prep Time: 30 minutes

Ingredients:

3 tablespoons extra virgin olive oil, plus more for garnish

1 medium onion, chopped

2 ribs celery, cut into 1/2-inch slices

2 carrots with green leafy tops; carrots cut into 1/2-inch cubes, leafy tops roughly chopped

Salt, to taste

2–3 cloves garlic, finely chopped

1/2 teaspoon crushed red pepper flakes or 1 fresh chile pepper split halfway down the middle (optional)

2–3 sprigs fresh oregano, marjoram, or thyme, or any combination

I cup tomato puree (see Fresh Tomato Sauce, p. 332) (can substitute 4–6 fresh plum tomatoes, peeled, seeded, and chopped or I small can chopped tomatoes)

I medium zucchini, cut into ½-inch cubes

2 medium purple potatoes, cut into ½-inch cubes

I small sweet potato, cut into ½-inch cubes

I quart vegetable stock

I dry or 2–3 fresh bay leaves

2 cups dinosaur kale (cavolo nero), chopped

I can cannellini beans, drained and rinsed

10–12 leaves fresh mint or basil, chopped

Toasted sourdough bread

Preparation:

Heat the olive oil in a large stockpot over medium-high heat. Add the onion, celery, and carrots, sprinkle with salt, and cook 3–4 minutes. Add the garlic, red pepper flakes, and oregano. Cook 2–3 minutes longer. Add the tomato puree, season with salt, and simmer for about 5 minutes. Add the zucchini, purple potatoes, sweet potatoes, and the stock. Bring to a boil. Add the bay leaf, reduce the heat, and simmer about 20–25 minutes, until the potatoes are fork-tender. Add the kale, carrot tops, and beans; cook an additional 10 minutes. Remove from the heat. Add the mint and stir. Serve in bowls with a drizzle of extra virgin olive oil and toasted sourdough bread.

Note: Use any combination of preferred herbs and vegetables. Sage and cilantro are other herb options. Other vegetables that work well are summer squash, butternut squash, green beans, golden potatoes, and corn. For a heartier stew, you can add cooked pasta, quinoa, or farro. You can top the stew with fresh avocado cubes and/or your favorite cheese.

Basic Pesto with Trofie

This traditional pasta from Liguria, Italy, simply can't be beat for its amazing taste, simplicity, and its unique combination of bioactives from basil, pine nuts, garlic, olive oil. The pasta is often made with chestnut flour, which gives it an additional health twist.

Servings: 2–3
Cooking Time: 0 minutes
Prep Time: 5 minutes

Ingredients:

2 cups fresh basil leaves, stems removed

¼ cup pine nuts or walnuts

2 small cloves garlic

⅔ cup extra virgin olive oil, divided

⅔ cup grated Parmigiano-Reggiano cheese, plus more for garnish

Sea salt, to taste

1 pound trofie pasta, made with chestnut flour (can be ordered online if your market does not carry it)

Preparation:

In a food processor, combine the basil, nuts, garlic, half of the oil, and half of the cheese. Pulse to combine well. With the processor running slowly, pour in the remaining olive oil in a slow and steady stream. Once it is well incorporated, stop processing and transfer to a bowl. Fold in the remaining cheese. Add a pinch of sea salt to taste, if desired.

Meanwhile, bring a large pot of salted water to a boil. Add the pasta to the boiling water and cook al dente, 1 minute less than package directions. Reserve 1 cup of pasta cooking water before draining pasta in a colander. In a large serving bowl, mix the pasta, pesto, and enough cooking water to evenly coat the pasta. Serve immediately, garnished with additional Parmigiano-Reggiano.

Walnut Pesto

If you thought basil pesto was the best, you should try making it with walnut. Think about all the clinical studies showing that eating walnuts improves health and fights disease.

Servings: 4
Cooking Time: 5 minutes
Prep Time: 15 minutes

Ingredients:

1 slice sourdough bread, crusts removed
½ cup whole milk
1 cup shelled walnuts
2 tablespoons pine nuts
1 clove garlic, peeled and roughly chopped
¼ cup grated Parmigiano-Reggiano
Sprig of fresh marjoram
3 tablespoons extra virgin olive oil
Salt, to taste
Black pepper, to taste

Preparation:

Place the bread in a small bowl. Add the milk and allow the bread to soak for 1–2 minutes. Squeeze the bread gently and add to the bowl of a food processor. Reserve the leftover milk.

To the bowl of the food processor add the walnuts, pine nuts, garlic, cheese, and marjoram. Turn on the food processor and slowly pour in the olive oil. Add the reserved milk as needed to obtain a thick but creamy consistency. Add salt and pepper to taste.

Walnut pesto can be served over pasta or used as a topping on fish, chicken, or vegetables. It can be stored tightly sealed in the refrigerator for 3–4 days; do not freeze.

Note: Walnuts may also be toasted lightly in a sauté pan or in a 375°F oven for 5 minutes for a nuttier flavor. The skins may also be rubbed off toasted walnuts with a clean kitchen towel if desired.

Purple Potato Gnocchi

Another way to make pasta work on behalf of your health. Purple potatoes. Gnocchi. Targets cancer stem cells. Enough said.

Servings: 4
Cooking Time: 40–50 minutes
Prep Time: 30 minutes

Ingredients:
2 pounds purple potatoes
2 cups flour, plus more for dusting
I egg, lightly beaten
½ teaspoon salt
Parmigiano-Reggiano cheese, for garnish

Preparation:
Wash the potatoes. In a large pot with enough water to cover them, boil the potatoes with their skins on until easily pierced with a fork, about 30–40 minutes, depending on the size of the potatoes. Remove the potatoes and drain well. Allow to cool on a clean dishtowel or paper towels.

When the potatoes are cool enough to handle, remove the skins and mash the potatoes. For best results and light, fluffy gnocchi, use a potato ricer or food mill. Spread the mashed potatoes on a large floured surface and allow to cool. Sprinkle about two-thirds of the flour over the potatoes and form a well in the center. Add the egg and salt to the center of the well. Use your hands to combine the ingredients and begin forming the dough. Knead the dough gently, adding the remaining flour a little at a time as needed until the dough sticks together well. Do not overwork the dough or add any extra flour.

Shape the dough into a rectangular loaf. Cut the loaf into 8–10 pieces. Roll each piece on a lightly floured surface into a long rope about ½-inch thick. Cut each rope into 1-inch pieces and set aside.

Gently shake away the excess flour and add the gnocchi to a large pot of boiling salted water. Cook the gnocchi until they float to the top, about 2–4 minutes. Gently remove with a slotted spoon and drain well. Reserve 1 cup of pasta cooking water. Place the gnocchi in a warm serving bowl. Top with walnut pesto or another sauce and mix gently. Add a few spoonfuls of pasta cooking water if needed.

Top with additional grated Parmigiano-Reggiano, if desired.

Note: Gnocchi should be cooked within 30–45 minutes of making them or they will become sticky. If not using immediately, arrange on a floured cookie sheet to prevent sticking and freeze for 2 hours or until completely frozen. Once frozen, move to a freezer-safe container and store in the freezer until ready to use.

Fresh Tomato Sauce with Pasta

This classic tomato and pasta dish emphasizes the freshness of the tomatoes, which have antiangiogenic, microbiome-enhancing, and DNA-protective benefits. Add some grated Parmigiano-Reggiano cheese to garnish.

Servings: 4–6
Cooking Time: 30 minutes
Prep Time: 30–40 minutes

Ingredients:

2–3 pounds firm ripe tomatoes, preferably San Marzano, Roma, or other plum-type tomato

1–2 tablespoons extra virgin olive oil, plus more for garnish

½ small onion, finely chopped

1–2 cloves garlic, finely chopped

½ teaspoon crushed red pepper (optional)

Salt, to taste

3–4 fresh basil leaves, julienned, divided

1 pound whole wheat pasta

Parmigiano-Reggiano cheese, grated (optional)

Preparation—Tomato Puree Method 1 (using a food mill):

Bring a large pot of water to a boil. Wash the tomatoes and cut in half lengthwise. Remove and discard the stems and any loose seeds. Add the tomatoes to boiling water and cook for 4–6 minutes, until tomatoes soften but do not break apart.

Drain the tomatoes in a colander for several minutes, shaking the colander to remove as much excess water as possible.

Place a food mill over a large bowl. Working in batches, scoop the tomatoes into the food mill. Turn the handle of the food mill clockwise to extract tomato puree through the bottom. When finished with each batch, turn the handle counterclockwise to clear out the skins and seeds and discard.

Preparation—Tomato Puree Method 2 (using food processor or blender):

Bring a large pot of water to a boil. Prepare a large bowl of ice water and place next to the stove. Working in batches, add 3–4 tomatoes at a time to the boiling water. Boil for 45–90 seconds, until the skins start to crack. Remove with a slotted spoon and drop into the ice water.

Peel the tomatoes, cut in half lengthwise, and remove stems and all seeds and discard. Place the tomatoes in a colander to drain as much excess water as possible. In batches, add the tomatoes to a food processor or blender and process until smooth.

Preparation—Basic Tomato Sauce:

Heat the olive oil in a large skillet or wide heavy saucepan over medium-high heat. Add the onion and sauté 2–3 minutes. Add the garlic and crushed red pepper, if using, and sauté until the garlic becomes fragrant, but be careful not to brown. Add about 2 cups of tomato puree. Season with salt. Cook the sauce for 20–30 minutes. Add half of the fresh basil. Serve with your favorite pasta (spaghetti suggested). Drizzle a little extra virgin olive oil over the top, sprinkle with the remaining basil, and top with freshly grated Parmigiano-Reggiano, if desired.

Variations:

Mushroom sauce: Add a variety of fresh mushrooms of your choice to the onion-garlic mixture and sauté 2–3 minutes before adding the tomato puree.

Eggplant sauce: Add eggplant cubes (preferably with skin on, but it can be removed if preferred) to the onion-garlic mixture. Add ½ cup water and sauté covered for 4–5 minutes, until the water evaporates, before adding the tomato puree.

Note: You can make bigger batches of tomato puree and store in mason jars following proper canning instructions. Season with salt before adding the sauce to the jars. In a pinch, extra tomato puree can also be frozen. Tomato puree can be used as a quick pizza sauce—just add some olive oil, salt, and oregano to taste.

Pasta with Garlic Scapes and Cherry Tomatoes

Garlic scapes are a summer treat. When caramelized and combined with lycopene-containing cherry tomatoes, they make a light and tasty pasta dish. A squeeze of fresh lemon juice lights up the taste buds and provides a hit of citrus bioactives.

Serves: 2–4

Cooking Time: 15 minutes

Prep Time: 10 minutes

Ingredients:

12 garlic scapes (approximately 6 ounces), cleaned and trimmed into 2-inch pieces, including flowers

4 tablespoons extra virgin olive oil, divided

Salt, to taste

2 pounds cherry tomatoes

12 ounces linguine or other long pasta

Freshly squeezed lemon juice, to taste

1 tablespoon lemon zest

Black pepper, to taste

Fresh whole basil leaves, hand torn in half

Fresh mozzarella, cut into 1-inch cubes (optional)

Preparation:

Preheat oven to 425°F.

Place the cut garlic scapes into a mixing bowl with 2 tablespoons of the olive oil and pinch of salt, and toss to coat thoroughly. Spread evenly in a single layer on a lipped baking sheet or roasting pan. Roast for 10–13 minutes to caramelize the scapes and make them crispy. Be careful not to burn them. Set aside to cool.

Meanwhile, bring a large pot of water to a boil and season generously with salt. Boil the pasta until al dente, 1 minute less than package directions. Drain and set aside.

Heat the remaining 2 tablespoons of extra virgin olive oil in a skillet. Add the cherry tomatoes to sear them, allowing them to break open and collapse, releasing their juices.

In a mixing bowl, combine the cooked linguine and roasted scapes until well integrated. Place a serving of the pasta into a pasta bowl and top generously with the seared tomatoes. Squeeze fresh lemon juice over the top, sprinkle with lemon zest, and add freshly ground black pepper to taste. Top with torn basil leaves and mozzarella (optional).

Serve at room temperature.

Spaghetti with Cocoa, Calamari, and Chili Spices

This healthful recipe may seem adventurous, but it pays off on your taste buds. The combination of cocoa and chili spices coats the pasta with amazing flavor. The calamari adds the perfect taste combination.

Servings: 4
Cooking Time: 15–20 minutes
Prep Time: 10 minutes

Ingredients:
2 tablespoons extra virgin olive oil
½ shallot, finely chopped
1 small clove garlic, minced
¼ teaspoon crushed red pepper
8 ounces baby calamari or sliced calamari rings and tentacles
Salt, to taste
2 tablespoons cocoa nibs
2 tablespoons dark cocoa powder
6 ounces fish stock
2 ounces freshly squeezed orange juice
12 ounces spaghetti
80% dark chocolate, shaved
1 tablespoon grated orange zest
Chili powder, to taste

Preparation:
Heat the olive oil in a large sauté pan over medium-high heat. Add the shallots, garlic, and crushed red pepper. Add the calamari pieces,

season with salt, and sauté for 2–3 minutes. Remove the calamari from pan and keep warm.

To the sauté pan add the cocoa nibs, cocoa powder, fish stock, and orange juice. Stir until well combined and the cocoa powder is completely dissolved. Reduce the heat to low.

Cook the spaghetti in well-salted water until al dente, 1 minute less than package directions. Drain the pasta and add to the sauce. Heat 1 minute to combine.

Plate the spaghetti, add the calamari, and top with shaved dark chocolate, orange zest, and chili powder.

Chicken Coconut Curry

A good go-to curry dish is a must in every household and delivers the benefits of turmeric in the curry powder. This one adds chicken thighs and chile peppers for antiangiogenic and immune-enhancing benefits.

Servings: 4
Cooking Time: 45 minutes
Prep Time: 15 minutes

Ingredients (sauce):
1 13.5-ounce can coconut milk
⅓ cup chicken broth (homemade or organic)
¼ cup orange marmalade
2 tablespoons Thai fish sauce
1 tablespoon curry powder
½ jalapeño or serrano chile, seeded and finely minced
Fresh cracked black pepper, to taste

Ingredients (chicken):
1 tablespoon cooking oil
2½ pounds boneless chicken thighs, cut in halves

1 medium onion, cut into 1-inch pieces

1 tablespoon minced garlic

2 medium thin-skinned potatoes, cut into 1-inch chunks

1 medium sweet potato, peeled and cut into 1-inch chunks

¾ pound whole peeled baby carrots

2 teaspoons grated orange peel

Salt, to taste

3 tablespoons chopped fresh Thai or regular basil

Preparation:

Combine the sauce ingredients in a metal bowl and whisk until evenly blended. Set aside.

Heat the oil in a wok or large sauté pan over medium-high heat. Add the chicken and cook, turning once, until lightly browned, about 5 minutes total. Remove the chicken from the pan. Discard all but 2 tablespoons of pan drippings. Add the onion and cook for 1–2 minutes. Add the garlic and cook for 15 seconds. Return the chicken to the pan; add the potatoes, carrots, and orange peel and pour in the sauce. Bring to a boil; reduce the heat, cover, and simmer until the chicken is no longer pink when cut in the thickest part and potatoes and carrots are tender, about 45 minutes. Add salt to taste. Stir in the basil just before serving.

Chicken with Mint in Fish Sauce

Chicken thighs, with their antiangiogenic benefits, never tasted so good as in this mouthwatering dish made with mint and Thai fish sauce.

Servings: 4
Cooking Time: 15 minutes
Prep Time: 15 minutes

Ingredients (sauce):

½ cup dry white wine

2 tablespoons soy sauce

2 tablespoons Thai fish sauce

2 tablespoons chopped mint

2 teaspoons demerara sugar

1/4 teaspoon black pepper

Ingredients (chicken):

1/4 cup cooking oil

6–8 fresh mint leaves, washed and patted dry

1 jalapeño or serrano chile, thinly sliced

2 teaspoons minced garlic

1/2 teaspoon crushed red pepper, or to taste

1 pound boneless, skinless chicken thighs, thinly sliced crosswise

Preparation:

Combine the sauce ingredients in a small bowl, mix well. Set aside.

Heat the oil in a wok until hot but not smoking. Place a mint leaf in the oil until it is glossy, transparent, and emerald green, about 30 seconds. If the oil temperature is too high, the leaf will turn olive green and become bitter. Lift out the leaf and drain on a paper towel. Repeat with the remaining leaves.

Pour off all but 2 tablespoons of the oil. Add the chile, garlic, and red pepper, and stir-fry for 15 seconds. Do not let burn. Immediately add the sliced chicken and stir-fry for 2–3 minutes. Pour the sauce in the wok, and turn the chicken in the sauce until fully cooked, about 2 minutes. Serve immediately over brown rice.

Clams a la Plancha

The simplicity of fresh clams, olive oil, garlic, and white wine creates a sublime dish guaranteed to please shellfish lovers and health seekers alike.

Servings: 4

Cooking Time: 15 minutes

Prep Time: 10 minutes

Ingredients:

¼ cup extra virgin olive oil

3 cloves garlic, finely chopped

2 pounds fresh clams (littlenecks, razor clams, cockles, or Manila clams), cleaned

1 cup dry white wine

Flaky sea salt, to taste

Crusty bread

Preparation:

Heat a plancha or heavy-bottomed pan on a grill or gas burner until very hot (if indoors, make sure you turn on the exhaust fan). Pour the olive oil on the pan after the pan is hot, so the oil doesn't smoke. Add garlic and stir for 10 seconds, then immediately add the clams in a single layer and cook for 5 minutes, turning once, until most are opened and have released their juices. Add the wine and shake pan briskly. Cook for another 5–6 minutes, until all clams have opened. Discard any clams that did not open.

Spoon the clams into a large bowl, pour in the juices, and season with sea salt. Serve immediately with lots of bread to soak up the juices.

Steamed Fish with Ginger

Steaming fish makes a delicious and healthy meal easy and quick to prepare. Add some mushrooms, soy, and scallions, and you are activating multiple health defenses in one fell swoop.

Serves: 4
Cooking Time: 20 minutes
Prep Time: 10 minutes

Ingredients:
2 shiitake mushrooms

6 tablespoons soy sauce

1/8 teaspoon sugar

4 fillets sea bass

2 tablespoons sesame oil

2 scallions, sliced lengthwise julienne-style, white and green parts separated

3-inch piece fresh ginger, peeled and julienned, divided

1 small bunch cilantro, hand ripped to have small groups of leaves

3 tablespoons Shaoxing rice wine

Preparation:

Slice the mushrooms wafer thin and set aside. Combine the soy sauce, salt, sugar, and 2 tablespoons of water in a small bowl, and set aside. Add 2 inches of water to the bottom of a wok, place a metal cover on it, and wait for the water to come to a boil. Remove the cover and place a bamboo steamer in the wok.

Rinse the fish and pat dry. Place the fish on a heatproof plate or a Pyrex dish. Pour the rice wine on the fish. Place the plate in the steamer and cover. Steam for 10–12 minutes. Test the fish for doneness by probing with a sharp knife to see if it penetrates through the fish completely. Remove from the steamer and place the fish on a serving platter. Arrange the green scallions, half the ginger, and all of the cilantro and mushrooms running lengthwise on the fish.

Heat the sesame oil in a skillet to hot but not smoking. Turn off the heat and pour the oil on top of the fish. Then, pour the soy sauce mixture over the fish. Serve immediately.

Dark Chocolate Chestnut Truffles

These truffles are a great way to get the benefits of chocolate in small quantities combined with the ellagic acid in chestnuts—enjoy this European-style treat.

Servings: approx. 3 dozen truffles
Cooking Time: 5 minutes
Prep Time: 20 minutes, 30 minutes rest time

Ingredients:
1 pound cooked chestnuts
4 ounces dark chocolate (70% or greater cacao), chopped into 1-inch pieces
3 tablespoons honey
1 teaspoon vanilla extract
⅓ cup dark cocoa powder
Finely grated zest of 1 orange (optional)
Almond, coconut, or whole milk, as needed
Paper truffle cups (optional)

To coat the truffles—select as many coatings as you like, and place in small individual bowls:
Dark cocoa powder
Coconut flour
Pure cane sugar
Finely chopped walnuts
Finely chopped chocolate chips

Preparation:

Using a food mill, potato ricer, or fork, mash the cooked chestnuts and place in a large mixing bowl. Over a double boiler, melt the chocolate. Remove from the heat and add to the chestnuts. Add the honey, vanilla, cocoa powder, and grated orange zest, if using, to the chestnut mixture. Mix all ingredients well to combine. If the mixture is too dry to hold together, add milk one tablespoon at a time until the mixture holds together. If the mixture is sticky when handling, allow to rest in the refrigerator for 20–30 minutes. Scoop a spoonful of the mixture and roll in the palms of your hands to form a ball. Roll the ball in one of the coatings above and place on a serving tray or in a paper truffle cup. Store in a covered container in the refrigerator.

Variations:

Add finely chopped walnuts or other nuts to truffle mixture.

Healthy Chocolate Mousse

Chocolate for dessert is always a hit, especially if it's dark chocolate to help your blood vessels and stem cells. This recipe also gives you the benefits of soy protein.

Serves: 4
Cooking Time: 5 minutes, 30 minutes set time
Prep Time: 5 minutes

Ingredients:

4 ounces dark chocolate (70% cacao or greater), chopped into 1-inch pieces
12 ounces silken tofu
2 tablespoons maple syrup
Chopped tree nuts (walnuts, hazelnuts, pecans), for garnish
Blueberries, strawberries, and/or blackberries, for garnish
Fresh mint or lavender, for garnish (optional)

Preparation:

In a double boiler, melt the chocolate over medium heat, stirring periodically to prevent scorching. When the chocolate has completely melted, add the silken tofu and maple syrup. Stir to combine. Transfer the mixture to a food processor and whip until fluffy. Spoon the mousse into individual ramekins or serving cups. Place in the refrigerator to cool and set for at least 30 minutes. To serve, garnish with crushed nuts, berries, and mint leaves, if desired.

* * *

Next up is a very special chapter for readers who are battling disease or care for someone who is. I hope these past four chapters have given you new ways to think about your food choices and how you prepare your meals. Now, in the last chapter, I'm going to take the conversation about food to the next level. While other books are filled with advice on what to eat, I'm going to tell you about the actual amounts you need to eat to achieve health benefits: the food doses.

CHAPTER 15

Food Doses

In this final chapter, I'd like to introduce an important new concept: food doses. If we are to approach food as medicine, then food must have doses. Just like the (bio)chemical constituents of drugs, the bioactives in the foods you eat have specific pharmacological-like effects on your cells. As you've seen throughout this book, foods are being studied using some of the same methods as those employed in drug development. I want to bring you to the forefront of the "food as medicine" movement and show you how the concept of food doses is shaping the future of how we will use food to fight disease. The first step is to discover the right doses for the foods that will help us improve our health.

When it comes to medicines, doctors know that it's important to know the right drug to use, and the right dose needed to achieve the best outcomes. Dose is the quantity of a drug that is taken in a certain way at a certain frequency. Before a new drug can be approved by the FDA for widespread use, pharmaceutical companies invest heavily (more than $2.6 billion on average per drug) in development and testing to find the right dose for the best response. Yet doctors don't have conversations with patients about food doses in the way that they talk about doses of pharmaceuticals.

A food dose is the amount of any food or beverage consumed that is associated with or leads to a specific health outcome. For example, how many apples do you need to eat to reduce the risk of a given disease? This dose can be relevant for disease prevention or treatment, long-term management, or suppression to keep the disease from returning. A mountain of research has been revealing how specific foods and beverages can influence health and disease, and the amount associated to achieve it.

I talk about food doses every time I discuss dietary health with a patient. I explain how specific foods can be useful because, like medicines, the bioactives in them can influence our cells and the biological systems in our body in ways that resemble drugs. I share what I know about the importance of selecting the food, as well as how to prepare it to get the most out of its health benefits. And I share any dose information that has been published by researchers, so my patients can think about how to incorporate the food in their lives. Most doctors are sorely in need of more training about food and health, and how to discuss these kinds of topics with patients. We need to do much more and invest in educating medical students, practicing doctors, and nutritionists about food doses. The goal of comprehensive health care should include helping each patient match their needs with the tools of diet they can access.

The Science of Food Doses

Food dosing is a logical idea being developed by researchers like myself and my team at the Angiogenesis Foundation, where we examine foods, food extracts, and bioactives with rigorous scientific methods. We start with quantities of a food identified through clinical studies or epidemiological research of real-life dietary patterns reported from large populations, and analyze their beneficial health effect. We analyze the data to see if the benefits found to be associated with the food match what we know about the bioactive constituents of the food across the health defense systems, and they act to help maintain health and repel disease.

We then translate the amount of the food or beverage that was reported as consumed and its frequency into doses.

In cases where a dietary factor is being measured, we calculate the amount of that factor present in actual foods using government databases. We also analyze the actual bioactives in the food and look for their effects in laboratory studies using molecular, genetic, and biochemical tests that are commonly used for biopharmaceutical research. The activities of these substances are then translated back to their amounts in food to determine if the dose of the food required would be realistic to consume. This is how we study food as medicine.

In my TED Talk, some of the biggest audience reactions came when I showed the results of a study where we did a head-to-head comparison of the potency of different foods versus drugs on angiogenesis. We examined four cancer drugs, seven other common medications (anti-inflammatory drugs, statins, a blood pressure medication, and an antibiotic), and sixteen dietary factors from foods associated with lowering the risk of various cancers. Remarkably, fifteen of the dietary factors were more potent than one of the cancer drugs in the experiment we did. Most of the foods held their own ground or were more potent than the common medications. Some of the oldest cancer drugs originally were discovered from natural sources like tree bark, medicinal plants, and even marine organisms. While this study does not equate the effect of the food with drug effects in humans, the results force even the most hard-boiled adherent to the pharmaceutical model of health to pause and marvel at the potency of what Mother Nature has laced into foods.

Up until now, most references to the amount of a "healthy" food have been focused on portion size (usually connected to a weight loss goal). But today, we can apply new tools of molecular and cell biology and genomics to explore how food can support health in ways that weren't possible even a few years ago. And we already have some extraordinary clinical and epidemiological findings that give us new perspectives to think about the quantities of food that we eat and how often.

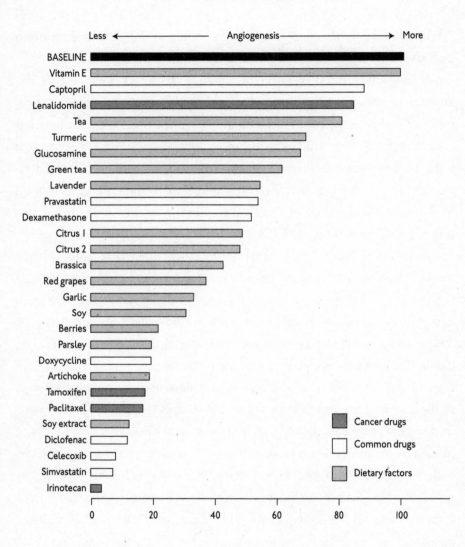

Below is a chart that summarizes many of the foods that have been described in this book, and the doses found with disease-fighting benefits. Take a look: it's quite remarkable that you can find specific foods with a published associated impact on diseases like colon cancer, kidney cancer, lupus, and arthritis, among many others.

This is by no means a complete list, nor could it be, since the research is ongoing and new discoveries are being published every week. Also, be advised that the foods that made the cut to be listed here have been identified through the research into specific food doses for specific diseases. There are many more foods that can combat disease by promoting sustained health through their support and activation of the health defense systems. See the chart in appendix A for a reminder of which foods affect which defense systems, and which diseases are impacted when you feed your defense, as a way to build into your diet a diverse arsenal of disease-fighting foods.

FOOD DOSE CHART

Foods, Their Doses, and Diseases Impacted

Food/Beverage	Human Dose	Disease
Apples	1–2 per day	Bladder cancer
	1–2 per day	Colorectal cancer
Apricots	2 fruits per day	Esophageal cancer
	2 fruits per day	Head and neck cancer
Bamboo shoots	⅓ cup per day*	Metabolic syndrome/obesity
Beer	1 beer per day	Colorectal cancer
	1 beer per day	Coronary artery disease
	5 beers per week	Kidney cancer
	1–2 beers per day	Dementia
Black raspberries	2 cups per day	Barrett's esophagus
	7 cups per day*	Bladder cancer
	4 berries per day	Cardiovascular disease
Black tea	2 cups per day	Hypertension
Blackberries	5½ cups per day*	Bladder cancer
Blueberries	1 cup per week	Breast cancer
Bluefish	1+ servings per week	Age-related macular degeneration
	3½ ounces per day	Colorectal cancer
Broccoli	1–2 cups per week	Breast cancer
	1–2 cups per week	Esophageal cancer
	2 cups per day	Systemic lupus erythematosus
Cashews	26 nuts per day	Colorectal cancer
Cherries	2 fruits per day	Esophageal cancer
	2 fruits per day	Head and neck cancer

Foods, their Doses, and Diseases Impacted (cont.)

Food/Beverage	Human Dose	Disease
Cherry tomatoes	8 cups uncooked per day	Systemic lupus erythematosus
Chestnuts	1.7 ounces per day*	Bladder cancer
Coffee	2+ cups per day	Myocardial infarction
Dark chocolate	375 milligrams flavonoids (1 pack CocoaPro) per day	Coronary artery disease
Dark meat chicken	~1 drumstick/thigh (100 grams) per day	Colorectal cancer
Edam cheese	2 slices per day	Colorectal cancer
Edamame	1.2 cups per day	Breast cancer
Fermented kimchi	1.2 cups per day	Metabolic syndrome/ obesity
Fish/shellfish high in PUFAs	3 ounces per day	Colorectal cancer
	3 ounces per day	Breast cancer
Green tea	2–3 cups per day	Colorectal cancer
	4 cups per day	Cardiovascular disease[7]
	4–5 cups per day	Systemic lupus erythematosus
	4–5 cups per day	Multiple sclerosis
	4–5 cups per day	Rheumatoid arthritis
Kimchi	1⅕ cups per day	Hypertension
Macadamia	17 nuts per day	Colorectal cancer
Mackerel	1+ servings per week	Age-related macular degeneration
	3½ ounces per day	Colorectal cancer
Mango	2 fruits per day	Esophageal cancer
	2 fruits per day	Head and neck cancer
Nectarines	2 fruits per day	Esophageal cancer
	2 fruits per day	Head and neck cancer
Olive oil	3–4 tablespoons per day	Breast cancer
	3–4 tablespoons per day	Colorectal cancer
	3–4 tablespoons per day	Laryngeal cancer
Oranges	1½ oranges per day	Systemic lupus erythematosus
Peaches	2 fruits per day	Esophageal cancer
	2 fruits per day	Head and neck cancer
Pine nuts	¼ cup per day	Colorectal cancer

Plums	2 fruits per day	Esophageal cancer
	2 fruits per day	Head and neck cancer
Purple potatoes	5 small potatoes per day*	Colorectal cancer
Red wine	1 glass per day	Colorectal cancer
	½ glass per day	Atherosclerosis
Salmon	1+ servings per week	Age-related macular degeneration
	3½ ounces per day	Colorectal cancer
Sardines	1+ servings per week	Age-related macular degeneration
	3½ ounces per day	Colorectal cancer
Soy milk	1 cup per day	Breast cancer
	1 cup per day	Atherosclerosis
Strawberries	1½ cups per day	Systemic lupus erythematosus
Swordfish	1+ servings per week	Age-related macular degeneration
	3½ ounces per day	Colorectal cancer
Tuna	1+ servings per week	Age-related macular degeneration
	3½ ounces per day	Colorectal cancer
Walnut	22 halves per day	Colorectal cancer (risk)
	29 halves per week	Stage 3 colorectal cancer (death from)
Whole wheat	2.7 servings per day	Cardiovascular disease
	2.7 servings per day	Type 2 diabetes
Yogurt	>1 serving per day	Cardiovascular disease

Indicates dose is an equivalent, calculated from a preclinical study.

For people who want to start eating to prevent or halt a disease, the central question was once "What foods should I avoid?" What I am telling you now: the better question to ask is "Which foods can I add?"

This positive shift in thinking is a more encouraging approach that will get you thinking about the foods I've shown you throughout this book that you actually enjoy. It will prompt you to look at the data and ask new questions, such as "How much?" "How many?" "How often?"

I've found the concept of food doses to be particularly impactful for a patient, friend, or family member who is battling cancer. For example, as discussed in part 2, studies in people with colon cancer have shown that eating two servings of tree nuts (fourteen walnuts) per week is associated with a 42 percent lowered risk of having the disease return. That leads to a no-brainer recommendation for a low-cost lifestyle change. For breast cancer, consuming ten grams of soy protein (equivalent to one cup of soy milk) per day is associated with a 29 percent decrease in the risk of death from the disease. You can't ignore this kind of information once you've seen the evidence. And it is definitely helpful in guiding your dietary choices if you are trying to prevent a disease like cancer.

No Magic Bullets

As with everything in health and disease, when it comes to food doses, things are not always as simple as they seem. Yes, food dose is a pretty incredible concept, but there are five important caveats to keep in mind.

First, most of the studies are done using epidemiological research, which is a way of using real-world populations made up of people like you and me, to look for the associations between dietary patterns reported or tracked by researchers, and specific health outcomes. Statisticians and nutrition scientists will tell you that this type of research does not nail down cause and effect the same way a drug study using mice or a clinical trial would. But it's a powerful method, and the associations that emerge can be incredibly informative—especially when hundreds, thousands, or hundreds of thousands of people are involved.

Second, most clinical studies on food and specific health outcomes (high blood pressure, blood sugar control, heart disease) are small studies, meaning they involve relatively few people, perhaps only a few dozen or even fewer. This means the studies are not as robust as the studies involving hundreds or thousands of people in pharmaceutical trials. But the data that emerges is part of our knowledge base about diet and health. It is flawed thinking to discount the value of clinical research that is not conducted at the pharmaceuticals scale. Data is data. And more research is always needed to get at the truth. Even with drugs.

Third, we are learning from the cutting edge of personalized medicine that every individual is different. We all have our own unique microbiomes, genetics, and epigenetics. We each metabolize food differently. When we eat combinations of foods, their bioactives combine in our body to produce different effects than what you'd predict with a single food. This means, even when a large number of individuals are studied, we cannot predict whether an individual will respond to a particular food in exactly the same way. Individual responses need to be studied at the individual level. This gets back to the flawed thinking that every study on food needs to enroll hundreds of patients in order to get any meaningful information.

Fourth, remember that if you are currently battling a disease, you should definitely consult your doctor before changing how you eat. Foods can interact with drugs, like blood thinners, chemotherapy, antibiotics, and many others too numerous to list here. Arm yourself with new knowledge on the health benefits of specific foods and food doses, and then you and your doctor or health team can decide together on the best way to eat.

Fifth, the biggest reason why you should take a broader, more flexible approach to diet and health is because there are no magic bullets that will ward off all disease. As I showed you in part 3, the human body operates as a collection of interconnected systems. What affects one organ or system can affect the whole body. In terms of choosing which healthy foods to eat, this interconnectedness is a good thing. Foods can be viewed in many ways with the same lens as medicines, but the complex nature of food means it can achieve health in ways drugs cannot. We don't take a medicine to stay healthy, we take it to cure or manage a disease—but we can eat foods for our health.

Many people live their lives according to the principle that bigger is better, more is more, and therefore when you eat for health, it's best to consume as much as you can of a single food. That doesn't work with complicated biological systems in the body. Health is about a state of balance, not a state of excess. Just because two cups of tomato sauce per week is beneficial for lowering prostate cancer risk doesn't mean that you gain more protection by drinking a gallon of it each day. Paracelsus, the Swiss pioneer of toxicology, once said, "All things are poisons, for there is nothing without poisonous qualities. It is only the dose which makes a thing poison." More is not always more. Sometimes less is more.

Balance is your goal when it comes to health. You want to aim to keep your health defense systems in a state of balance. In biology there is an important concept that everyone should know about called hormesis. In simplest terms, hormesis describes the response of a complex system, where a small amount of a stimulus (like food) is beneficial, and a bit more is a bit better. But, there is a peak amount of stimuli where more doesn't result in further benefit. In fact, a lot more can lead to loss of the benefit and even a harmful effect. This is sometimes called the U-shaped curve. Familiar examples for humans include exercise, fasting, and even drinking water. All are beneficial to your health, but there comes a point of excess where overexertion, starvation, or water intoxication can destroy your health and even be fatal.

What this means is that you have to take reasonable care when it comes to using the data on food doses. Don't go out and eat only one thing all the time at one dose like a robot! Diet faddists like to find a formula and slavishly stick with it as long as they can to extract the most benefit. But maintaining good health through food should come naturally. New good habits can take time to stick, and you may have to unlearn or replace a few bad habits of the past. I recommend that you eat to beat disease by following a diverse diet, following the principles and patterns I've shown you in this book. Incorporate food doses into your diet for foods you prefer that have evidence for a health benefit.

Protecting Yourself from the Top Killers

Cardiovascular disease. Cancer. Diabetes. Obesity. Autoimmune disease. Diseases of aging.

These are the chronic conditions that take millions of lives each year, cause untold suffering, and burden our health-care systems. Many of these diseases are directly related to lifestyle. As you can see from the risk assessment I've included for you in appendix B, there are many risk factors that can affect your overall risk of disease. But whatever your level of risk, if you develop chronic illness, chances are good that it will be one (or several) of these major killers. Why not then just use the food doses chart and pick one food to target each condition?

The reason is: in order to eat to beat the big diseases, we need to take a more holistic view. Each of these diseases has many dimensions in which multiple health defenses are malfunctioning and need to be boosted. The fact is that if your body's health defenses are fully geared up and functioning, you will stand a good chance of avoiding them. Success requires we engage multiple defense systems to properly prevent or modify the disease. No single food does it all. You need to rally all the defense systems in your body. I'll show you why this is the case in six devastating diseases. Once armed with this information, you can refer to the convenient tables in appendix A to see which foods impact which defense systems. Once you see the connections with the defense systems, you will want to consider how to build your own personal plan to fend off these killers.

Cardiovascular Diseases

Heart disease is one of the world's biggest killers. You almost certainly know someone who has suffered a heart attack. But cardiovascular diseases don't just affect the heart. They involve circulatory problems that cause malfunctions of the heart, brain, leg muscles, and other organs. Bad genetics, high cholesterol (specifically the "bad" kind), inflammation, obesity, diabetes, and smoking are all factors that contribute. These put a big strain on the body's health defense systems to maintain balance and health. Diet clearly plays a major role in preventing and modifying the effects of these risk factors.

Here is how eating to activate the health defense systems would be game-changing for anyone worried about cardiovascular disease:

- Eating foods that stimulate angiogenesis can grow blood vessels to improve blood flow to cardiovascular organs.
- Foods that recruit stem cells can help build new blood vessels as well as regenerate heart muscle, brain cells, and other muscles.
- Eating foods that lower inflammation will lessen the chances that plaque-clogging blood vessels will rupture to cause a heart attack or stroke.
- Cardiologists are now finding key links between the gut microbiome and blood cholesterol, so a diet that improves the microbiome may prove to be heart healthy in more ways than one.

Cancer

Cancer is a global killer, and its toxic treatments have long been as feared as much as the disease itself. One in three people in the United States will be diagnosed with some form of cancer during their lifetime,[1] and cancer is the second leading cause of death behind heart disease.[2] In the United Kingdom, the risk is even higher: one in two will develop cancer.[3] The next time you're at a dinner party, look at the people sitting around you and count those statistics (don't forget to include yourself).

While it was once thought that the sole goal for cancer treatment was killing the cancer cells, the modern understanding of cancer is that it is a disease of mutated cells that the body's defenses have failed to thwart and get rid of. Genetics, lifestyle, and high-risk exposures all threaten your defenses, and some of the most revolutionary treatments for cancer of the twenty-first century are aimed at activating immunity. The food you eat can play a role in this goal.

Many of the cancers we've discussed have been solid tumors whose names refer to the organ in which they arise, like colon cancer, ovarian cancer, lung cancer, and the like. There is another category that is referred to as blood or liquid cancers, which includes leukemias, lymphomas, and multiple myeloma. These are cancers that arise from white blood cells in the bone marrow. Rather than existing as tumors in specific organs, the cells of liquid cancers course through the whole body. If you are facing or have a history of one of these cancers, know that the exact same basic principles of health defense apply to liquid cancers as to solid tumors. Liquid cancers also depend on angiogenesis to grow, have stem cells that need to be destroyed, are riddled with DNA mutations, and can be wiped out by immune defenses. As you'll see shortly, there are ways to find foods that can help tackle liquid cancers.

A poor diet has long been tied to increased cancer risk. The emphasis has been on identifying carcinogenic elements in foods and removing them from food. That is only part of the solution. Now, it's time to look at how diet can decrease the risk by boosting your health defense, which also can improve your odds of survival if you have the disease.

- Foods with antiangiogenic activity can starve a tumor by cutting off its blood supply.
- Foods that help get rid of tenacious and dangerous cancer stem cells can improve the odds the cancer won't come back after treatment.

- A diet that activates the immune system, which can also occur by eating foods that promote a healthier microbiome, can assist in cancer control and elimination.

- Eating foods that protect DNA serves as both a shield and a repair mechanism to make sure errors in our DNA don't lead to even more cancer.

Diabetes

Diabetes is a growing health problem in which the body's failure to properly control metabolism leads to catastrophic problems in many organs. While type 1 diabetes is an autoimmune disease, type 2 diabetes is regarded as a lifestyle disease in which the body develops insulin resistance that can often be reversed with exercise and a healthy diet. In fact, the best opportunity to beat this disease is at its inception, during a stage called prediabetes. One study showed that by age forty-five, people who were otherwise healthy have a 49 percent chance of developing prediabetes, and among those, 74 percent will eventually go on to develop full-on type 2 diabetes.

Diabetes is a disease to avoid at all costs. While reducing carbohydrates, red meat intake, and sugary drinks is fundamental to preventing diabetes, actively eating foods that fortify the health defense systems is known to reduce your diabetes risk.

There is evidence that whole grains, nuts, plant-based foods, and fish can help prevent diabetes. Even if you already have diabetes, your diet is a crucial opportunity for you to lower the risk of the many serious complications of the disease, which ultimately wreaks havoc on your heart, eyes, brain, nerves, kidneys, feet, and immune system.

- Foods that stimulate angiogenesis can help your body compensate for the slower blood vessel growth that occurs in diabetes. Better angiogenesis is important for improving blood flow in the heart as well as growing more circulation in wounds that need to heal. Foods that inhibit angiogenesis in the eye can ward off problems causing vision loss. (The body will know how to partition the effects to help good blood vessels and not the bad ones, so consuming both types of angiogenesis-modifying foods is fine.)

- Stem cells are fewer in number and less active in people with diabetes, so eating foods that invigorate stem cells can help improve circulation, regenerate nerves, restore the heart, and repair damaged eyes.

- People with diabetes have a disrupted microbiome, so a diet that rebuilds healthy gut bacteria can be essential.

- Eating the right foods to counteract inflammation is important because diabetes causes inflammation throughout the body.

- As every doctor learned early in medical school, diabetes also lowers immune defenses, so foods that activate the immune system can help people with diabetes avoid infection.

- The metabolic chaos of diabetes leads to biochemical shrapnel in the body that can damage DNA and accelerate aging. DNA-protective foods can help defend the body against this damage.

Obesity

As many as 40 percent of adults worldwide are overweight or obese, leading to more than 3 million deaths. China and the United States are the leaders in the problem of excess weight, in part, as the consequence of poor dietary choices and insufficient exercise. And the greater danger lurking alongside being overweight is metabolic syndrome, a condition of having multiple risk factors for heart disease: abdominal obesity, high cholesterol and triglyceride levels, high blood pressure, and elevated blood glucose. As many as one-third of American adults have metabolic syndrome.[4] The wisest way to lose weight is to eat better, eat less, and exercise more.

Here's how eating to boost your health defenses can fight obesity:

- Because fat tissue grows like a tumor and needs a blood supply, eating antiangiogenic foods can literally starve fat and restrict its growth.
- Foods that promote a healthy microbiome can lower blood cholesterol and foster weight loss.
- Being obese causes DNA damage in your cells, so foods that repair DNA are beneficial for individuals who are overweight.[5]
- Studies have shown that obesity is essentially a state of whole body inflammation. So, eating anti-inflammatory foods can help lessen that inflammatory state.
- The weapons of the immune system are also blunted in people who are obese, and this has implications for many other chronic diseases. A diet containing immunity-activating foods can help counteract this weakness.

Autoimmune Diseases

Autoimmune diseases are conditions in which the body's immune system attacks its own cells. This category of diseases encompasses more than eighty different conditions, including type 1 diabetes, lupus, rheumatoid arthritis, multiple sclerosis, and inflammatory bowel disease (Crohn's disease and ulcerative colitis), among others. The immune attack against self causes severe and chronic inflammation throughout the body, and medical interventions like steroids and biological therapies can be effective at combating inflammation but have major side effects. Steroids in particular have terrible side effects, such as glaucoma, weight gain, increased risk for infections, and even psychosis.

A dietary approach for autoimmune diseases involves all defense systems.

- Any foods that calm the immune system can be useful, including foods with anti-inflammatory properties.
- Chronic inflammation usually causes undesirable blood vessels to form. These vessels can invade and destroy healthy tissues, like the joints in rheumatoid arthritis, so foods with antiangiogenic activity can help lessen that damage.
- An abnormal gut microbiome triggers some autoimmune diseases, so it can be helpful to eat foods that restore healthy gut bacteria. For example, foods like walnuts, beans (black and navy), kiwifruit, and cocoa increase bacteria production of butyrate, which has anti-inflammatory properties shown to reduce the bone and joint destruction of arthritis.[6]
- Strong evidence from clinical trials shows that some autoimmune diseases, like scleroderma, multiple sclerosis, and myesthenia gravis, can be eliminated by rebuilding the immune system with stem cell transplants.[7] Another approach is to use fasting to reboot the immune system. Foods that foster the regeneration of a healthy immune system will be useful in keeping order and preventing the chaos of autoimmune diseases.

Diseases of Aging

As we get older, our body shows the inevitable signs of aging, like graying hair and wrinkles. But some diseases seen in elderly people are overwhelmingly destructive to health and well-being, and everyone wants to avoid them.

Neurodegenerative conditions like Alzheimer's disease and Parkinson's disease involve loss of normal brain function over time.[8] Some diets, such as the MIND Diet, which is a combination of the Mediterranean and the DASH diet, and the Canadian Brain Health Food Guide, can help maintain mental function and delay the inevitable progression of neurodegenerative disease.

Eating foods that improve health defenses may be even more important as we age.

- For neurodegenerative diseases, stimulating angiogenesis through foods can improve blood flow and lower inflammation to benefit cognitive function.
- Diets that activate stem cells can improve regeneration of nerves and brain tissue.
- Taming the microbiome with diet helps healthy gut bacteria send proper messages to the brain.
- Foods that protect DNA can shield the aging brain from DNA damage that can impair mental function.
- Brain inflammation is seen in virtually all neurodegenerative diseases, so eating foods with anti-inflammatory benefits calms the immune system.

Another disease of aging is age-related macular degeneration (AMD), which is the most common cause of vision loss in people age fifty or older. In the most destructive form for this condition, called "wet" AMD, abnormal leaky blood vessels grow under the nerve layer that is responsible for vision. Blindness eventually results. While not fatal, an elderly person who cannot see loses his or her independence and must depend on others for routine life activities. As their quality of life declines, they become depressed and isolated and have difficulty managing other medical conditions that they may have, showing up at medical appointments, and taking needed medications.

Dietary factors are clearly important for prevention of AMD. Leafy green vegetables and fish as well as dietary supplements called AREDS (a specific combination of certain vitamins, minerals, and plant-based bioactives) are recommended.[9]

- An even more comprehensive approach to wet AMD can be taken as a person ages by including foods with antiangiogenic properties to keep those destructive blood vessels from growing.
- Because key nerves in the back of the eye degenerate in wet AMD, eating foods that prompt retinal stem cells to regenerate tissues can help.
- There is clear evidence that microbiome disruptions are seen in people with AMD, so foods that restore healthy gut bacteria are important.[10]
- DNA-protecting and anti-inflammatory foods can be useful because in AMD fatty deposits build up and cause inflammation and oxidative damage that wrecks DNA.

Final Word

As I've shown you throughout this book, health is much more than the absence of disease. It is the presence of your five health defense systems working together in complex ways to keep your body functioning normally, while at the same time responding to the assault of life and aging in order to prevent disease. As they exist today, the health-care systems of most countries fail in their mission of protecting public health. Rather than improving health defense, the health systems are made up of doctors, hospitals, and payers who focus their primary efforts on delivering disease care, not health care. Modern medicine as I see it has become a reactive system designed to eradicate disease with man-made technologies and other blunt instruments once disease has declared its presence. While surgery is still often a life-saving act, the knee-jerk response to prescribe drugs to try to wipe out disease without harming the patient is limited in what it can do to make societies healthier. The system winds up treating diseases instead of protecting people, and keeping them healthy and vibrant.

The medical establishment will argue that the conventional approach to health care can lead to resounding successes in disease fighting. I can vouch for that—I have had many patients who have been pulled back from the brink and are leading fulfilling lives today that would not have been possible without drugs, surgery, or radiation. But if you look at the big picture, the inadequate focus on health and disease prevention has generated a huge body count of people who rely on costly medications that never quite achieve the goal of giving them back their health. And as the burden of disease rises, health-care systems around the world are buckling under the tremendous financial strain.

The costs of treating disease are unsustainable and have gone beyond astronomical—they have grown to a breaking point. One of the most important drugs for leukemia, for example, costs $475,000 *per dose.*[11] As remarkable as some breakthroughs are in transforming modern medicine, even by being able to put cancer patients into complete remission, they are so expensive that most people who need them will never be able to access them. This inequity flies in the face of the real progress of medical research.

Amid our planet's own declining health, we are all exposed to more chemical toxins, pollutants, radiation, and infectious diseases, no matter where we live. It's remarkable that we don't get sick more often and that we live as long as we do. While advances like immunotherapy, gene editing, robotic surgery, precision medicine, tissue regeneration, and health-care big data mining will indeed change modern medicine, these innovations merely extend the current model of health care while retaining its siloed focus on treating disease.

At the same time, we are discovering how much we barely know about our health. We know that DNA errors occur daily, but not why we do not develop more cancer as a result. We know the microbiome is critical, but we don't understand how we can be infected with bacteria and not get sick. We've discovered two new organs, the interstitium (a connected network of fluid-filled spaces everywhere throughout the whole body between organs) and the mesentery (a web of tissue that attaches the intestines to the back wall inside the belly), but we are still defining what they do (probably help our immune system).[12] From advances in cancer immunotherapy, we know that an elderly person's immune system is perfectly capable of wiping out metastatic cancer, but we do not know how to make this happen for most cancer patients yet. We've discovered that certain gut bacteria can be crucial brokers of our immune response to cancer and that antibiotics that wipe out these bacteria may doom a patient's chance to respond to cancer-reversing immune treatments (certain foods can help restore these critical bacteria).

So many important and exciting questions about health loom. Like explorers of the ocean abyss or astrobiologists searching distant galaxies for signs of life, we medical researchers need to approach our task of discovering the secrets of health with a sense of wonderment and humility.

As a doctor who has treated thousands of patients and as a scientist who works at the forefront of medicine, I've come to the conclusion that the most powerful way to beat disease is to prevent it in the first place. This requires promoting more scientific research and better public health efforts aimed at health and prevention. It involves putting the power where it belongs: in the hands of the individual who can take actions to preserve their own health.

Eating to beat disease empowers you to help yourself and the people you care about. So, look at all the foods listed throughout this book. See the myriad choices. Decide what you enjoy eating. It is all about you. Any health-promoting food that supports one of your defense systems will point you in the right direction. Have a reasonable approach. The 5 × 5 × 5 framework guides you to select five foods (more if you like) off the preferred food list to eat each day. Mix it up, so you don't get into a rut, and don't overdo it with any single food.

Eating to beat disease is an important part of the solution to the health-care crisis. With a global effort in research that is gaining momentum and a growing body of scientific evidence showing our health can be influenced and optimized by food, you should expect to see even more data coming out in the years ahead. Unlike pharmaceutical research, which takes billions of dollars and decades before a new pill becomes available, the results of food and health research has immediacy. We don't have to wait for lengthy clinical trials to finish or FDA approval to recommend eating a tangerine or a turnip.

When I participated in an extraordinary medical research conference titled Unite to Cure convened by the Vatican in April 2018, Pope Francis delivered a private address to our gathering in which he said, "The true measure of progress is the ability to help every person." May what you've learned here be a new beginning for your health, and may you share it with the people around you.

A Note on the Science

Throughout this book, I have highlighted the science behind how specific foods can help our bodies defend our health. My goal is to share this information in a way that allows you to turn this knowledge into action which, I suspect, is why you picked up this book in the first place. You might want to understand how I chose the scientific data. After all, anyone interested in health news knows there is a lot of information out there about food and health that sometimes is contradictory.

Translating science news for the public can be a real challenge. But here are the take-home messages I want to leave you with. First, no single research study is ever the final word on a topic. Good science is a rigorous, exacting process that examines, considers, concludes, and confirms its results through repetition and improvement of methodology. This is how we continually evolve and refine our understanding of the world, including food and our health. There are many exciting findings from the hundreds of research studies I've discussed throughout this book, but the results of each study inevitably lead to new questions. Such is the nature of science. When it comes to food and health-defense systems, this is an exciting new area of human exploration, with enough data for us to know it is important to pursue, but still with so much to learn.

The studies that I've selected for this book generally come from one of four methodologies: clinical studies on humans, large-scale epidemiological studies of real-world human populations, animal studies, and laboratory studies examining the effect of food factors on human cells. I've tried to focus on the human data at every possible turn, because that's what matters most. Studies involving animals and cells, however, can provide deep insights into how and why things work. The findings are most meaningful if they can help clarify and make sense of the human data that also exists.

The studies themselves use methods similar to those used in drug development: genomic sequencing, proteomics, cell culture, animal models, randomized placebo-controlled human clinical trials, and real-world studies of large populations. I've chosen to highlight the studies that have some specific hypothesis or result that makes them stand out. These are the kinds of studies I talk about with scientists and doctors who are working at the leading edge of medical research.

More research is essential to further develop the scientific foundations on which specific dietary recommendations can be made at an individual level. Food scientists, life scientists, nutritionists, agricultural experts, doctors, behavioral scientists, and epidemiologists need to unite their efforts to continue to investigate how foods impact our body.

A few final points.

The food recommendations in this book are not meant to be taken as gospel. Each person has their own dietary health needs, and the 5 × 5 × 5 framework is designed so that you can develop the regimen that works best for you. Much more data on foods will be published in the future, and I encourage you to stay up-to-date by using PubMed as an ongoing resource. Or visit http://drwilliamli.com to sign up for periodic updates.

Second, exercise common sense in consuming any food or drink mentioned in this book. I have not suggested that you incorporate any item in limitless quantities into your diet. Consuming any natural substance at unnatural levels is bound to have a deleterious effect. Health is defined by a state of balance, or homeostasis. Taking anything in excess, whether alcohol, sugar, or even plain old water, disrupts this balance. When it comes to your body, more isn't always better. And no food is a magic bullet.

Finally, food is not a substitute for medical treatment. I believe in using all the best resources at your disposal. Medicines can be lifesaving. But foods are part of the health toolbox, and they are interventions that do not require a prescription or an intravenous line. Combinations of foods and drugs have been widely studied for their potential harmful interactions, but how they might interact in beneficial ways is also an exciting new area to be explored.

No whole food is universally good or bad. The impact of food on each person is unique depending upon a number of factors, including their genetic makeup. This book was deliberately written to highlight foods that can be beneficial because of their positive effects on the health-defense systems, but there are other factors on an individual level to consider when you are choosing what to eat. Always check with your doctor before making any major changes to your diet, especially if you are sick or taking medications. You should also factor in considerations that are best for your situation, which might include diabetes, cardiovascular disease, or other chronic diseases.

I encourage you to use this book as a launchpad. You've seen throughout the book that there is scientific evidence showing the health benefits of many more foods than the ingredients in a salad. Everyone can eat to beat disease using easily accessible and highly appealing foods found across many cultures and traditions. I set out to tell you about the exciting new insights on how the body heals itself through its defense systems. I will consider my efforts a success if you go on from here, choosing foods every day with an informed mind and a clear intent to eat to beat disease.

5 × 5 × 5 Daily Worksheet— Preferred Foods List

Choose one item from each defense category to eat each day.

Defense: Angiogenesis

Antiangiogenic

- Almonds
- Anchovies
- Apple peel
- Apples (Granny Smith, Red Delicious, Reinette)
- Apricot
- Arctic char
- Arugula
- Bamboo shoots
- Barley
- Beer
- Belgian endive
- Bigeye tuna
- Black bass
- Black beans
- Black plums
- Black raspberries
- Black tea
- Blackberries
- Blueberries
- Blueberries (dried)
- Bluefin tuna
- Bluefish
- Bok choy
- Bottarga
- Broccoli
- Broccoli rabe
- Cabbage
- Camembert cheese
- Capers
- Carrots
- Cashews
- Cauliflower
- Caviar (sturgeon)
- Chamomile tea
- Cherries
- Cherries (dried)
- Cherry tomatoes
- Chestnuts
- Chia seeds

- Chicken (dark meat)
- Chile peppers
- Cinnamon
- Cloudy apple cider
- Cockles (clam)
- Coffee
- Cranberries
- Cranberries (dried)
- Dark chocolate
- Eastern oysters
- Edam cheese
- Eggplant
- Emmenthal cheese
- Escarole
- Fiddleheads
- Fish roe (salmon)
- Flax seeds
- Frisee
- Ginseng
- Gouda cheese
- Gray mullet
- Green tea
- Guava
- Hake
- Halibut
- Jamón iberico de bellota

- Jarlsberg cheese
- Jasmine green tea
- John Dory (fish)
- Kale
- Kimchi
- Kiwifruit
- Licorice root
- Lychee
- Macadamia nuts
- Mackerel
- Mangoes
- Manila clams
- Mediterranean sea bass
- Muenster cheese
- Navy beans
- Nectarine
- Olive oil (EVOO)
- Onions
- Oolong tea
- Oregano
- Pacific oysters
- Peaches
- Pecans
- Peppermint
- Pine nuts
- Pink grapefruit
- Pistachios
- Plums
- Pomegranates
- Pompano

- Proscuitto di Parma
- Pumpkin seeds
- Puntarelle
- Radicchio
- Rainbow trout
- Raspberries
- Red black-skin tomatoes
- Redfish
- Red-leaf lettuce
- Red mullet
- Red wine (Cabernet, Cabernet Franc, Petit Verdot)
- Romanesco
- Rosemary
- Rutabaga
- Salmon
- San Marzano tomatoes
- Sardine
- Sauerkraut
- Sea bream
- Sea cucumber
- Sencha green tea
- Sesame seeds
- Soy
- Spiny lobster
- Squash blossoms

- Squid ink
- Stilton cheese
- Strawberries
- Sultana raisins
- Sunflower seeds
- Swordfish

- Tangerine tomatoes
- Tardivo di Treviso
- Tieguanyin green tea
- Tuna

- Turmeric
- Turnips
- Walnuts
- Watermelon
- Yellowtail (fish)

Angiogenesis Stimulating

- Apple peel
- Apples (Granny Smith, Red Delicious, Reinette)
- Asparagus
- Barley
- Belgian endive
- Black plums
- Blueberries (dried)

- Capers
- Cherries (dried)
- Chia seeds
- Chile peppers
- Cranberries
- Cranberries (dried)
- Escarole
- Flax seeds
- Frisee
- Ginseng

- Onions
- Peppermint
- Pumpkin seeds
- Puntarelle
- Radicchio
- Red-leaf lettuce
- Rosemary
- Sesame seeds
- Sultana raisins
- Sunflower seeds
- Tardivo di Treviso

Defense: Regeneration

- Anchovies
- Apple peel
- Apples (Granny Smith, Red Delicious, Reinette)
- Apricots
- Arctic char
- Bamboo shoots

- Barley
- Beer
- Belgian endive
- Bigeye tuna
- Bitter melon
- Black bass
- Black chokeberry
- Black plums
- Black raspberries

- Black tea
- Blackberries
- Blueberries
- Blueberries (dried)
- Bluefin tuna
- Bluefish
- Bottarga
- Capers
- Carrots

- Caviar (sturgeon)
- Celery
- Chamomile tea
- Cherries
- Cherries (dried)
- Chestnuts
- Chia seeds
- Chile peppers
- Chinese celery
- Cockles (clam)
- Coffee
- Collard greens
- Concord grape juice
- Cranberries
- Cranberries (dried)
- Dark chocolate
- Eastern oysters
- Eggplant
- Escarole
- Fiddleheads
- Fish roe (salmon)
- Flax seeds
- Frisee
- Ginseng
- Goji berries
- Grapes
- Gray mullet
- Green beans
- Green tea
- Hake

- Halibut
- John Dory (fish)
- Kale
- Kiwifruit
- Lychee
- Mackerel
- Mangoes
- Manila clams
- Mediterranean sea bass
- Mustard greens
- Nectarines
- Olive oil (EVOO)
- Onions
- Oregano
- Pacific oysters
- Peaches
- Peanuts
- Peppermint
- Persimmon
- Pistachios
- Plums
- Pomegranates
- Pompano (fish)
- Pumpkin seeds
- Puntarelle
- Purple potatoes
- Radicchio
- Rainbow trout
- Raspberries
- Razor clams

- Red-leaf lettuce
- Red mullet
- Red wine (Cabernet, Cabernet Franc, Petit Verdot)
- Redfish
- Rice bran
- Rosemary
- Saffron
- Salmon
- Sardine
- Sea bass
- Sea bream
- Sea cucumber
- Sesame seeds
- Soy
- Spinach
- Spiny lobster
- Squash blossoms
- Squid ink
- Strawberries
- Sultana raisins
- Sunflower seeds
- Swiss chard
- Swordfish
- Tardivo di Treviso
- Thyme
- Truffles
- Tuna
- Turmeric

- Walnuts
- Wasabi
- Watercress
- Whole grains
- Yellowtail (fish)

Defense: Microbiome

- Apricots
- Arugula
- Asparagus
- Bamboo shoots
- Black beans
- Black tea
- Blueberries
- Bok choy
- Broccoli
- Cabbage
- Camembert cheese
- Carrots
- Cauliflower
- Chamomile tea
- Chanterelle mushrooms
- Cherries
- Chia seeds
- Chickpeas
- Chile peppers
- Coffee
- Concord grape juice
- Cranberries
- Cranberry juice
- Dark chocolate
- Eggplant
- Enoki mushrooms
- Escarole
- Fiddleheads
- Flax seeds
- Frisee
- Gouda cheese
- Green tea
- Kale
- Kimchi
- Kiwifruit
- Lentils
- Lion's mane mushrooms
- Lychee
- Maitake mushrooms
- Mangoes
- Morel mushrooms
- Navy beans
- Nectarines
- Olive oil (EVOO)
- Oolong tea
- Oyster mushrooms
- Pao cai
- Parmigiano-Reggiano
- Peaches
- Peas
- Plums
- Pomegranate juice
- Porcini mushrooms
- Pumpernickel bread
- Pumpkin seeds
- Puntarelle
- Radicchio
- Red wine (Cabernet, Cabernet Franc, Petit Verdot)
- Rutabaga
- Sauerkraut
- Sesame seeds
- Shiitake mushrooms
- Sourdough bread
- Squid ink
- Sunflower seeds

- Tardivo di Treviso
- Tomatoes
- Turnips
- Walnuts
- White button mushrooms
- Whole grains
- Yogurt

Defense: DNA Protection

- Acerola
- Almond butter
- Almonds
- Anchovies
- Apricots
- Arctic char
- Arugula
- Bamboo shoots
- Basil
- Bigeye tuna
- Black bass
- Black tea
- Blueberries
- Bluefin tuna
- Bluefish
- Bok choy
- Bottarga
- Brazil nuts
- Broccoli
- Broccoli rabe
- Broccoli sprouts
- Cabbage
- Camu camu
- Carrots
- Cashew butter
- Cashews
- Cauliflower
- Caviar (sturgeon)
- Chamomile tea
- Cherries
- Cherry tomatoes
- Chestnuts
- Cockles (clam)
- Coffee
- Concord grape juice
- Dark chocolate
- Eastern oysters
- Eggplant
- Fiddleheads
- Fish roe (salmon)
- Flax seeds
- Grapefruit
- Gray mullet
- Green tea
- Guava
- Hake
- Halibut
- Hazelnuts
- John Dory (fish)
- Kale
- Kiwifruit
- Lychee
- Macadamia nuts
- Mackerel
- Mangoes
- Manila clams
- Marjoram
- Mediterranean sea bass
- Mixed berry juice
- Nectarines
- Olive oil (EVOO)
- Oolong tea
- Orange juice
- Oranges
- Oyster sauce
- Pacific oysters
- Papaya
- Peaches
- Peanut butter
- Peanuts
- Pecans
- Peppermint
- Pine nuts

- Pink grapefruit
- Pistachios
- Plums
- Pompano
- Pumpkin seeds
- Rainbow trout
- Red black-skin tomatoes
- Red mullet
- Redfish
- Romanesco
- Rosemary
- Rutabaga
- Sage
- Salmon
- San Marzano tomato
- Sardine
- Sea bass
- Sea bream
- Sea cucumber
- Sesame seeds
- Soy
- Spiny lobster
- Squash blossoms
- Squash seeds
- Squid ink
- Strawberries
- Sunflower seeds
- Swordfish
- Tahini
- Tangerine tomatoes
- Thyme
- Truffles
- Tuna
- Turmeric
- Turnips
- Walnuts
- Watermelon
- Yellowtail (fish)

Defense: Immunity

- Acerola
- Aged garlic
- Apple peel
- Apples (Granny Smith, Red Delicious, Reinette)
- Apricots
- Arugula
- Bamboo shoots
- Barley
- Belgian endive
- Black plums
- Black raspberries
- Black tea
- Blackberries
- Blackberries (dried)
- Blueberries
- Blueberries (dried)
- Bok choy
- Broccoli
- Broccoli rabe
- Broccoli sprouts
- Cabbage
- Camu camu
- Capers
- Carrots
- Cauliflower
- Chamomile tea
- Chanterelle mushrooms
- Cherries
- Cherries (dried)
- Cherry tomatoes
- Chestnuts
- Chia seeds
- Chile peppers
- Coffee
- Collard greens

- Concord grape juice
- Cranberries
- Cranberries (dried)
- Cranberry juice
- Dark chocolate
- Eggplant
- Enoki mushrooms
- Escarole
- Fiddleheads
- Flax seeds
- Frisee
- Ginseng
- Goji berries
- Grapefruit
- Green tea
- Guava
- Kale
- Kimchi
- Kiwifruit
- Licorice root
- Lychee
- Maitake mushrooms

- Mangoes
- Morel mushrooms
- Mustard greens
- Nectarines
- Olive oil (EVOO)
- Onions
- Orange juice
- Oranges
- Oyster mushrooms
- Pacific oysters
- Peaches
- Peppermint
- Plums
- Pomegranates
- Porcini mushrooms
- Pumpkin seeds
- Puntarelle
- Radicchio
- Raspberries
- Razor clams
- Red-leaf lettuce
- Red wine (Cabernet, Cabernet Franc, Petit Verdot)

- Romanesco
- Rosemary
- Rutabaga
- Saffron
- Sauerkraut
- Sesame seeds
- Shiitake mushrooms
- Spinach
- Squash blossoms
- Squid ink
- Strawberries
- Sultana raisins
- Swiss chard
- Tardivo di Treviso
- Truffles
- Turmeric
- Turnips
- Walnuts
- Watercress
- White button mushrooms

Assess Your Risks

Now that you've had a deep dive on your health defense systems and learned how foods can be used in an everyday framework to enhance them, I've created an additional tool that you can use to calculate how much risk you face with your health, adapted from an algorithm that's used by medical doctors around the world.

The Health Risk Score system that I've developed is designed to help you assess your current health situation and future risks and apply this knowledge to making smart decisions to protect your health. Understanding your personal risk can be a highly motivating factor for changing your diet and lifestyle. The foods and beverages you choose to consume every day can help change your risks.

Face it, everyone has his or her own personal health risks. Many factors can impact your body and affect your risk of developing a serious disease over your lifetime. From childhood through adolescence, and from adulthood and into your golden years, where you live, what you do for work, what you eat, and how you spend your leisure time can increase or decrease those risks. Your genes set the stage for the diseases you might eventually develop, but you can change your fate by understanding and lowering some risks.

You've probably noticed that your primary care doctor, also called general practitioner, assesses your health risk every time you go in for a checkup. During your very first appointment, your doctor interviews you in some depth about your personal history, your family's history, your lifestyle, your concerns and fears, all before the stethoscope comes out. He or she asks you what you do for work, your hobbies, the health of your parents and siblings, and a myriad of other questions that physicians are trained to ask. Your doctor is getting to know you as an individual with these questions, while also doing a health risk assessment—gathering and mentally analyzing your information to generate a picture of how likely you are to develop a serious, life-threatening condition while at the same time devising a plan to help you avoid a future health calamity.

The Health Risk Score

For this assessment, I've designed an easy scoring system that helps you calculate how much risk to your health you currently face. My system is based on three levels of health risk: low risk, moderate risk, and high risk. You can find out which category you are in based on your answers to a series of eighteen questions that are part of a formula that generates your Health Risk Score. Each answer generates a partial score. When you add up the scores, you have a total composite score.

Scoring systems in health assessments are an important way to help people understand their risks for diseases as well as mortality. The Centers for Disease Control, the Agency for Health Research and Quality, and insurance companies all use various instruments to measure health risks.[1] In my system, which is based on known health risk factors from personal and family history, your total score is not a predictor for any specific disease but is designed to show you the weight of your risk factors stacked together, reflecting the increased danger of having more risks compared to fewer risks in any individual person.

I'll take you through each question in my Health Risk Score system and show you examples of scoring and how to calculate the composite score.

QUESTION I: How Old Are You?

Your risk for a large number of preventable chronic diseases increases as you get older.

Scoring: If you are under thirty, give yourself a score of 0. If you are between thirty and fifty years old, give yourself a score of +1. If you are older than fifty, you are at higher risk for most chronic diseases from this point onward, so give yourself a score of +2.

QUESTION 2: What Is Your Sex?

This question doesn't get a numerical score. The purpose of this question is to help you focus on specific dietary factors that have evidence for reducing the risk of gender-specific conditions.

If you are a female, as you age, your risk increases for specific conditions, like breast, ovarian, cervical, endometrial, and uterine cancer. If you are male, you are at increasing risk for prostate cancer as you get older.

QUESTION 3: What Is Your Body Mass Index?

Your body mass index correlates with your risk for disease. The higher your body mass index, the greater your risk for conditions ranging from diabetes to cancer to cardiovascular disease.[2] Body Mass Index is a measure of how much fat is in the body based on your weight and height. The formula for BMI[3] is:

In kilograms and meters:
Weight (kilograms) / Height (meters)^2 = BMI

In pounds and inches:
Weight (pounds) / Height (inches)^2 × 703 = BMI

So, for example, someone who is 5 feet 7 inches tall (67 inches) and weighs 120 pounds has a BMI of 18.79.

The normal healthy range for BMI is considered to be between 18 and 25. If your BMI is below 18, you are considered underweight. A BMI between 25 and 30 is overweight. Any number above 30 is considered obese. Morbid obesity is defined as a BMI greater than 40. The risk associated with all the diseases linked to obesity goes way up if your BMI is over 30. An elevated BMI is going to increase your Health Risk Score. Keep in mind there are several variations of BMI scoring and interpretations adapted for children and for people of Asian origin. The calculation used in this algorithm is the one accepted by the World Health Organization.

Scoring: If your BMI is normal (18–25), your score is 0. For BMI 26–30, score yourself +1. For BMI over 30, give yourself a score of +2.

QUESTION 4: What Is Your Past Medical History?

As with so many things in life, your past can predict the future in terms of health. The more diseases you've had in the past, the greater the risk of potential future problems, regardless of the past conditions. This relates to diseases, not surgery or trauma. If you actively take any prescription medications, you probably have at least one medical condition. If you've ever been hospitalized for anything other than surgery for an accident or childbirth, you likely have a history of one or more medical conditions. Mental health conditions, such as depression, bipolar disorder, and schizophrenia, are an important part of your medical history. If you have any questions about this, just ask your primary care doctor to give you a list of the conditions reflecting your medical history, or you can get a copy of your medical record and look for notes your doctor has written under "past medical history." When you review all the medical conditions you've had, you'll want to label them either "active," which means it's an ongoing condition you are dealing with, or "inactive," meaning it was present in the past but no longer requiring attention or treatment.

Scoring: If you have had a clean bill of health and never been diagnosed with a disease, congratulations, score yourself a 0. If you have had one prior disease but it is inactive (not requiring attention and not being treated), score yourself a +1. This means your body may have recovered but there may still be lingering damage that increases your risk for future conditions. If you have at least one active medical condition for which you are currently being treated, or if you have had more than one prior disease diagnoses, whether they are active or inactive, then give yourself a score of +2.

QUESTION 5: Do You Have Any Super-High-Risk Medical Conditions That Predispose You for Developing Other Complications or Diseases in the Future?

Certain conditions are known by doctors to put a patient at high risk for developing future problems associated with disease as a downstream consequence. Some examples of super-high-risk conditions are:

- Actinic keratosis
- Autoimmune diseases such as inflammatory bowel disease, celiac disease, scleroderma, lupus, rheumatoid arthritis, multiple sclerosis
- Alcoholic liver disease
- Barrett's esophagus
- Cardiovascular disease, such as hypertension, coronary artery disease, carotid artery disease, or peripheral vascular disease
- Endometriosis
- Hepatitis
- HPV exposure
- Hyperlipidemia, including familial hypercholesterolemia
- Periodontitis
- Preeclampsia
- Renal insufficiency
- Traumatic head injury
- Type 1, type 2, or gestational diabetes

Scoring: If you have no super high-risk diseases in your medical history, your score is 0. If you have one high-risk disease, give yourself +1. If you have more than one high-risk condition, give yourself +2.

QUESTION 6: What Is Your Family History?

A family history of a certain medical condition can increase your own risk for developing that disease. Ask yourself if someone in your family—your mother, father, sibling, grandparents—had a disease that can be passed down across generations. This is a legacy you can't do anything about genetically (yet), but knowing you have this risk should guide you to taking swift actions on your diet to lower it. Some family history to risk assess for are:

- Cancer-associated syndromes, such as familial polyposis coli (FAP), Li-Fraumeni syndrome, Lynch syndrome, Von Hippel–Lindau Syndrome, or polycystic ovary syndrome
- Crohn's disease
- Familial hypercholesterolemia (high cholesterol)
- Heritable cancers, such as breast, ovarian, colon, prostate, stomach, melanoma, pancreatic, uterine, or retinoblastoma
- Neurodegenerative diseases such as Alzheimer's disease, Huntington's disease, and Parkinson's disease
- Type 1, type 2, or gestational diabetes

Scoring: If you have no family history of a heritable condition, score yourself 0. If you have one or more conditions, score yourself +2.

QUESTION 7: Where Do You Live?

Where you live can kill you. Even if you don't live near radioactive Chernobyl or Fukushima, some locations around the world have rates of diseases, like cancer, that are disproportionately higher than elsewhere—yet people live there without this knowledge or knowing what they can do to counteract their risks. Among U.S. locales, the top ten states with highest risk of cancer, in rank order, are Kentucky, Delaware, Louisiana, Pennsylvania, New York, Maine, New Jersey, Iowa, Rhode Island, and Connecticut.[4] Public health specialists speculate that there are environmental or other exposures present in these locales that are responsible for the elevated risk. If you reside in one of these states, you definitely need to do something to lower your risk. Around the world, the countries with the highest cancer rates are Denmark, France (metropolitan), Australia, Belgium, Norway, Ireland, Korea, Netherlands, and New Caledonia. If you live in one of these areas, you are in high-risk territory.

For diabetes, the locations with highest rates in the United States are Puerto Rico, Guam, Mississippi, West Virginia, Kentucky, Alabama, Louisiana, Tennessee, Texas, and Arkansas.[5] Worldwide, the areas with the highest diabetes rates are the Marshall Islands, Micronesia, Kiribati, French Polynesia, Saudi Arabia, Vanuatu, Kuwait, Bahrain, Mauritius, and New Caledonia.[6]

For highest cardiovascular disease risk, the states are Kentucky, West Virginia, Louisiana, Oklahoma, Alabama, Mississippi, Michigan, Arkansas, Tennessee, and Texas. Around the world, the countries with the highest death rates from cardiovascular disease are Russia, Ukraine, Romania, Hungary, Cuba, Brazil, Czech Republic, Argentina, and Mexico.

Keep in mind, deaths can be associated with the lack of access to modern medical care and a shortage of physicians in some areas. Nonetheless, these are some of the deadliest locales in the world. If you live in one of them, you are at higher risk than those living elsewhere.

These three major diseases—cancer, diabetes, and cardiovascular disease—represent the lion's share of largely preventable chronic diseases that not only can be reversed in many cases, but also can be prevented with improved diet and lifestyle.

Scoring: If you live in a top-ten high-risk area for one of these three killer diseases, give yourself a score of +1. If you do not, give yourself a score of 0.

QUESTION 8: What Is Your Genetic Risk?

A growing number of companies offer DNA testing on body fluids that can determine your risk for hereditary diseases. These services are part of a precision medicine revolution that became possible as increased computing power developed that can analyze millions of genetic data points. Your saliva contains DNA, and you can send it away to test for risk markers of cancers, Parkinson's disease, late-onset Alzheimer's disease, celiac disease, and rare disorders (hereditary thrombophilia, hereditary hemochromatosis, glucose-6-phosphate dehydrogenase deficiency, Gaucher's disease type 1, Factor XI deficiency, early-onset primary dystonia, and alpha-1-antitrysin deficiency).[7]

While only 5–10 percent of cancers are hereditary in nature, they can be identified through genetic testing. These are breast (female and male), colorectal, melanoma, ovarian, pancreatic, prostate, stomach, and uterine. The risk for some heart conditions can also be detected through DNA tests. Familial hypercholesterolemia, arteriopathies, arrhythmias, and cardiomyopathies are all detectable. If you've had your DNA analyzed and test positive for a genetic risk of disease, you can take immediate lifestyle actions, including changing your diet, to help lower your risks, especially for cancer, autoimmune diseases, neurodegenerative diseases, and heart disease.

Scoring: If you have not yet had a DNA test, score 0. If you've had a DNA test and no increased risks are detected, score 0. If your DNA test reveals one disease for which you are at higher risk, score +1. If the test reveals two or more conditions for which you are at risk, give yourself a score of +2.

QUESTION 9: Have You Had Any Toxic Exposures?

Toxic exposures in the environment increase your risk for a disease, and there are so many potential sources that it's impossible to list them all. You could have been exposed from where you live, from your work environment, from your home, and even from your hobbies.[8] Check to see if you've ever had significant contact with any of these common toxins that can pose a health threat:

- Arsenic (old toys)
- Asbestos (old buildings)
- Benzene (gasoline)
- Carbon tetrachloride (formerly used in dry cleaning solvents)
- Dioxin and the pesticide DDT
- Formaldehyde (auto exhaust)
- Industrial dyes (aromatic amines and aniline dyes)
- Lead
- Mercury (old dental fillings)
- Methylene chloride (paint thinner)
- Paradichlorobenzene (moth balls, toilet bowl deodorizer, room fresheners)
- Perfluorinated chemicals (found in old nonstick pans)
- Radiation (you were not shielded from)
- Radon (radiation from the ground that seeps into your home)
- Toluene (paint thinner)
- Vape smoke (from e-cigarettes)
- Vinyl chloride (water pipes)

Scoring: If you answered no to any history of significant exposure, then give yourself a 0. If you've had one significant exposure, score yourself +1. If you've had exposure to more than one toxin, give yourself a +2.

QUESTION 10: *Have You Ever or Do You Currently Use Tobacco?*

It's a no-brainer. Tobacco use (cigarettes, cigars, pipes, snuff, chew) is a deadly habit, but not everyone realizes that this holds true even if the exposure was years ago. This is true whether it is smoked or chewed. In fact, even though tobacco is a toxic exposure, it increases the danger to your health so much that it merits its own risk score. And being in the household or regular company of an active smoker is almost as bad as smoking yourself. Even pet cats that live with smokers develop oral cancers, because they lick the smoke off their fur.[9]

Scoring: If you have never smoked, give yourself a 0. If you are a former habitual smoker, previously lived in a smoker's household, or worked in or spent any significant time in an environment filled with tobacco smoke (restaurant, bar, club)—but you do not now—give yourself a +1. If you are an active smoker—including vaping—or live, work, or spend significant time in an environment where other people smoke, score yourself a +2.

QUESTION 11: *Do You Drink Alcohol?*

Mild to moderate consumption of red wine and beer, as you've read about in this book, can be beneficial to your health. Heavy consumption places you at risk for a number of chronic diseases, especially of the gastrointestinal system, because alcohol is a toxin. This is true for every type of alcoholic drink.

Score: If you don't drink at all, give yourself a 0. If you drink modestly (one or fewer glasses of red wine or beer per day, but not liquor), give yourself a −1 (subtract a point) because your disease risk is lowered. If you routinely drink more than one glass of wine or a beer or take a shot of distilled spirits each day, score yourself a +1. If you regularly drink hard liquor, then score yourself a +2.

QUESTION 12: What Is Your Lifelong Dietary Pattern?

Most people don't think about their diet in the context of their lifetime, but how you were raised and what you've consumed over years eating in specific patterns either builds or reduces your health risks. What you suddenly do to change course may be a good new start toward a healthier future, but your overall Health Risk Score is, in fact, based on lifetime exposures and long-standing behaviors when it comes to food.

So, over the course of your life, how would you describe your overall dietary pattern? Think of which of the following three broad patterns your life has generally followed: a Mediterranean or Asian diet made with fresh ingredients and abundant in vegetables and dietary fiber; a Western-style diet that is often referred to as a "meat and potatoes" plan with a heavy emphasis on meat and light on fresh vegetables; or a junk food diet made of mostly prepared and packaged industrially processed foods, fast foods and fried foods from restaurants, saturated fats, soft drinks, and rampant snacking.

Scoring: If you are in the first category, give yourself a −1 (this favors health, so you subtract a risk point). If you once had an unhealthy diet but are now eating a healthier, mostly plant-based diet, give yourself a 0. If you answered Western-style diet, give yourself a +1. If you answered junk food diet, give yourself a +2.

QUESTION 13: What Is Your Level of Physical Activity?

Being physically active is central to health at any age. Exercise is key for strength and fitness, but even regular brisk walking is beneficial. You don't need to belong to a gym or have a trainer. Perhaps you enjoy the outdoors and regularly go for hikes. Or maybe your work keeps you in physical motion, requiring muscle strength and some exertion.

On the other hand, if your job involves sitting at a desk staring at a computer screen the entire workday and then you drive home and sit on the couch watching television, let's face it—you live a sedentary lifestyle.

People who have lower levels of physical activity tend to spend almost all of their time indoors. Living a sedentary life is itself a health risk and a setup for future disease.

Scoring: If you have an active physical activity program, such as regular exercise, give yourself a score of −2 (subtract two points). If you have occasional exercise and rate yourself as being physically active, give yourself a 0. If you have absolutely no exercise and are not physically active, give yourself a +2.

QUESTION 14: Do You Own a Pet?

Owning a pet decreases stress and anxiety, helps mental health, and can increase your physical activity. Do you have a pet dog, cat, bird, lizard, horse, or other companion animal? Even having owned a pet in years past can leave a beneficial mark on your health destiny.

Scoring: If you have a pet or have ever had one, give yourself a −1 (subtract a point). If you don't have a pet, give yourself a 0.

QUESTION 15: Were You Breastfed as an Infant?

Breastfeeding not only bonds an infant with his or her mother but it also gives the infant's immunity a head start in life. Studies have shown that breastfeeding as an infant benefits the immune system for the rest of an individual's life. In addition to the mother's antibodies, breast milk also contains healthy bacteria and is a probiotic delivery system that builds the infant's healthy microbiome. And it increases telomere length. Simply put, if you were breastfed, you have an advantage over someone who was not.

Scoring: If you know you were breastfed, give yourself a −1. If you are not certain, score yourself a 0. If you are certain you were not breastfed, give yourself a +1.

QUESTION 16: Do You Work a Night Shift?

Many important jobs require people to work overnight shifts. Medicine, law enforcement, security, military, and tech all are examples of fields where night shifts are common. During my medical residency training, I was regularly assigned overnight shifts for weeks on end. While it's still possible to get the right number of hours of sleep each day, there's a caveat: your body was designed to follow cues from the sun. Your hormones, cardiovascular system, microbiome, and immunity all are coordinated to follow a circadian rhythm. Staying up all night forces these systems to be out of sync with their innate schedule, and your health defenses become weaker. Pulling an all-nighter for a few nights here or there while you are a student is not a problem, but your body pays for it afterward. You not only feel terrible for days, but you might also get sick more easily. These are signs your body's defenses are out of kilter. Being a professional night shift worker amplifies the disruption big time. Studies show that people who work night shifts are at increased risk for chronic diseases ranging from cardiovascular disease to several types of cancer.[10]

Scoring: If you are currently working a night shift job, give yourself a +1. If you do not currently work a nightshift job, give yourself a score of 0.

QUESTION 17: What Is the Level of Stress in Your Life?

A little stress in life is fine and might even give you an edge to succeed in your work and hobbies. But chronic stress places a huge and harmful burden on your health defenses. It increases cortisol secretion from your adrenal glands, places undue demands on your heart, alters your microbiome for the worse, disrupts angiogenesis, impairs the function of your stem cells, and lowers your immunity.[11] Stress can be linked to emotional, behavioral, physical, social, or financial factors. Do you live in a constant state of unrelieved stress, anxiety, fear, or anger? Or do you tend to flow through life's periodic stressors with minimal angst? Rate your daily stress level as low, moderate, or high.

Scoring: If you rate yourself as low stress, give yourself a 0. If you are moderately stressed, give yourself a +1. If you live in a state of chronic high stress, give yourself +2.

QUESTION 18: Did One or Both of Your Parents Die at an Early Age (before the Age of Fifty) from a Health Problem?

The health of your parents can be a predictive factor for the fate of your own health. In addition to genetics, our parents pass on traits and behaviors that influence our lifestyle choices, which can create exposures at an early age. These epigenetic influences can be beneficial or harmful, and we carry them with us for the rest of our lives. When parents die at an early age from ill health (as opposed to accidental death), it can be a signal of a problem that has been passed down genetically or epigenetically. Some of the common causes of premature death in parents are cancer, cardiovascular disease, and complications from diabetes. If one or both of your parents died from one of these multifactorial killers before the age of fifty, you may be at higher risk than average, too.

Scoring: If both your parents lived beyond the age of fifty, score yourself 0. If one of your parents died before fifty, give yourself a +1. If both did, score yourself +2.

Totaling Your Health Risk Score

Now that you've finished the health risk assessment questionnaire, add up your individual scores to get your overall Health Risk Score. The higher the number, the greater your risk. The highest possible score is 29. Based on your total score, you will land in one of three color-coded zones: red, yellow, or green. To interpret your health risk and your need to take action, find where your final score falls in the groups below.

Total Score: 19–29. You Are in the Red Zone

HIGHEST RISK

If your score puts you in this category, you are squarely in the danger zone. Without some deliberate changes in your life, the odds are stacked against you—there's every chance you are on a collision course with a major illness in the future. It's time to take a serious look at what you can do to lower your risks, especially when it comes to your diet and lifestyle. If you look at the questions that generate the score, there are at least nine places where you could make a deliberate change to lower your risk score. Here's how it could work: lose weight, move to a lower-risk locale (not easy, but worth considering), quit smoking or vaping, reduce alcohol intake, lower stress, quit the night shift, get a pet, take a daily brisk walk. Very importantly, change your diet immediately by using the 5 × 5 × 5 framework to get the benefits of foods described in this book.

Total Score: 10–18. You Are in the Yellow Zone

MODERATE RISK

If your score puts you in this category, you are not in imminent danger, but you need to actively reduce risks so your score doesn't increase further. Pay close attention to your diet in order to lower your health risks. Remember, if you don't smoke and do exercise regularly, you can reduce the risk of some cancers by 70 percent, diabetes by 90 percent, and heart disease by as much as 80 percent using diet.[12] You are not yet in danger, but don't let your guard down. Build health-defensive eating into your life on a daily basis.

By the way, you may think of yourself as a healthy person, but you are still in the Yellow Zone. The reason why may be, in part, because of factors you can't control, such as where you live or your age. Age in particular can elevate your score because as you get older, the risk for many diseases simply increases. Add to that a family history, a bad habit, or an occupational hazard, and you can see how you wound up in the yellow zone. You should make it a priority to start decreasing the risks you can control.

Total Score: 0–9. You Are in the Green Zone

LOWEST RISK

Congratulations! You are in the lowest possible risk category. This probably means you are younger, slimmer, haven't had many harmful exposures in your life, never smoked, made healthy decisions in your diet (whether you knew it or not), have good genetics, and are physically active. The green zone is where you want to stay. You are in the best possible position to make this happen. Recognize that as you get older and continue to encounter harmful toxins in the environment, you'll be adding numbers to your score. This is where diet comes in. Start by deliberately eating foods that boost your health defense systems. Try new foods described throughout the book. See how many food and beverage choices you can make each week based on one of the items in part 2. Keep a log of these choices so you can refer to previous weeks, and see if you can best yourself. Keep up the good work, and power up your health defenses so you can fight the assaults of aging and living in our modern world.

The research on food and health defenses is taking place at such a fast pace that new information is emerging on a regular basis. To get updated checklists with new preferred foods that impact the health defenses, visit www.drwilliamli.com/checklist.

Acknowledgments

Writing this book was far from a solo journey—it was a team effort. *Eat to Beat Disease* is the result of the hard work, persistence, and dedication of an amazing group of individuals to whom I owe my gratitude. I'd like to thank my longtime friend and advisor Robin Colucci, who encouraged me, rather insistently, to translate my knowledge into the pages of a book. She gave me a road map, then served as my coach, copilot, and copyeditor as I set off on the odyssey of writing. I must thank my outstanding research team—Catherine Ward, Dasha Agoulnik, Bridget Gayer, Rachel Chiaverelli, Samantha Stone, and Michelle Hutnik—who helped me to critically review and analyze hundreds of complex scientific, clinical, and public health studies described in this book. They provided perspective as I translated the findings into an understandable and accurate narrative for the nonscientist reader. I want to thank Maria Aufiero for working with me on developing recipes, as well as testing them in her kitchen. To Katrina Markoff, thank you for providing your talent with chocolate and the hot cocoa recipe. Many thanks to Liz Alverson for providing me with the perspectives of a motivated health seeker and helping me translate my ideas into practical everyday applications for readers.

I am truly grateful to my extraordinary agents—Celeste Fine, Sarah Passick, John Maas, Andrea Mei, and Emily Sweet—at Park & Fine Literary and Media. They are not only the best team any author could hope for, but they are also fun to work with while being laser focused on getting the highest quality results at every level. Celeste provided me with sage advice at every critical step as this book took shape. John became a key member of my writing team and lent his editorial experience to make complex content easier to understand and more enjoyable to read. To my editor, Karen Murgolo, and the team at Grand Central Publishing/Hachette, Ben Sevier, Leah Miller, Amanda Pritzker, and Matthew Ballast, who saw my vision and gave me the freedom to put into words how I believe the world can become a healthier place, I give my thanks and deep appreciation. I would also like to thank Ike Williams and Brian Carey, who were always there to support me with their counsel.

I'd like to acknowledge the many mentors and colleagues in science and medicine who have inspired and contributed to my career over the years: Anthony Vagnucci, Shang J. Yao, Franklin Fuchs, Winton Tong, Karel Liem, Judah Folkman, Pat D'Amore, Bob Langer, Chuck Watson, David Steed, Cesare Lombroso, Les Fang, Michael Maragoudakis, Moritz Konerding, Adriana Albini, Doug Losordo, Richard Beliveau, and Max Ackermann. Some of these individuals are no longer with us, but their influence burns bright and is still strongly felt.

A few people deserve special mention. Vincent Li, my brother, colleague, and fellow trailblazer, is an equal partner in the development of many of the ideas about food and health in this book, some of which took place in extraordinary locales and with amazing friends. Eric Lowitt, fellow author, friend, and social-impact expert, encouraged me with useful advice, humor, and wit during the book development process. Courtney Martel, my chief of staff, always made sure everything got done seamlessly and properly. Dean Ornish, with whom I share a similar career path, camaraderie, research, and intellectual passions, was an inspiration for bringing my message to the public. The Edge, my friend, ally, and compatriot for advancing medicine, has always generously given me his time, great ideas, and enthusiasm for finding better ways to beat disease.

Finally, I could not have written this book without the support of Shawna, Madeleine, and Oliver, who gave me the time away to put this all together to share with the world.

Notes

Chapter 1: Angiogenesis

1. J. Folkman and R. Kalluri, "Cancer without Disease," *Nature* 427, no. 6977 (2004): 787.
2. B. N. Ames, M. K. Shigenaga, and T. M. Hagen, "Oxidants, Antioxidants, and the Degenerative Diseases of Aging," *Proceedings of the National Academy of Sciences USA* 90, no. 17 (1993): 7915–7922; S. Clancy, "DNA Damage and Repair: Mechanisms for Maintaining DNA Integrity," *Nature Education* 1, no. 1 (2008): 103.
3. J. Folkman and R. Kalluri, "Cancer without Disease," *Nature* 427, no. 6977 (2004): 787.
4. M. Lovett, K. Lee, A. Edwards, and D. L. Kaplan, "Vascularization Strategies for Tissue Engineering," *Tissue Engineering Part B: Reviews* 15, no. 3 (2009): 353–370.
5. Robyn D. Pereira et al., "Angiogenesis in the Placenta: The Role of Reactive Oxygen Species Signaling," *BioMed Research International* (2015): 814543.
6. L. A. DiPietro, "Angiogenesis and Wound Repair: When Enough Is Enough," *Journal of Leukocyte Biology* 100, no. 5 (2016): 979–984.
7. A. Orlidge and P. A. D'Amore, "Inhibition of Capillary Endothelial Cell Growth by Pericytes and Smooth Muscle Cells," *Journal of Cell Biology* 105, no. 3 (1987): 1455–1462.
8. M. A. Gimbrone, S. B. Leapman, R. S. Cotran, and J. Folkman, "Tumor Dormancy In Vivo by Prevention of Neovascularization," *Journal of Experimental Medicine* 136 (1974): 261.
9. C. W. White et al., "Treatment of Pulmonary Hemangiomatosis with Recombinant Interferon Alfa-2a," *New England Journal of Medicine* 320, no. 18 (1989): 1197–1200.
10. Y. Cao and R. Langer, "A Review of Judah Folkman's Remarkable Achievements in Biomedicine," *Proceedings of the National Academy of Sciences USA* 105, no. 36 (2008): 13203–13205.
11. A. H. Vagnucci Jr. and W. W. Li, "Alzheimer's Disease and Angiogenesis," *Lancet* 361, no. 9357 (2003): 605–608.
12. J. V. Silha, M. Krsek, P. Sucharda, and L. J. Murphy, "Angiogenic Factors Are Elevated in Overweight and Obese Individuals," *International Journal of Obesity* 29, no. 11 (2005): 1308–14.
13. M. A. Rupnick et al., "Adipose Tissue Mass Can Be Regulated through the Vasculature," *Proceedings of the National Academy of Sciences USA* 99, no. 16 (2002): 10730–10735.
14. P. Schratzberger et al., "Reversal of Experimental Diabetic Neuropathy by VEGF Gene Transfer," *Journal of Clinical Investigation* 107, no. 9 (2001): 1083–1092.

15. R. Kirchmair et al., "Therapeutic Angiogenesis Inhibits or Rescues Chemotherapy-Induced Peripheral Neuropathy: Taxol- and Thalidomide-Induced Injury of Vasa Nervorum Is Ameliorated by VEGF," *Molecular Therapy* 15, no. 1 (2007): 69–75.

16. S. R. Nussbaum et al., "An Economic Evaluation of the Impact, Cost, and Medicare Policy Implications of Chronic Nonhealing Wounds" *Value Health* 21, no. 1 (2018): 27–32; D. G. Armstrong, J. Wrobel, and J. M. Robbins, "Guest Editorial: Are Diabetes-Related Wounds and Amputations Worse than Cancer?" *International Wound Journal* 4, no. 4 (2007): 286–287.

17. Emiko Jozuka and Yoko Ishitani, "World's Oldest Person Dies at 117," CNN, https://www.cnn.com/2018/07/26/health/japan-centenarian-longevity/index.html.

Chapter 2: Regeneration

1. R. J. Kara et al., "Fetal Cells Traffic to Injured Maternal Myocardium and Undergo Cardiac Differentiation," *Circulation Research* 110, no. 1 (2012): 82–93.

2. Ron Milo and Rob Phillips, "How Quickly Do Different Cells in the Body Replace Themsleves?" Cell Biology by the Numbers, http://book.bionumbers.org/how-quickly-do-different-cells-in-the-body-replace-themselves; "Lifespan of a Red Blood Cell," Bionumbers, http://bionumbers.hms.harvard.edu/bionumber.aspx?&id=107875.

3. "Determination of Adipose Cell Size in Eight Epididymal Fat Pads by Four Methods," Bionumbers, http://bionumbers.hms.harvard.edu/bionumber.aspx?&id=107076.

4. J. E. Till and E. A. McCulloch, "A Direct Measurement of the Radiation Sensitivity of Normal Mouse Bone Marrow Cells," *Radiation Research* 14, no. 2 (1961): 213–222.

5. Eva Bianconi et al., "An Estimation of the Number of Cells in the Human Body," *Annals of Human Biology* 40, no. 6 (2013).

6. S. Y. Rabbany, B. Heissig, K. Hattori, and S. Rafii, "Molecular pathways regulating mobilization of marrow-derived stem cells for tissue revascularization," *Trends in Molecular Medicine* 9, no. 3 (2003): 109–17.

7. I. Petit, D. Jin, and S. Rafii, "The SDF-1-CXCR4 Signaling Pathway: A Molecular Hub Modulating Neo-Angiogenesis," *Trends in Immunology* 28, no. 7 (2007): 299–307.

8. E. T. Condon, J. H. Wang, and H. P. Redmond, "Surgical Injury Induces the Mobilization of Endothelial Progenitor Cells," *Surgery* 135, no. 6 (2004): 657–661.

9. G. D. Kusuma, J. Carthew, R. Lim, and J. E. Frith, "Effect of the Microenvironment on Mesenchymal Stem Cell Paracrine Signaling: Opportunities to Engineer the Therapeutic Effect," *Stem Cells and Development* 26, no. 9 (2017): 617–631; S. Keshtkar, N. Azarpira, and M. H. Ghahremani, "Mesenchymal Stem Cell-Derived Extracellular Vesicles: Novel Frontiers in Regenerative Medicine," *Stem Cell Research and Therapy* 9, no. 1 (2018): 63.

10. I. Linero and O. Chaparro, "Paracrine Effect of Mesenchymal Stem Cells Derived from Human Adipose Tissue in Bone Regeneration," *PLOS One* 9, no. 9 (2014): e107001.

11. F. Mobarrez et al., "The Effects of Smoking on Levels of Endothelial Progenitor Cells and Microparticles in the Blood of Healthy Volunteers," *PLOS One* 9, no. 2 (2014): e90314; S. Beyth et al., "Cigarette Smoking Is Associated with a Lower Concentration of CD105(+) Bone Marrow Progenitor Cells," *Bone Marrow Research* 2015 (2015): 914935.

12. S. E. Michaud et al., "Circulating Endothelial Progenitor Cells from Healthy Smokers Exhibit Impaired Functional Activities," *Atherosclerosis* 187, no. 2 (2006): 423–432.

13. C. Heiss et al., "Brief Secondhand Smoke Exposure Depresses Endothelial Progenitor Cells Activity and Endothelial Function: Sustained Vascular Injury and Blunted Nitric Oxide Production," *Journal of the American College of Cardiology* 51, no. 18 (2008): 1760–1771.

14. T. E. O'Toole et al., "Episodic Exposure to Fine Particulate Air Pollution Decreases Circulating Levels of Endothelial Progenitor Cells," *Circulation Research* 107, no. 2 (2010): 200–203.

15. J. K. Williams et al., "The Effects of Ethanol Consumption on Vasculogenesis Potential in Nonhuman Primates," *Alcoholism: Clinical and Experimental Research* 32, no. 1 (2008): 155–161.

16. H. Wang et al., "In Utero Exposure to Alcohol Alters Cell Fate Decisions by Hematopoietic Progenitors in the Bone Marrow of Offspring Mice during Neonatal Development," *Cell Immunology* 239, no. 1 (2006): 75–85.

17. J. A. McClain, D. M. Hayes, S. A. Morris, and K. Nixon, "Adolescent Binge Alcohol Exposure Alters Hippocampal Progenitor Cell Proliferation in Rats: Effects on Cell Cycle Kinetics," *Journal of Comparative Neurology* 519, no. 13 (2011): 2697–2710.

18. At the University of Colorado in Boulder, researchers studied this by comparing the stem cells of healthy, non-obese older men (in their sixties) to those found in younger men in their twenties. There were striking differences. EPCs from older people produced 60 percent fewer factors that help the cells survive compared to stem cells from the young group.

19. M. Pirro et al., "Hypercholesterolemia-Associated Endothelial Progenitor Cell Dysfunction," *Therapeutic Advances in Cardiovascular Disease* 2, no. 5 (2008): 329–339.

20. D. R. Pu and L. Liu, "HDL Slowing Down Endothelial Progenitor Cells Senescence: A Novel Anti-Atherogenic Property of HDL," *Medical Hypotheses* 70, no. 2 (2008): 338–342.

21. H. Kang et al., "High Glucose-Induced Endothelial Progenitor Cell Dysfunction," *Diabetes and Vascular Disease Research* 14, no. 5 (2017): 381–394; G. P. Fadini, M. Albiero, S. Vigili de Kreutzenberg, E. Boscaro, R. Cappellari, M. Marescotti, N. Poncina, C. Agostini, and A. Avogaro, "Diabetes Impairs Stem Cell and Proangiogenic Cell Mobilization in Humans," *Diabetes Care* 36, no. 4 (2013): 943–949.

22. K. Aschbacher et al., "Higher Fasting Glucose Levels Are Associated with Reduced Circulating Angiogenic Cell Migratory Capacity among Healthy Individuals," *American Journal of Cardiovascular Disease* 2, no. 1 (2012): 12–19.

23. O. M. Tepper et al., "Human Endothelial Progenitor Cells from Type II Diabetics Exhibit Impaired Proliferation, Adhesion, and Incorporation into Vascular Structures," *Circulation* 106, no. 22 (2002): 2781–2786.

24. C. J. Loomans et al., "Endothelial Progenitor Cell Dysfunction: A Novel Concept in the Pathogenesis of Vascular Complications of Type 1 Diabetes," *Diabetes* 53, no. 1 (2004): 195–199.

25. "Diabetes," World Health Organization, http://www.who.int/mediacentre/factsheets/fs312/en.

26. G. P. Fadini et al., "Circulating Endothelial Progenitor Cells Are Reduced in Peripheral Vascular Complications of Type 2 Diabetes Mellitus," *Journal of the American College of Cardiology* 45, no. 9 (2005): 1449–1457.

27. T. Kusuyama et al., "Effects of Treatment for Diabetes Mellitus on Circulating Vascular Progenitor Cells," *Journal of Pharmacological Sciences* 102, no. 1 (2006): 96–102.

28. N. Werner et al., "Circulating Endothelial Progenitor Cells and Cardiovascular Outcomes," *New England Journal of Medicine* 353, no. 10 (2005): 999–1007.

29. H. Björkbacka et al., "Plasma Stem Cell Factor Levels Are Associated with Risk of Cardiovascular Disease and Death," *Journal of Internal Medicine* 282, no. 2 (2017): 508–521.

30. A. Rivera, I. Vanzuli, J. J. Arellano, and A. Butt, "Decreased Regenerative Capacity of Oligodendrocyte Progenitor Cells (NG2-Glia) in the Ageing Brain: A Vicious Cycle of Synaptic Dysfunction, Myelin Loss, and Neuronal Disruption?" *Current Alzheimer Research* 13, no. 4 (2016): 413–418.

31. Q. Wang et al., "Stromal Cell-Derived Factor 1α Decreases β-Amyloid Deposition in Alzheimer's Disease Mouse Model," *Brain Research* 1459 (2012): 15–26.

32. O. Fernández et al., Adipose-Derived Mesenchymal Stem Cells (AdMSC) for the Treatment of Secondary-Progressive Multiple Sclerosis: A Triple Blinded, Placebo Controlled, Randomized Phase I/II Safety and Feasibility Study," *PLOS One* 13, no. 5 (2018): e0195891; C. G. Song et al., "Stem Cells: A Promising Candidate to Treat Neurological Disorders," *Neural Regeneration Research* 13, no. 7 (2018): 1294–1304; G. Dawson et al., "Autologous Cord Blood Infusions Are Safe and Feasible in Young Children with Autism Spectrum Disorder: Results of a Single-Center Phase I Open-Label Trial," *Stem Cells Translational Medicine* 6, no. 5 (2017): 1332–1339.

33. J. H. Houtgraaf et al., "First Experience in Humans Using Adipose Tissue-Derived Regenerative Cells in the Treatment of Patients with ST-Segment Elevation Myocardial Infarction," *Journal of the American College of Cardiology* 59, no. 5 (2012): 539–540.

34. Peter Dockrill, "Japanese Scientists Have Used Skin Cells to Restore a Patient's Vision for the First Time," https://www.sciencealert.com/japanese-scientists-have-used-skin-cells-to-restore-a-patient-s-vision-for-the-first-time.

35. Cura Foundation, "Cellular Horizons Day 2: Using Adult Stem Cells to Treat Autoimmune Disorders," https://www.youtube.com/watch?v=Iafkr-qRnm0.

36. C. M. Zelen et al., "A Prospective, Randomised, Controlled, Multi-Centre Comparative Effectiveness Study of Healing Using Dehydrated Human Amnion/Chorion Membrane Allograft, Bioengineered Skin Substitute, or Standard of Care for Treatment of Chronic Lower Extremity Diabetic Ulcers," *International Wound Journal* 12, no. 6 (2015): 724–732; T. E. Serena et al., "A Multicenter, Randomized, Controlled Clinical Trial Evaluating the Use of Dehydrated Human Amnion/Chorion Membrane Allografts and Multilayer Compression Therapy vs. Multilayer Compression Therapy Alone in the Treatment of Venous Leg Ulcers," *Wound Repair and Regeneration* 22, no. 6 (2014): 688–693.

37. Z. N. Maan et al., "Cell Recruitment by Amnion Chorion Grafts Promotes Neovascularization," *Journal of Surgical Research* 193, no. 2 (2015): 953–962.

38. E. Keelaghan, D. Margolis, M. Zhan, and M. Baumgarten, "Prevalence of Pressure Ulcers on Hospital Admission among Nursing Home Residents Transferred to the Hospital," *Wound Repair and Regeneration* 16, no. 3 (2008): 331–336.

Chapter 3: Microbiome

1. P. Hartmann et al., "Normal Weight of the Brain in Adults in Relation to Age, Sex, Body Height, and Weight." *Pathologe* 15, no. 3 (1994): 165–170; Alison Abbott, "Scientists Bust Myth That Our Bodies Have More Bacteria than Human Cells," *Nature*, Jan. 8, 2016, http://www.nature.com/news/scientists-bust-myth-that-our-bodies-have-more-bacteria-than-human-cells-1.19136.

2. G. Clarke et al., "Minireview: Gut Microbiota: The Neglected Endocrine Organ," *Molecular Endocrinology* 28, no. 8 (2014): 1221–1238.

3. Jane A. Foster, Linda Rinaman, and John F. Cryan, "Stress and the Gut-Brain Axis: Regulation by the Microbiome," *Neurobiology of Stress* 7 (2017): 124–136.

4. C. M. Schlebusch et al., "Southern African Ancient Genomes Estimate Modern Human Divergence to 350,000 to 260,000 Years Ago," *Science* 358, no. 6363 (2017): 652–655; C. M. Schlebusch et al., "Southern African Ancient Genomes Estimate Modern Human Divergence to 350,000 to 260,000 Years Ago," *Science* 358, no. 6363 (2017): 652–655.

5. C. Menni et al., "Gut Microbiome Diversity and High Fibre Intake Are Related to Lower Long-Term Weight Gain," *International Journal of Obesity* 41, no. 7 (2017): 1099–1105.

6. I. Semmelweis, *Die Aetiologie, der Begriff und die Prophylaxis des Kindbettfiebers* [The Etiology, Concept, and Prophylaxis of Childbed Fever] (Pest: C. H. Hartleben's Verlag-Expedition, 1861).

7. Joseph Lister, "On the Antiseptic Principle in the Practice of Surgery," *Lancet* 90, no. 2299 (1867): 353–356.

8. Lina Zeldovich, "The Man Who Drank Cholera and Launched the Yogurt Craze," *Nautilus*, Apr. 23, 2015, http://nautil.us/issue/23/dominoes/the-man-who-drank-cholera-and-launched-the-yogurt-craze.

9. Bill Landers, "Oral Bacteria: How Many? How Fast?" RDHmag.com, July 1, 2009, https://www.rdhmag.com/articles/print/volume-29/issue-7/columns/the-landers-file/oral-bacteria-how-many-how-fast.html.

10. https://www.hmpdacc.org/hmp.

11. Human Microbiome Project Consortium, "Structure, Function, and Diversity of the Healthy Human Microbiome," *Nature* 486, no. 7402 (2012): 207–214.

12. "The Precise Reason for the Health Benefits of Dark Chocolate: Mystery Solved," American Chemical Society, Mar. 18, 2014, https://www.acs.org/content/acs/en/press room/newsreleases/2014/march/the-precise-reason-for-the-health-benefits-of-dark-chocolate-mystery-solved.html; D. J. Morrison and T. Preston, "Formation of Short Chain Fatty Acids by the Gut Microbiota and Their Impact on Human Metabolism," *Gut Microbes* 7, no. 3 (2016): 189–200.

13. H. J. Kim, J. S. Noh, and Y. O. Song, "Beneficial Effects of Kimchi, a Korean Fermented Vegetable Food, on Pathophysiological Factors Related to Atherosclerosis," *Journal of Medicinal Food* 21, no. 2 (2018): 127–135.

14. C. Nastasi et al., "The Effect of Short-Chain Fatty Acids on Human Monocyte-Derived Dendritic Cells," *Scientific Reports* 5 (2015): 16148.

15. D. Liu et al., "Low Concentration of Sodium Butyrate from Ultrabraid+NaBu Suture, Promotes Angiogenesis and Tissue Remodelling in Tendon-Bones Injury," *Scientific Reports* 6 (2016): 34649.

16. E. S. Chambers, D. J. Morrison, and G. Frost, "Control of Appetite and Energy Intake by SCFA: What Are the Potential Underlying Mechanisms?" *Proceedings of the Nutrition Society* 74, no. 3 (2015): 328–336.

Notes

17. A. F. Athiyyah et al., "Lactobacillus Plantarum IS-10506 Activates Intestinal Stem Cells in a Rodent Model," *Beneficial Microbes* (May 4, 2018): 1–6.

18. M. K. Kwak et al., "Cyclic Dipeptides from Lactic Acid Bacteria Inhibit Proliferation of the Influenza A Virus," *Journal of Microbiology* 51, no. 6 (2013): 836–43.

19. C. Carreau, G. Flouriot, C. Bennetau-Pelissero, and M. Potier, "Enterodiol and Enterolactone, Two Major Diet-Derived Polyphenol Metabolites Have Different Impact on ERalpha Transcriptional Activation in Human Breast Cancer Cells," *Journal of Steroid Chemistry and Molecular Biology* 110, no. 1–2 (2008): 176–185.

20. F. P. Martin et al., "Metabolic Effects of Dark Chocolate Consumption on Energy, Gut Microbiota, and Stress-Related Metabolism in Free-Living Subjects," *Journal of Proteome Research* 8, no. 12 (2009): 5568–5579.

21. "Intestinal Bacteria May Protect against Diabetes," Science Daily, Apr. 11, 2017, https://www.sciencedaily.com/releases/2017/04/170411090159.htm.

22. J. Loubinoux et al., "Sulfate-Reducing Bacteria in Human Feces and Their Association with Inflammatory Bowel Diseases," *FEMS Microbiology Ecology* 40, no. 2 (2002): 107–112.

23. Cassandra Willyard, "Could Baby's First Bacteria Take Root before Birth?" *Nature*, Jan. 17, 2018, https://www.nature.com/articles/d41586-018-00664-8.

24. E. Jašarević, C. L. Howerton, C. D. Howard, and T. L. Bale, "Alterations in the Vaginal Microbiome by Maternal Stress Are Associated with Metabolic Reprogramming of the Offspring Gut and Brain," *Endocrinology* 156, no. 9 (2015): 3265–3276.

25. Ashley P. Taylor, "Breast Milk Contributes Significantly to Babies' Bacteria," The Scientist, May 10, 2017, https://www.the-scientist.com/?articles.view/articleNo/49400/title/Breast-Milk-Contributes-Significantly-to-Babies-Bacteria.

26. Pia S. Pannaraj et al., "Association between Breast Milk Bacterial Communities and Establishment and Development of the Infant Gut Microbiome," *JAMA Pediatrics* 171, no. 7 (2017): 647–654.

27. J. C. Madan et al., "Association of Cesarean Delivery and Formula Supplementation With the Intestinal Microbiome of 6-Week-Old Infants," *JAMA Pediatrics* 170, no. 3 (2016): 212–219.

28. G. Bian et al., "The Gut Microbiota of Healthy Aged Chinese Is Similar to That of the Healthy Young," *mSphere* 2, no. 5 (2017): e00327-17.

29. E. Thursby and N. Juge, "Introduction to the Human Gut Microbiota," *Biochemical Journal* 474, no. 11 (2017): 1823–1836.

30. R. Kort et al., "Shaping the Oral Microbiota through Intimate Kissing," *Microbiome* 17, no. 2 (2014): 41.

31. O. Firmesse et al., "Fate and Effects of Camembert Cheese Micro-Organisms in the Human Colonic Microbiota of Healthy Volunteers after Regular Camembert Consumption," *International Journal of Food Microbiology* 125, no. 2 (2008): 176–181.

32. E. D. Sonnenburg et al., "Diet-Induced Extinctions in the Gut Microbiota Compound over Generations," *Nature* 529, no. 7585 (2016): 212–215.

33. Y. Su et al., "Ecological Balance of Oral Microbiota Is Required to Maintain Oral Mesenchymal Stem Cell Homeostasis," *Stem Cells* 36, no. 4 (2018): 551–561; A. Khandagale and C. Reinhardt, "Gut Microbiota—Architects of Small Intestinal Capillaries," *Frontiers in Bioscience* 23 (2018): 752–766; X. Sun and M. J. Zhu, "Butyrate Inhibits Indices of Colorectal Carcinogenesis via Enhancing α-Ketoglutarate-Dependent DNA Demethylation of Mismatch Repair Genes," *Molecular Nutrition and Food Research* 62, no. 10 (2018): e1700932.

34. Moises Velasquez-Manoff, "Microbes, a Love Story," *New York Times*, Feb. 10, 2017, https://www.nytimes.com/2017/02/10/opinion/sunday/microbes-a-love-story.html.

35. S. Carding et al., "Dysbiosis of the Gut Microbiota in Disease," *Microbial Ecology in Health and Disease* 26 (2015): 10.3402/mehd.v26.26191; J. Lu et al., "The Role of Lower Airway Dysbiosis in Asthma: Dysbiosis and Asthma," *Mediators of Inflammation* 2017 (2017): 3890601; A. C. R. Tanner et al., "The Caries Microbiome: Implications for Reversing Dysbiosis," *Advances in Dental Research* 29, no. 1 (2018): 78–85; F. Lv et al., "The Role of Microbiota in the Pathogenesis of Schizophrenia and Major Depressive Disorder and the Possibility of Targeting Microbiota as a Treatment Option," *Oncotarget* 8, no. 59 (2017): 100899–100907.

36. "FDA in Brief: FDA Issues Final Rule on Safety and Effectiveness for Certain Active Ingredients in Over-the-Counter Health Care Antiseptic Hand Washes and Rubs in the Medical Setting," U.S. Food and Drug Administration, Dec. 19, 2017, https://www.fda.gov/newsevents/newsroom/fdainbrief/ucm589474.htm; C. S. Bever et al., "Effects of Triclosan in Breast Milk on the Infant Fecal Microbiome," *Chemosphere* 203 (2018): 467–473; H. Yang et al., "A Common Antimicrobial Additive Increases Colonic Inflammation and Colitis-Associated Colon Tumorigenesis in Mice," *Science Translational Medicine* 10, no. 443 (2018).

37. "Probiotics Market to Exceed $65bn by 2024," Global Market Insights, Oct. 10, 2017, https://globenewswire.com/news-release/2017/10/10/1143574/0/en/Probiotics-Market-to-exceed-65bn-by-2024-Global-Market-Insights-Inc.html.

Chapter 4: DNA Protection

1. B. N. Ames, M. K. Shigenaga, and T. M. Hagen, "Oxidants, Antioxidants, and the Degenerative Diseases of Aging," *Proceedings of the National Academy of Sciences USA* 90, no. 17 (1993): 7915–7922.

2. "Deciphering the Genetic Code," Office of NIH History, https://history.nih.gov/exhibits/nirenberg/HS1_mendel.htm.

3. R. Dahm, "Friedrich Miescher and the Discovery of DNA," *Developmental Biology* 278, no. 2 (2005): 274–288.

4. "International Consortium Completes Human Genome Project," National Human Genome Research Institute, Apr. 14, 2003, https://www.genome.gov/11006929/2003-release-international-consortium-completes-hgp.

5. Eva Bianconi et al., "An Estimation of the Number of Cells in the Human Body," *Annals of Human Biology* 40, no. 6 (2013).

6. Stephen P. Jackson and Jiri Bartek, "The DNA-Damage Response in Human Biology and Disease," *Nature* 461, no. 7267 (2009): 1071–1078.

7. S. Premi et al., "Photochemistry: Chemiexcitation of Melanin Derivatives Induces DNA Photoproducts Long after UV Exposure," *Science* 347, no. 6224 (2015): 842–847.

8. M. Sanlorenzo et al., "The Risk of Melanoma in Pilots and Cabin Crew: UV Measurements in Flying Airplanes," *JAMA Dermatology* 151, no. 4 (2015): 450–452.

9. "Health Risk of Radon," U.S. Environmental Protection Agency, https://www.epa.gov/radon/health-risk-radon.

10. "Carcinogens in Tobacco Smoke," Government of Canada, https://www.canada.ca/en/health-canada/services/publications/healthy-living/carcinogens-tobacco-smoke.html.

11. P. Mikeš et al., "3-(3,4-Dihydroxyphenyl)adenine, a Urinary DNA Adduct Formed in Mice Exposed to High Concentrations of Benzene," *Journal of Applied Toxicology* 33, no. 6 (2013): 516–520.

12. M. S. Estill and S. A. Krawetz, "The Epigenetic Consequences of Paternal Exposure to Environmental Contaminants and Reproductive Toxicants," *Current Environmental Health Reports* 3, no. 3 (2016): 202–213.

13. R. H. Waring, R. M. Harris, and S. C. Mitchell, "In Utero Exposure to Carcinogens: Epigenetics, Developmental Disruption, and Consequences in Later Life," *Maturitas* 86 (2016): 59–63.

14. "What Are Genome Editing and CRISPR-Cas9?" Genetics Home Reference, U.S. National Library of Medicine, https://ghr.nlm.nih.gov/primer/genomicresearch/geno meediting.

15. L. A. Macfarlane and P. R. Murphy, "MicroRNA: Biogenesis, Function and Role in Cancer," *Current Genomics* 11, no. 7 (2010): 537–561.

16. Elisa Grazioli et al., "Physical Activity in the Prevention of Human Diseases: Role of Epigenetic Modifications," *BMC Genomics* 18, suppl. 8 (2017): 802.

17. J. Denham, "Exercise and Epigenetic Inheritance of Disease Risk," *Acta Physiologica* 222, no. 1 (2018).

18. C. Spindler et al., "Treadmill Exercise Alters Histone Acetyltransferases and Histone Deacetylases Activities in Frontal Cortices from Wistar Rats," *Cellular and Molecular Neurobiology* 34, no. 8 (2014): 1097–1101.

19. Lars R. Ingerslev et al., "Endurance Training Remodels Sperm-Borne Small RNA Expression and Methylation at Neurological Gene Hotspots," *Clinical Epigenetics* 2018; 10: 12.

20. G. V. Skuladottir, E. K. Nilsson, J. Mwinyi, and H. B. Schiöth, "One-Night Sleep Deprivation Induces Changes in the DNA Methylation and Serum Activity Indices of Stearoyl-CoA Desaturase in Young Healthy Men," *Lipids in Health and Disease* 15, no. 1 (2016): 137.

21. L. Li, S. Zhang, Y. Huang, and K. Chen, "Sleep Duration and Obesity in Children: A Systematic Review and Meta-analysis of Prospective Cohort Studies." *Journal of Paediatrics and Child Health* 53, no. 4 (2017): 378–385.

22. Emil K. Nilsson, Adrian E. Bostrom, Jessica Mwinyi, and Helgi B. Schioth, "Epigenomics of Total Acute Sleep Deprivation in Relation to Genome-Wide DNA Methylation Profiles and RNA Expression," *OMICS* 20, no. 6 (2016): 334–342; S. Lehrer, S. Green, L. Ramanathan, and K. E. Rosenzweig, "Obesity and Deranged Sleep Are Independently Associated with Increased Cancer Mortality in 50 US States and the District of Columbia," *Sleep and Breathing* 17, no. 3 (2013): 1117–1118.

23. P. Kaliman et al., "Rapid Changes in Histone Deacetylases and Inflammatory Gene Expression in Expert Meditators," *Psychoneuroendocrinology* 40 (2014): 96–107.

24. A. K. Smith et al., "Differential Immune System DNA Methylation and Cytokine Regulation in Post-Traumatic Stress Disorder," *American Journal of Medical Genetics Part B: Neuropsychiatric Genetics* 156B, no. 6 (2011): 700–708.

25. B. C. J. Dirven, J. R. Homberg, T. Kozicz, and M. J. A. G. Henckens, "Epigenetic Programming of the Neuroendocrine Stress Response by Adult Life Stress," *Journal of Molecular Endocrinology* 59, no. 1 (2017): R11–R31.

26. Elizabeth Blackburn, "The Science of Cells That Never Get Old," TED, Apr. 2017, https://www.ted.com/talks/elizabeth_blackburn_the_science_of_cells_that_never_get_old.

27. J. Wojcicki et al., "Exclusive Breastfeeding Is Associated with Longer Telomeres in Latino Preschool Children," *American Journal of Clinical Nutrition* 104, no. 2 (2016): 397–405.

28. M. A. Shammas, "Telomeres, Lifestyle, Cancer, and Aging," *Current Opinion in Clinical Nutrition and Metabolic Care* 14, no. 1 (2011): 28–34.

29. D. F. Terry et al., "Association of Longer Telomeres with Better Health in Centenarians," *Journal of Gerontology Series A: Biological Sciences and Medical Sciences* 63, no. 8 (2008): 809–812.

30. L. A. Tucker, "Physical Activity and Telomere Length in U.S. Men and Women: An NHANES Investigation," *Preventive Medicine* 100 (2017): 145–151.

31. H. Lavretsky et al., "A Pilot Study of Yogic Meditation for Family Dementia Caregivers with Depressive Symptoms: Effects on Mental Health, Cognition, and Telomerase Activity," *International Journal of Geriatric Psychiatry* 28, no. 1 (2013): 57–65; N. S. Schutte and J. M. Malouff, "A Meta-Analytic Review of the Effects of Mindfulness Meditation on Telomerase Activity," *Psychoneuroendocrinology* 42 (2014): 45–48; S. Duraimani et al., "Effects of Lifestyle Modification on Telomerase Gene Expression in Hypertensive Patients: A Pilot Trial of Stress Reduction and Health Education Programs in African Americans," *PLOS One* 10, no. 11 (2015): e0142689.

32. D. Ornish et al., "Increased Telomerase Activity and Comprehensive Lifestyle Changes: A Pilot Study," *Lancet Oncology* 9, no. 11 (2008): 1048–1057; D. Ornish et al., "Effect of Comprehensive Lifestyle Changes on Telomerase Activity and Telomere Length in Men with Biopsy-Proven Low-Risk Prostate Cancer: 5-Year Follow-Up of a Descriptive Pilot Study," *Lancet Oncology* 14, no. 11 (2013): 1112–1120.

33. J. M. Wojcicki, R. Medrano, J. Lin, and E. Epel, "Increased Cellular Aging by 3 Years of Age in Latino, Preschool Children Who Consume More Sugar-Sweetened Beverages: A Pilot Study," *Childhood Obesity* 14, no. 3 (2018): 149–157.

Chapter 5: Immunity

1. C. Ceci et al., "Ellagic Acid Inhibits Bladder Cancer Invasiveness and In Vivo Tumor Growth," *Nutrients* 8, no. 11 (2016).

2. "The Smallpox Eradication Programme—SEP (1966–1980)," World Health Organization, May 2010, http://www.who.int/features/2010/smallpox/en.

3. C. Chang, "Time Frame and Reasons of Kangxi Emperor Adopted Variolation" [in Chinese], *Zhonghua Yi Shi Za Zhi* 26, no. 1 (1996): 30–32.

4. For an excellent TED-Ed animation describing smallpox eradication, see Simona Zompi, "How We Conquered the Deadly Smallpox Virus," YouTube, Oct. 28, 2013, https://www.youtube.com/watch?v=yqUFy-t4MlQ.

5. T. Araki et al., "Normal Thymus in Adults: Appearance on CT and Associations with Age, Sex, BMI and Smoking," *Eur Radiol.* 26, no. 1 (2016): 15–24.

6. Suzanne Wu, "Fasting Triggers Stem Cell Regeneration of Damaged, Old Immune System," USC News, June 5, 2014, https://news.usc.edu/63669/fasting-triggers-stem-cell-regeneration-of-damaged-old-immune-system; C. W. Cheng et al., "Prolonged Fasting Reduces IGF-1/PKA to Promote Hematopoietic-Stem-Cell-Based Regeneration and Reverse Immunosuppression," *Cell Stem Cell* 14, no. 6 (2014): 810–823.

7. John Travis, "On the Origin of the Immune System," *Science* 324, no. 5927 (2009): 580–582, http://science.sciencemag.org/content/324/5927/580.

8. For science buffs: the beacon is called a class 2 major histocompatability complex (MHC). This is found on a variety of immune cells, such as macrophages, dendritic cells, cytotoxic T cells, and B cells. These cells will combine the particles from invaders with class 2 MHC, and the group will be presented on the surface of the

immune cell, signaling that they are in the heat of battle and could use some guidance and backup. This draws in the helper T cell to help coordinate and amplify the response.

9. For science buffs: the beacon here is a class 1 MHC. An infected cell will combine the foreign antigen of its invader with class 1 MHC and move this group to the surface of the cell, effectively "presenting" it to cytoxic T cells to signal for their own destruction.

10. J. Yang and M. Reth, "Receptor Dissociation and B-Cell Activation," *Current Topics in Microbiology and Immunology* 393 (2016): 27–43.

11. B. Alberts et al. "B Cells and Antibodies," in *Molecular Biology of the Cell*, 4th ed. (New York: Garland Science, 2002), https://www.ncbi.nlm.nih.gov/books/NBK 26884.

12. T. D. Noakes et al., "Semmelweis and the Aetiology of Puerperal Sepsis 160 Years On: An Historical Review," *Epidemiology and Infection* 136, no. 1 (2008): 1–9.

13. J. D. de Sousa, C. Alvarez, A. M. Vandamme, and V. Müller, "Enhanced Heterosexual Transmission Hypothesis for the Origin of Pandemic HIV-1," *Viruses* 4, no. 10 (2012): 1950–1983.

14. P. E. Serrano, S. A. Khuder, and J. J. Fath, "Obesity as a Risk Factor for Nosocomial Infections in Trauma Patients," *Journal of the American College of Surgeons* 211, no. 1 (2010): 61–67.

15. G. V. Bochicchio et al., "Impact of Obesity in the Critically Ill Trauma Patient: A Prospective Study," *Journal of the American College of Surgeons* 203, no. 4 (2006): 533–538.

16. J. Suvan et al., "Association between Overweight/Obesity and Periodontitis in Adults: A Systematic Review," *Obesity Reviews* 12, no. 5 (2011): e381–404; M. J. Semins et al., "The Impact of Obesity on Urinary Tract Infection Risk," *Urology* 79, no. 2 (2012): 266–269; J. C. Kwong, M. A. Campitelli, and L. C. Rosella, "Obesity and Respiratory Hospitalizations during Influenza Seasons in Ontario, Canada: A Cohort Study," *Clinical Infectious Diseases* 53, no. 5 (2011): 413–421.

17. S. V. Aguayo-Patrón and A. M. Calderón de la Barca, "Old Fashioned vs. Ultra-Processed-Based Current Diets: Possible Implication in the Increased Susceptibility to Type 1 Diabetes and Celiac Disease in Childhood," *Foods* 6, no. 11 (2017).

18. E. Y. Huang et al., "The Role of Diet in Triggering Human Inflammatory Disorders in the Modern Age," *Microbes and Infection* 15, no. 12 (2013): 765–774.

Chapter 6: Starve Your Disease, Feed Your Health

1. T. Fotsis et al., "Genistein, a Dietary-derived Inhibitor of Vitro Angiogenesis," *Proceedings of the National Academy of Sciences USA* 90, no. 7 suppl. (1993): 2690–4.

2. F. Tosetti, N. Ferrari, S. De Flora, and A. Albini, "Angioprevention: Angiogenesis Is a Common and Key Target for Cancer Chemopreventive Agents," *FASEB Journal* 16, no. 1 (2002): 2–14.

3. A. Albini et al., "Cancer Prevention by Targeting Angiogenesis," *Nature Reviews Clinical Oncology* 9, no. 9 (2012): 498–509.

4. J. Liu et al., "Balancing between Aging and Cancer: Molecular Genetics Meets Traditional Chinese Medicine," *Journal of Cellular Biochemistry* 118, no. 9 (2017): 2581–2586.

5. E. R. O'Brien et al., "Angiogenesis in Human Coronary Atherosclerotic Plaques," *American Journal of Pathology* 145, no. 4 (1994): 883–894.

6. P. R. Moreno et al., "Plaque Neovascularization Is Increased in Ruptured Atherosclerotic Lesions of Human Aorta: Implications for Plaque Vulnerability," *Circulation* 110, no. 14 (2004): 2032–2038.

7. Preetha Anand et al., "Cancer Is a Preventable Disease That Requires Major Lifestyle Changes," *Pharmaceutical Research* 25, no. 9 (2008): 2097–2116.

8. X. O. Shu et al., "Soy Food Intake and Breast Cancer Survival," *JAMA* 302, no. 22 (2009): 2437–2443; C. C. Applegate et al., "Soy Consumption and the Risk of Prostate Cancer: An Updated Systematic Review and Meta-Analysis," *Nutrients* 10, no. 1 (2018); Z. Yan et al., "Association between Consumption of Soy and Risk of Cardiovascular Disease: A Meta-Analysis of Observational Studies," *European Journal of Preventive Cardiology* 24, no. 7 (2017): 735–747.

9. S. H. Lee, J. Lee, M. H. Jung, and Y. M. Lee, "Glyceollins, a Novel Class of Soy Phytoalexins, Inhibit Angiogenesis by Blocking the VEGF and bFGF Signaling Pathways," *Molecular Nutrition and Food Research* 57, no. 2 (2013): 225–234.

10. D. L. Bemis et al., "A Concentrated Aglycone Isoflavone Preparation (GCP) That Demonstrates Potent Anti-Prostate Cancer Activity In Vitro and In Vivo," *Clinical Cancer Research* 10, no. 15 (2004): 5282–5292; J. L. McCall, R. A. Burich, and P. C. Mack, "GCP, a Genistein-Rich Compound, Inhibits Proliferation and Induces Apoptosis in Lymphoma Cell Lines," *Leukeumia Research* 34, no. 1 (2010): 69–76.

11. G. C. Meléndez et al., "Beneficial Effects of Soy Supplementation on Postmenopausal Atherosclerosis Are Dependent on Pretreatment Stage of Plaque Progression," *Menopause* 22, no. 3 (2015): 289–296.

12. Z. Yan et al., "Association between Consumption of Soy and Risk of Cardiovascular Disease: A Meta-Analysis of Observational Studies," *European Journal of Preventive Cardiology* 24, no. 7 (2017): 735–747.

13. S. Lecomte, F. Demay, F. Ferrière, and F. Pakdel, "Phytochemicals Targeting Estrogen Receptors: Beneficial Rather than Adverse Effects?" *International Journal of Molecular Sciences* 18, no. 7 (2017): E1381.

14. X. O. Shu et al., "Soy Food Intake and Breast Cancer Survival," *Journal of the American Medical Association* 302, no. 22 (2009):2437–2443.

15. J. Shi, M. Le Maguer, Lycopene in Tomatoes: Chemical and Physical Properties Affected by Food Processing," *Critical Reviews in Food Science and Nutrition* 40, no. 1 (2000): 1–42.

16. N. Z. Unlu et al., "Lycopene from Heat-Induced Cis-Isomer-Rich Tomato Sauce Is More Bioavailable than from All-Trans-Rich Tomato Sauce in Human Subjects," *British Journal of Nutrition* 98, no. 1 (2007): 140–146.

17. J. L. Rowles III et al., "Processed and Raw Tomato Consumption and Risk of Prostate Cancer: A Systematic Review and Dose-Response Meta-analysis," *Prostate Cancer and Prostatic Diseases* 21 (2018): 319–336.

18. R. E. Graff et al., "Dietary Lycopene Intake and Risk of Prostate Cancer Defined by ERG Protein Expression," *American Journal of Clinical Nutrition* 103, no. 3 (2016): 851–860.

19. K. Zu et al., "Dietary Lycopene, Angiogenesis, and Prostate Cancer: A Prospective Study in the Prostate-Specific Antigen Era," *Journal of the National Cancer Institute* 106, no. 2 (2014): djt430.

20. S. R. Bhandari, M.-C. Cho, and J. G. Lee, "Genotypic Variation in Carotenoid, Ascorbic Acid, Total Phenolic, and Flavonoid Contents, and Antioxidant Activity in Selected Tomato Breeding Lines," *Horticulture, Environment, and Biotechnology* 57, no. 5 (2016): 440–452.

21 J. L. Cooperstone et al., "Enhanced Bioavailability of Lycopene When Consumed as Cis-Isomers from Tangerine Compared to Red Tomato Juice, a Randomized, Cross-over Clinical Trial," *Molecular Nutrition and Food Research* 59, no. 4 (2015): 658–669.

22. N. Z. Unlu et al., "Carotenoid Absorption in Humans Consuming Tomato Sauces Obtained from Tangerine or High-Beta-Carotene Varieties of Tomatoes," *Journal of Agricultural and Food Chemistry* 55, no. 4 (2007): 1597–1603.

23. P. Flores, E. Sánchez, J. Fenoll, and P. Hellín, "Genotypic Variability of Carotenoids in Traditional Tomato Cultivars," *Food Research International* 100, pt. 3 (2017): 510–516.

24. B. C. Chiu et al., "Dietary Intake of Fruit and Vegetables and Risk of Non-Hodgkin Lymphoma," *Cancer Causes and Control* 22, no. 8 (2011): 1183–1195; K. A. Steinmetz, J. D. Potter, and A. R. Folsom, "Vegetables, Fruit, and Lung Cancer in the Iowa Women's Health Study," *Cancer Research* 53, no. 3 (1993): 536–543; L. I. Mignone et al., "Dietary Carotenoids and the Risk of Invasive Breast Cancer," *International Journal of Cancer* 124, no. 12 (2009): 2929–2937; M. A. Gates et al., "A Prospective Study of Dietary Flavonoid Intake and Incidence of Epithelial Ovarian Cancer," *International Journal of Cancer* 121, no. 10 (2007): 2225–2232; N. D. Freedman et al., "Fruit and Vegetable Intake and Esophageal Cancer in a Large Prospective Cohort Study," *International Journal of Cancer* 121, no. 12 (2007): 2753–2760; E. L. Richman, P. R. Carroll, and J. M. Chan, "Vegetable and fruit intake after diagnosis and risk of prostate cancer progression. *International Journal of Cancer* 131, no. 1 (2012): 201–210; A. E. Millen et al., "Diet and Melanoma in a Case-Control Study," *Cancer Epidemiology, Biomarkers, and Prevention* 13, no. 6 (2004): 1042–1051.

25. N. D. Freedman et al., "Fruit and Vegetable Intake and Esophageal Cancer in a Large Prospective Cohort Study," *International Journal of Cancer* 121, no. 12 (2007): 2753–2760; M. E. Wright et al., "Intakes of Fruit, Vegetables, and Specific Botanical Groups in Relation to Lung Cancer Risk in the NIH-AARP Diet and Health Study," *American Journal of Epidemiology* 168, no. 9 (2008): 1024–1034.

26. S. Katayama, H. Ogawa, and S. Nakamura, "Apricot Carotenoids Possess Potent Anti-Amyloidogenic Activity In Vitro," *Journal of Agricultural and Food Chemistry* 59, no. 23 (2011): 12691–12696.

27. S. Erdoğan and S. Erdemoğlu, "Evaluation of Polyphenol Contents in Differently Processed Apricots Using Accelerated Solvent Extraction Followed by High-Performance Liquid Chromatography-Diode Array Detector," *International Journal of Food Sciences and Nutrition* 62, no. 7 (2011): 729–739.

28. F. L. Büchner et al., "Consumption of Vegetables and Fruit and the Risk of Bladder Cancer in the European Prospective Investigation into Cancer and Nutrition," *International Journal of Cancer* 125 (2009): 2643–2651; S. Gallus et al., "Does an Apple a Day Keep the Oncologist Away?" *Annals of Oncology* 16, no. 11 (2005): 1841–1844; M. E. Wright et al., "Intakes of Fruit, Vegetables, and Specific Botanical Groups in Relation to Lung Cancer Risk in the NIH-AARP Diet and Health Study," *American Journal of Epidemiology* 168, no. 9 (2008): 1024–1034.

29. D. A. Hyson, "A Comprehensive Review of Apples and Apple Components and Their Relationship to Human Health," *Advances in Nutrition* 2, no. 5 (2011): 408–420.

30. C. A. Thompson et al., "Antioxidant Intake from Fruits, Vegetables, and Other Sources and Risk of Non-Hodgkin's Lymphoma: The Iowa Women's Health Study," *International Journal of Cancer* 126, no. 4 (2010): 992–1003.

31. F. L. Büchner et al., "Fruits and Vegetables Consumption and the Risk of Histological Subtypes of Lung Cancer in the European Prospective Investigation into Cancer and Nutrition (EPIC)," *Cancer Causes and Control* 21, no. 3 (2010): 357–371.

32. L. A. Kresty, S. R. Mallery, and G. D. Stoner, "Black Raspberries in Cancer Clinical Trials: Past, Present, and Future," *Journal of Berry Research* 6, no. 2 (2016): 251–261.

33. S. Lamy et al., "Delphinidin, a Dietary Anthocyanidin, Inhibits Vascular Endothelial Growth Factor Receptor-2 Phosphorylation," *Carcinogenesis* 27, no. 5 (2006): 989–996.

34. T. T. Fung et al., "Intake of Specific Fruits and Vegetables in Relation to Risk of Estrogen Receptor-Negative Breast Cancer among Postmenopausal Women," *Breast Cancer Research and Treatment* 138, no. 3 (2013): 925–930.

35. J. Kowshik et al., "Ellagic Acid Inhibits VEGF/VEGFR2, PI3K/Akt and MAPK Signaling Cascades in the Hamster Cheek Pouch Carcinogenesis Model," *Anticancer Agents in Medicinal Chemistry* 14, no. 9 (2014): 1249–1260.

36. S. Muthukumaran et al., "Ellagic Acid in Strawberry (*Frangaria* spp.): Biological, Technological, Stability, and Human Health Aspects," *Food Quality and Safety* 1, no. 4 (2017): 227–252.

37. K. K. Kim et al., "Anti-Angiogenic Activity of Cranberry Proanthocyanidins and Cytotoxic Properties in Ovarian Cancer Cells," *International Journal of Oncology* 40, no. 1 (2012): 227–235.

38. D. Mozaffarian et al., "Plasma Phospholipid Long-Chain ω-3 Fatty Acids and Total and Cause-Specific Mortality in Older Adults: A Cohort Study," *Annals of Internal Medicine* 158, no. 7 (2013): 515–525.

39. J. X. Kang and A. Liu, "The Role of the Tissue Omega-6/Omega-3 Fatty Acid Ratio in Regulating Tumor Angiogenesis," *Cancer and Metastasis Reviews* 32, no. 1–2 (2013): 201–210.

40. A. P. Simopoulos, "The Importance of the Omega-6/Omega-3 Fatty Acid Ratio in Cardiovascular Disease and Other Chronic Diseases," *Experimental Biology and Medicine* 233, no. 6 (2008): 674–688.

41. M. Gago-Dominguez et al., "Opposing Effects of Dietary n-3 and n-6 Fatty Acids on Mammary Carcinogenesis: The Singapore Chinese Health Study," *British Journal of Cancer* 89, no. 9 (2003): 1686–1692.

42. T. Norat et al., "Meat, Fish, and Colorectal Cancer Risk: The European Prospective Investigation into Cancer and Nutrition," *Journal of the National Cancer Institute* 97, no. 12 (2005): 906–916.

43. W. G. Christen et al., "Dietary ω-3 Fatty Acid and Fish Intake and Incident Age-Related Macular Degeneration in Women," *Archives of Ophthalmology* 129, no. 7 (2011): 921–929.

44. W. Zhu et al., "Fish Consumption and Age-Related Macular Degeneration Incidence: A Meta-Analysis and Systematic Review of Prospective Cohort Studies," *Nutrients* 8, no. 11 (2016).

45. T. J. Koivu-Tikkanen, V. Ollilainen, and V. I. Piironen, "Determination of Phyllo-quinone and Menaquinones in Animal Products with Fluorescence Detection after Postcolumn Reduction with Metallic Zinc," *Journal of Agricultural and Food Chemistry* 48, no. 12 (2000): 6325–6331.

46. T. Kayashima et al., "1,4-Naphthoquinone Is a Potent Inhibitor of Human Cancer Cell Growth and Angiogenesis," *Cancer Letters* 278, no. 1 (2009): 34–40.

47. A. Samykutty et al., "Vitamin K2, a Naturally Occurring Menaquinone, Exerts Thera-peutic Effects on Both Hormone-Dependent and Hormone-Independent Prostate Cancer Cells," *Evidence-Based Complementary and Alternatative Medicine* 2013, article ID 287358.

48. J. M. Geleijnse et al., "Dietary Intake of Menaquinone Is Associated with a Reduced Risk of Coronary Heart Disease: The Rotterdam Study," *Journal of Nutrition* 134, no. 11 (2004): 3100–3105.

49. H. Kawashima et al. "Effects of Vitamin K2 (Menatetrenone) on Atherosclerosis and Blood Coagulation in Hypercholesterolemic Rabbits," *Japanese Journal of Pharmacol-ogy* 75, no. 2 (1997): 135–143.

50. "About Jamón Ibérico," Jamon.com, https://www.jamon.com/about-jamon-iberico .html.

51. M. R. Sartippour et al., "Green Tea Inhibits Vascular Endothelial Growth Factor (VEGF) Induction in Human Breast Cancer Cells," *Journal of Nutrition* 132, no. 8 (2002): 2307–2311; T. Nagao, T. Hase, and I. Tokimitsu, "A Green Tea Extract High in Catechins Reduces Body Fat and Cardiovascular Risks in Humans," *Obesity* 16, no. 6 (2007): 1473–1483; D. Wu, J. Wang, M. Pae, and S. N. Meydani, "Green Tea EGCG, T Cells, and T Cell-Mediated Autoimmune Diseases," *Molecular Aspects of Medicine* 33, no. 1 (2012): 107–118; A. Basu et al., "Green Tea Supplementation Increases Glu-tathione and Plasma Antioxidant Capacity in Adults with the Metabolic Syndrome," *Nutrition Research* 33, no. 3 (2013): 180–187.

52. G. Yang et al., "Prospective Cohort Study of Green Tea Consumption and Colorectal Cancer Risk in Women," *Cancer Epidemiology, Biomarkers, and Prevention* 16, no. 6 (2007): 1219–1223.

53. R. Guimarães et al., "Wild Roman Chamomile Extracts and Phenolic Compounds: Enzymatic Assays and Molecular Modelling Studies with VEGFR-2 Tyrosine Kinase," *Food and Function* 7, no. 1 (2016): 79–83.

54. M. M. Markoski et al., "Molecular Properties of Red Wine Compounds and Cardio-metabolic Benefits," *Nutrition and Metabolic Insights* 9 (2016): 51–57.

55. J. Y. Park et al., "Baseline Alcohol Consumption, Type of Alcoholic Beverage and Risk of Colorectal Cancer in the European Prospective Investigation into Cancer and Nutrition-Norfolk Study," *Cancer Epidemiology* 33, no. 5 (2009): 347–354.

56. S. D. Crockett et al., "Inverse Relationship between Moderate Alcohol Intake and Rectal Cancer: Analysis of the North Carolina Colon Cancer Study," *Diseases of the Colon and Rectum* 54, no. 7 (2011): 887–894.

57. A. Albini et al., "Mechanisms of the Antiangiogenic Activity by the Hop Flavonoid Xanthohumol: NF-kappaB and Akt as Targets," *FASEB Journal* 20, no. 3 (2006): 527–529.

58. S. Karami, S. E. Daugherty, and M. P. Purdue, "A Prospective Study of Alcohol Con-sumption and Renal Cell Carcinoma Risk," *International Journal of Cancer* 137, no. 1 (2015): 238–242.

59. S. D. Crockett et al., "Inverse Relationship between Moderate Alcohol Intake and Rectal Cancer: Analysis of the North Carolina Colon Cancer Study," *Diseases of the Colon and Rectum* 54, no. 7 (2011): 887–894.

60. A. Di Castelnuovo et al., "Meta-Analysis of Wine and Beer Consumption in Relation to Vascular Risk," *Circulation* 105, no. 24 (2002): 2836–2844.

61. S. Weyerer et al., "Current Alcohol Consumption and Its Relationship to Incident Dementia: Results from a 3-Year Follow-up Study among Primary Care Attenders Aged 75 Years and Older," *Age and Ageing* 40, no. 4 (2011): 456–463.

62. T. J. Koivu-Tikkanen, V. Ollilainen, and V. I. Piirnen, "Determination of Phylloquinone and Menaquinones in Animal Products with Fluorescence Detection after Postcolumn Reduction with Metallic Zinc," *Journal of Agricultural and Food Chemistry* 48, no. 12 (2000): 6325–6331; C. Vermeer et al., "Menaquinone Content of Cheese," *Nutrients* 10, no. 4 (2018).

63. K. Nimptsch, S. Rohrmann, and J. Linseisen, "Dietary Intake of Vitamin K and Risk of Prostate Cancer in the Heidelberg Cohort of the European Prospective Investigation into Cancer and Nutrition (EPIC-Heidelberg)," *American Journal of Clinical Nutrition* 87, no. 4 (2008): 985–992.

64. C. Bosetti, C. Pelucchi, and C. La Vecchia, "Diet and Cancer in Mediterranean Countries: Carbohydrates and Fats," *Public Health Nutrition* 12, no. 9A (2009): 1595–1600.

65. T. Fadelu et al., "Nut Consumption and Survival in Patients With Stage III Colon Cancer: Results from CALGB 89803 (Alliance)," *Journal of Clinical Oncology* 36, no. 11 (2018): 1112–1120.

66. M. Jenab et al., "Association of Nut and Seed Intake with Colorectal Cancer Risk in the European Prospective Investigation into Cancer and Nutrition," *Cancer Epidemiology, Biomarkers, and Prevention* 13, no. 10 (2004): 1595–1603.

67. M. G. Jain, G. T. Hislop, G. R. Howe, and P. Ghadirian, "Plant Foods, Antioxidants, and Prostate Cancer Risk: Findings from Case-Control Studies in Canada," *Nutrition and Cancer* 34, no. 2 (1999): 173–184.

68. T. P. Kenny et al., "Cocoa Procyanidins Inhibit Proliferation and Angiogenic Signals in Human Dermal Microvascular Endothelial Cells following Stimulation by Low-Level H_2O_2," *Experimental Biology and Medicine* 229, no. 8 (2004): 765–771.

69. T. Kayashima and K. Matsubara, "Antiangiogenic Effect of Carnosic Acid and Carnosol, Neuroprotective Compounds in Rosemary Leaves," *Bioscience, Biotechnology, and Biochemistry* 76, no. 1 (2012): 115–119; M. Saberi-Karimian et al., "Vascular Endothelial Growth Factor: An Important Molecular Target of Curcumin," *Critical Reviews in Food Science and Nutrition* (2017): 1–14; P. Kubatka et al., "Oregano Demonstrates Distinct Tumour-Suppressive Effects in the Breast Carcinoma Model," *European Journal of Nutrition* 56, no. 3 (2017): 1303–1316; S. Kobayashi, T. Miyamoto, I. Kimura, and M. Kimura, "Inhibitory Effect of Isoliquiritin, a Compound in Licorice Root, on Angiogenesis In Vivo and Tube Formation In Vitro," *Biological and Pharmaceutical Bulletin* 18, no. 10 (1995): 1382–1386; J. Lu et al., "Novel Angiogenesis Inhibitory Activity in Cinnamon Extract Blocks VEGFR2 Kinase and Downstream Signaling," *Carcinogenesis* 31, no. 3 (2010): 481–488.

70. S. Agostini et al., "Barley Beta-Glucan Promotes MnSOD Expression and Enhances Angiogenesis under Oxidative Microenvironment," *Journal of Cellular and Molecular Medicine* 19, no. 1 (2015): 227–238.

71. V. Casieri et al., "Long-Term Intake of Pasta Containing Barley (1–3)Beta-D-Glucan Increases Neovascularization Mediated Cardioprotection through Endothelial Upregulation of Vascular Endothelial Growth Factor and Parkin," *Scientific Reports* 7, no. 1 (2017): 13424.

72. S. V. Penumathsa et al., "Secoisolariciresinol Diglucoside Induces Neovascularization-Mediated Cardioprotection against Ischemia-Reperfusion Injury in Hypercholesterolemic Myocardium," *Journal of Molecular and Cellular Cardiology* 44, no. 1 (2008): 170–179.

73. A. W. Lee et al., "Ursolic Acid Induces Allograft Inflammatory Factor-1 Expression via a Nitric Oxide–Related Mechanism and Increases Neovascularization," *Journal of Agricultural and Food Chemistry* 58, no. 24 (2010): 12941–12949.

74. J. Lin et al., "Ursolic Acid Inhibits Colorectal Cancer Angiogenesis through Suppression of Multiple Signaling Pathways," *International Journal of Oncology* 43, no. 5 (2013): 1666–1674.

75. F. Zhang et al., "Oleanolic Acid and Ursolic Acid in Commercial Dried Fruits," *Food Science and Technology Research* 19, no. 1 (2013): 113–116.

76. M. Sumi et al., "Quercetin Glucosides Promote Ischemia-Induced Angiogenesis, but Do Not Promote Tumor Growth," *Life Sciences* 93, no. 22 (2013): 814–819.

77. A. K. Maurya and M. Vinayak, "Quercetin Attenuates Cell Survival, Inflammation, and Angiogenesis via Modulation of AKT Signaling in Murine T-Cell Lymphoma," *Nutrition and Cancer* 69, no. 3 (2017): 470–480; X. Zhao et al., "Quercetin Inhibits Angiogenesis by Targeting Calcineurin in the Xenograft Model of Human Breast Cancer," *European Journal of Pharmacology* 781 (2016): 60–68.

Chapter 7: (Re)generate Your Health

1. Y. Kim and Y. Je, "Flavonoid Intake and Mortality from Cardiovascular Disease and All Causes: A Meta-Analysis of Prospective Cohort Studies," *Clinical Nutrition ESPEN* 20 (2017): 68–77.

2. C. Heiss et al., "Improvement of Endothelial Function with Dietary Flavanols Is Associated with Mobilization of Circulating Angiogenic Cells in Patients with Coronary Artery Disease," *Journal of the American College of Cardiology* 56, no. 3 (2010): 218–224.

3. E. Shantsila, T. Watson, and G. Y. Lip, "Endothelial Progenitor Cells in Cardiovascular Disorders," *Journal of the American College of Cardiology* 49, no. 7 (2007): 741–752.

4. F. L'episcopo et al., "Neural Stem Cell Grafts Promote Astroglia-Driven Neurorestoration in the Aged Parkinsonian Brain via Wnt/β-Catenin Signaling," *Stem Cells* 36, no. 8 (2018); C. Beauséjour, "Bone Marrow-Derived Cells: The Influence of Aging and Cellular Senescence," Handbook of Experimental Pharmacology 180 (2007): 67–88; H. E. Marei et al., "Human Olfactory Bulb Neural Stem Cells Expressing hNGF Restore Cognitive Deficit in Alzheimer's Disease Rat Model," *Journal of Cell Physiology* 230, no. 1 (2015): 116–130.

5. L. da Cruz et al., "Phase 1 Clinical Study of an Embryonic Stem Cell-Derived Retinal Pigment Epithelium Patch in Age-Related Macular Degeneration," *Nature Biotechnology* 36, no. 4 (2018): 328–337.

6. B. Sui et al., "Allogeneic Mesenchymal Stem Cell Therapy Promotes Osteoblastogenesis and Prevents Glucocorticoid-Induced Osteoporosis," *Stem Cells Translational Medicine* 5, no. 9 (2016): 1238–1246.

7. C. De Bari and A. J. Roelofs, "Stem Cell-Based Therapeutic Strategies for Cartilage Defects and Osteoarthritis," *Current Opinion in Pharmacology* 40 (2018): 74–80.

8. H. H. Izmirli et al., "Use of Adipose-Derived Mesenchymal Stem Cells to Accelerate Neovascularization in Interpolation Flaps," *Journal of Craniofacial Surgery* 27, no. 1 (2016): 264–271; C. De Bari and A. J. Roelofs, "Stem Cell-Based Therapeutic Strategies for Cartilage Defects and Osteoarthritis," *Current Opinion in Pharmacology* 40 (2018): 74–80; J. Takahashi, "Stem Cells and Regenerative Medicine for Neural Repair," *Current Opinion in Biotechnology* 52 (2018): 102–108; M. Fernandes et al., "Bone Marrow–Derived Mesenchymal Stem Cells versus Adipose-Derived Mesenchymal Stem Cells for Peripheral Nerve Regeneration," *Neural Regeneration Research* 13, no. 1 (2018): 100–104; H. Fukuoka, K. Narita, and H. Suga, "Hair Regeneration Therapy: Application of Adipose-Derived Stem Cells," *Current Stem Cell Research and Therapy* 12, no. 7 (2017): 531–534; E. L. Matz et al., "Stem Cell Therapy for Erectile Dysfunction," *Sexual Medicine Reviews* (Apr. 6, 2018).

9. G. Dawson et al., "Autologous Cord Blood Infusions Are Safe and Feasible in Young Children with Autism Spectrum Disorder: Results of a Single-Center Phase I Open-Label Trial," *Stem Cells Translational Medicine* 6, no. 5 (2017): 1332–1339; F. Pischiutta et al., "Placenta-Derived Cells for Acute Brain Injury," *Cell Transplantation* 27, no. 1 (2018): 151–167.

10. J. Turgeon et al., "Fish Oil-Enriched Diet Protects against Ischemia by Improving Angiogenesis, Endothelial Progenitor Cell Function, and Postnatal Neovascularization," *Atherosclerosis* 229, no. 2 (2013): 295–303.

11. M. Lei et al., "Study of the Radio-Protective Effect of Cuttlefish Ink on Hemopoietic Injury," *Asia Pacific Journal of Clinical Nutrition* 16, suppl. 1 (2007): 239–243.

12. N. Okarter and R. H. Liu, "Health Benefits of Whole Grain Phytochemicals," *Critical Reviews in Food Science and Nutrition* 50, no. 3 (2010): 193–208.

13. D. Lucchesi et al., "Grain and Bean Lysates Improve Function of Endothelial Progenitor Cells from Human Peripheral Blood: Involvement of the Endogenous Antioxidant Defenses," *PLOS One* 9, no. 10 (2014): e109298.

14. D. Lucchesi et al., "Grain and Bean Lysates Improve Function of Endothelial Progenitor Cells from Human Peripheral Blood: Involvement of the Endogenous Antioxidant Defenses," *PLOS One* 9, no. 10 (2014): e109298.

15. A. Parzonko, A. Oświt, A. Bazylko, and M. Naruszewicz, "Anthocyans-Rich Aronia Melanocarpa Extract Possesses Ability to Protect Endothelial Progenitor Cells against Angiotensin II Induced Dysfunction," *Phytomedicine* 22, no. 14 (2015): 1238–1246.

16. C. Perez-Ternero et al., "Ferulic Acid, a Bioactive Component of Rice Bran, Improves Oxidative Stress and Mitochondrial Biogenesis and Dynamics in Mice and in Human Mononuclear Cells," *Journal of Nutritional Biochemistry* 48 (2017): 51–61.

17. C. Perez-Ternero et al., "Rice Bran Enzymatic Extract Reduces Atherosclerotic Plaque Development and Steatosis in High-Fat Fed ApoE-/- Mice," *Nutrition* 37 (2017): 22–29.

18. "How Much Arsenic Is in Your Rice?" *Consumer Reports*, Nov. 18, 2014, https://www.consumerreports.org/cro/magazine/2015/01/how-much-arsenic-is-in-your-rice/index.htm.

19. J. You et al., "Curcumin Induces Therapeutic Angiogenesis in a Diabetic Mouse Hindlimb Ischemia Model via Modulating the Function of Endothelial Progenitor Cell," *Stem Cell Research and Therapy* 8, no. 1 (2017): 182.

20. L. Ling, S. Gu, and Y. Cheng, "Resveratrol Activates Endogenous Cardiac Stem Cells and Improves Myocardial Regeneration following Acute Myocardial Infarction," *Molecular Medicine Reports* 15, no. 3 (2017): 1188–1194.

21. R. Liu et al., "Lutein and Zeaxanthin Supplementation and Association with Visual Function in Age-Related Macular Degeneration," *Investigative Ophthalmology and Visual Science* 56, no. 1 (2014): 252–258.

22. Y. Liu et al., "Precise Regulation of miR-210 Is Critical for the Cellular Homeostasis Maintenance and Transplantation Efficacy Enhancement of Mesenchymal Stem Cells in Acute Liver Failure Therapy," *Cell Transplantation* 26, no. 5 (2017): 805–820.

23. M. R. Olthof, P. C. Hollman, P. L. Zock, and M. B. Katan, "Consumption of High Doses of Chlorogenic Acid, Present in Coffee, or of Black Tea Increases Plasma Total Homocysteine Concentrations in Humans," *American Journal of Clinical Nutrition* 73, no. 3 (2001): 532–538.

24. S. Li, H. Bian et al., "Chlorogenic Acid Protects MSCs against Oxidative Stress by Altering FOXO Family Genes and Activating Intrinsic Pathway," *European Journal of Pharmacology* 674, no. 2–3 (2012): 65–72.

25. L.-S. Wang et al., "Abstract 163: Metabolomic Profiling Reveals a Protective Modulation on Fatty Acid Metabolism in Colorectal Cancer Patients following Consumption of Freeze-Dried Black Raspberries," *Cancer Research* 73 (2013): 163; J. H. An et al., "Effect of *Rubus occidentalis* Extract on Metabolic Parameters in Subjects with Prediabetes: A Proof-of-Concept, Randomized, Double-Blind, Placebo-Controlled Clinical Trial," *Phytotherapy Research* 30, no. 10 (2016): 1634–1640.

26. Q. S. Liu et al., "Ellagic Acid Improves Endogenous Neural Stem Cells Proliferation and Neurorestoration through Wnt/β-catenin Signaling In Vivo and In Vitro," *Molecular Nutrition and Food Research* 61, no. 3 (2017).

27. H. S. Jeong et al., "Black Raspberry Extract Increased Circulating Endothelial Progenitor Cells and Improved Arterial Stiffness in Patients with Metabolic Syndrome: A Randomized Controlled Trial," *Journal of Medicinal Food* 19, no. 4 (2016): 346–352.

28. Y. Kurobayashi et al., "Potent Odorants Characterize the Aroma Quality of Leaves and Stalks in Raw and Boiled Celery," *Bioscience, Biotechnology, and Biochemistry* 70, no. 4 (2006): 958–965.

29. I. A. Abdoulaye and Y. J. Guo, "A Review of Recent Advances in Neuroprotective Potential of 3-N-Butylphthalide and Its Derivatives," *BioMed Research International* (2016): 5012341.

30. P. Zhang et al., "DL-3-n-Butylphthalide Promotes Dendrite Development in Cortical Neurons Subjected to Oxygen-Glucose Deprivation/Reperfusion," *Cell Biology International* 42, no. 8 (2018): 1041–1049.

31. H. Zhao et al., "Mobilization of Circulating Endothelial Progenitor Cells by dl-3-n-Butylphthalide in Acute Ischemic Stroke Patients," *Journal of Stroke and Cerebrovascular Diseases* 25, no. 4 (2016): 752–760.

32. Q. Deng, Y. X. Tian, and J. Liang, "Mangiferin Inhibits Cell Migration and Invasion through Rac1/WAVE2 Signalling in Breast Cancer," *Cytotechnology* 70, no. 2 (2018): 593–601; M. Du et al., "Mangiferin Prevents the Growth of Gastric Carcinoma by Blocking the PI3K-Akt Signalling Pathway," *Anticancer Drugs* 29, no. 2 (2018): 167–175.

33. H. L. Wang et al., "Mangiferin Facilitates Islet Regeneration and β-Cell Proliferation through Upregulation of Cell Cycle and β-Cell Regeneration Regulators," *International Journal of Molecular Sciences* 15, no. 5 (2014): 9016–9035.

34. H. Li et al., "Preparation and Evaluations of Mangiferin-Loaded PLGA Scaffolds for Alveolar Bone Repair Treatment under the Diabetic Condition," *AAPS PharmSciTech* 18, no. 2 (2017): 529–538; Y. Bai et al., "Mangiferin Enhances Endochondral Ossification-Based Bone Repair in Massive Bone Defect by Inducing Autophagy through Activating AMP-Activated Protein Kinase Signaling Pathway," *FASEB Journal* 32, no. 8 (2018).

35. The red wine was Cabernet Sauvignon (Reserve Maison Nicholas 2009) from Languedoc Rousillon, France. The beer was Taiwan Beer. The vodka was Smirnoff.

36. P. H. Huang et al., "Intake of Red Wine Increases the Number and Functional Capacity of Circulating Endothelial Progenitor Cells by Enhancing Nitric Oxide Bioavailability" *Arteriosclerosis, Thrombosis, and Vascular Biology* 30, no. 4 (2010): 869–877.

37. A. Di Castelnuovo et al., "Meta-Analysis of Wine and Beer Consumption in Relation to Vascular Risk," *Circulation* 105, no. 24 (2002): 2836–2844.

38. P. E. Ronksley et al., "Association of Alcohol Consumption with Selected Cardiovascular Disease Outcomes: A Systematic Review and Meta-analysis," *BMJ* 342 (2011): d671.

39. G. Chiva-Blanch et al., "The Non-alcoholic Fraction of Beer Increases Stromal Cell Derived Factor 1 and the Number of Circulating Endothelial Progenitor Cells in High Cardiovascular Risk Subjects: A Randomized Clinical Trial," *Atherosclerosis* 233, no. 2 (2014): 518–524.

40. S. E. Michaud et al., "Circulating Endothelial Progenitor Cells from Healthy Smokers Exhibit Impaired Functional Activities," *Atherosclerosis* 187, no. 2 (2006): 423–432.

41. W. Kim et al., "Effect of Green Tea Consumption on Endothelial Function and Circulating Endothelial Progenitor Cells in Chronic Smokers," *Circulation Journal* 70, no. 8 (2006): 1052–1057.

42. Y. He et al., "Epigallocatechiomega-3-gallate Attenuates Cerebral Cortex Damage and Promotes Brain Regeneration in Acrylamide-Treated Rats," *Food and Function* 8, no. 6 (2017): 2275–2282; A. R. Kim et al., "Catechins Activate Muscle Stem Cells by Myf5 Induction and Stimulate Muscle Regeneration," *Biochemical and Biophysical Research Communications* 489, no. 2 (2017): 142–148; C. L. Shen et al., "Functions and Mechanisms of Green Tea Catechins in Regulating Bone Remodeling," *Current Drug Targets* 14, no. 13 (2013): 1619–1630; S. H. Zhou et al., "Allograft Pretreatment for the Repair of Sciatic Nerve Defects: Green Tea Polyphenols versus Radiation," *Neural Regeneration Research* 10, no. 1 (2015): 136–140; H. L. Kim et al., "Promotion of Full-Thickness Wound Healing Using Epigallocatechiomega-3-O-gallate/Poly (Lactic-co-glycolic Acid) Membrane as Temporary Wound Dressing," *Artificial Organs* 38, no. 5 (2014): 411–417.

43. D. Grassi et al., "Black Tea Increases Circulating Endothelial Progenitor Cells and Improves Flow Mediated Dilatation Counteracting Deleterious Effects from a Fat Load in Hypertensive Patients: A Randomized Controlled Study," *Nutrients* 8, no. 11 (2016).

44. C. Marin et al., "Mediterranean Diet Reduces Endothelial Damage and Improves the Regenerative Capacity of Endothelium," *American Journal of Clinical Nutrition* 93, no. 2 (2011): 267–274.

45. M. Igarashi and L. Guarente, "mTORC1 and SIRT1 Cooperate to Foster Expansion of Gut Adult Stem Cells during Calorie Restriction," *Cell* 166, no. 2 (2016): 436–450.

46. S. Periyasamy-Thandavan et al., "Caloric Restriction and the Adipokine Leptin Alter the SDF-1 Signaling Axis in Bone Marrow and in Bone Marrow Derived Mesenchymal Stem Cells," *Molecular and Cellular Endocrinology* 410 (2015): 64–72.

47. B. Xin et al., "Prolonged Fasting Improves Endothelial Progenitor Cell-Mediated Ischemic Angiogenesis in Mice," *Cell Physiology and Biochemistry* 40, no. 3–4 (2016): 693–706.

48. M. D. Mana, E. Y. Kuo, and Ö. H. Yilmaz, "Dietary Regulation of Adult Stem Cells," *Current Stem Cell Reports* 3, no. 1 (2017): 1–8.

49. H. R. Park et al., "A High-Fat Diet Impairs Neurogenesis: Involvement of Lipid Peroxidation and Brain-Derived Neurotrophic Factor," *Neuroscience Letters* 482, no. 3 (2010): 235–239.

50. L. Wei et al., "High-Fat Diet Aggravates Postoperative Cognitive Dysfunction in Aged Mice," *BMC Anesthesiology* 18, no. 1 (2018): 20.

51. Y. L. Chen et al., "Impact of Obesity Control on Circulating Level of Endothelial Progenitor Cells and Angiogenesis in Response to Ischemic Stimulation," *Journal of Translational Medicine* 10 (2012): 86.

52. A. W. Joe et al., "Depot-Specific Differences in Adipogenic Progenitor Abundance and Proliferative Response to High-Fat Diet," *Stem Cells* 27, no. 10 (2009): 2563–2570.

53. S. Beyaz et al., "High-Fat Diet Enhances Stemness and Tumorigenicity of Intestinal Progenitors," *Nature* 531, no. 7592 (2016): 53–58.

54. H. Kang et al., "High Glucose-Induced Endothelial Progenitor Cell Dysfunction," *Diabetes and Vascular Disease Research* 14, no. 5 (2017): 381–394; J. Wang et al., "High Glucose Inhibits Osteogenic Differentiation through the BMP Signaling Pathway in Bone Mesenchymal Stem Cells In Mice," *EXCLI Journal* 12 (2013): 584–597; H. Y. Choi et al., "High Glucose Causes Human Cardiac Progenitor Cell Dysfunction by Promoting Mitochondrial Fission: Role of a GLUT1 Blocker," *Biomolecules and Therapeutics* 24, no. 4 (2016): 363–370.

55. "Glycemic Index for 60+ Foods," Harvard Health Publishing, Harvard Medical School, Feb. 2015, updated Mar. 14, 2018, https://www.health.harvard.edu/diseases-and-conditions/glycemic-index-and-glycemic-load-for-100-foods.

56. J. R. Karcher and A. S. Greene, "Bone Marrow Mononuclear Cell Angiogenic Competency Is Suppressed by a High-Salt Diet," *American Journal of Physiology–Cell Physiology* 306, no. 2 (2014): C123–C131.

57. Charles A. Goldwater Jr., "Are Stem Cells Involved in Cancer?" Stem Cell Information, National Institutes of Health, https://stemcells.nih.gov/info/Regenerative_Medicine/2006chapter9.htm.

58. M. J. Munro et al., "Cancer Stem Cells in Colorectal Cancer: A Review," *Journal of Clinical Pathology* 71, no. 2 (2018): 110–116.

59. Y. Chen et al., "(-)-Epigallocatechiomega-3-Gallate Inhibits Colorectal Cancer Stem Cells by Suppressing Wnt/β-Catenin Pathway," *Nutrients* 9, no. 6, (2017).

60. G. Bonuccelli, F. Sotgia, and M. P. Lisanti, "Matcha Green Tea (MGT) Inhibits the Propagation of Cancer Stem Cells (CSCs), by Targeting Mitochondrial Metabolism, Glycolysis, and Multiple Cell Signalling Pathways," *Aging* 10, no. 8 (2018): 1867–1883.

61. V. Charepalli et al., "Anthocyanin-Containing Purple-Fleshed Potatoes Suppress Colon Tumorigenesis via Elimination of Colon Cancer Stem Cells," *Journal of Nutritional Biochemistry* 26, no. 12 (2015): 1641–1649.

62. T. Takayama et al., "Randomized Double-Blind Trial of Sulindac and Etodolac to Eradicate Aberrant Crypt Foci and to Prevent Sporadic Colorectal Polyps," *Clinical Cancer Research* 17, no. 11 (2011): 3803–3811; B. C. Sun et al., "Sulindac Induces Apoptosis and Protects against Colon Carcinoma in Mice," *World Journal of Gastroenterology* 11, no. 18 (2005): 2822–2826.

63. J. Lee et al., "Walnut Phenolic Extract and Its Bioactive Compounds Suppress Colon Cancer Cell Growth by Regulating Colon Cancer Stemness," *Nutrients* 8, no. 7 (2016).

64. "Chance of Colon Cancer Recurrence Nearly Cut in Half in People Who Eat Nuts," American Society of Clinical Oncology, May 17, 2017, https://www.asco.org/about -asco/press-center/news-releases/chance-colon-cancer-recurrence-nearly-cut-half-peop le-who-eat.

65. S. Silva et al., "High Resolution Mass Spectrometric Analysis of Secoiridoids and Metabolites as Biomarkers of Acute Olive Oil Intake—An Approach to Study Interindividual Variability in Humans," *Molecular Nutrition and Food Research* 62, no. 2 (2018).

66. B. Corominas-Faja et al., "Extra-Virgin Olive Oil Contains a Metabolo-Epigenetic Inhibitor of Cancer Stem Cells," *Carcinogenesis* 39, no. 4 (2018): 601–613.

67. L. Zhang et al., "Genistein Inhibits the Stemness Properties of Prostate Cancer Cells through Targeting Hedgehog-Gli1 Pathway," *Cancer Letters* 323, no. 1 (2012): 48–57; P. H. Tsai et al., "Dietary Flavonoids Luteolin and Quercetin Suppressed Cancer Stem Cell Properties and Metastatic Potential of Isolated Prostate Cancer Cells," *Anticancer Research* 36, no. 12 (2016): 6367–6380.

68. S. N. Tang et al., "The Dietary Bioflavonoid Quercetin Synergizes with Epigallocathechin Gallate (EGCG) to Inhibit Prostate Cancer Stem Cell Characteristics, Invasion, Migration, and Epithelial-Mesenchymal Transition," *Journal of Molecular Signaling* 5 (2010): 14.

69. K. Yamagata, Y. Izawa, D. Onodera, and M. Tagami, "Chlorogenic Acid Regulates Apoptosis and Stem Cell Marker-Related Gene Expression in A549 Human Lung Cancer Cells," *Molecular and Cellular Biochemistry* 441, no. 1–2 (2018): 9–19; S. Li et al., "Chlorogenic Acid Protects MSCs against Oxidative Stress by Altering FOXO Family Genes and Activating Intrinsic Pathway," *European Journal of Pharmacology* 674, no. 2–3 (2012): 65–72.

70. J. Suh, D. H. Kim, and Y. J. Surh, "Resveratrol Suppresses Migration, Invasion, and Stemness of Human Breast Cancer Cells by Interfering with Tumor-Stromal Cross-Talk," *Archives of Biochemistry and Biophysics* 643 (2018): 62–71.

71. N. Wang et al., "Direct Inhibition of ACTN4 by Ellagic Acid Limits Breast Cancer Metastasis via Regulation of β-catenin Stabilization in Cancer Stem Cells," *Journal of Experimental and Clinical Cancer Research* 36, no. 1 (2017): 172.

72. T. N. Seyfried et al., "Metabolic Therapy: A New Paradigm for Managing Malignant Brain Cancer," *Cancer Letters* 356, no. 2, pt. A (2015): 289–300.

73. R. T. Martuscello et al., "A Supplemented High-Fat Low-Carbohydrate Diet for the Treatment of Glioblastoma," *Clinical Cancer Research* 22, no. 10 (2016): 2482–2495.

Chapter 8: Feed Your Inner Ecosystem

1. R. Sender, S. Fuchs, and R. Milo, "Revised Estimates for the Number of Human and Bacteria Cells in the Body," *PLOS Biology* 14, no. 8 (2016): e1002533.

2. M. Schneeberger et al., "Akkermansia Muciniphila Inversely Correlates with the Onset of Inflammation, Altered Adiposetissue Metabolism, and Metabolic Disorders during Obesity in Mice," *Scientific Reports* 5 (2015): 16643.

3. B. Routy et al., "Gut Microbiome Influences Efficacy of PD-1-Based Immunotherapy against Epithelial Tumors," *Science* 359, no. 6371 (2018): 91–97.

4. T. Marrs and K. Sim, "Demystifying Dysbiosis: Can the Gut Microbiome Promote Oral Tolerance over IgE-Mediated Food Allergy?" *Current Pediatric Reviews* 14 (2018).

5. A. Kourosh et al., "Fecal Microbiome Signatures Are Different in Food Allergic Children Compared to Siblings and Healthy Children," *Pediatric Allergy and Immunology* 29, no. 5 (2018): 545–554.

6. A. M. Sheflin, A. K. Whitney, and T. L. Weir, "Cancer-Promoting Effects of Microbial Dysbiosis," *Current Oncology Reports* 16, no. 10 (2014): 406.

7. S. Ahmadmehrabi and W. H. W. Tang, "Gut Microbiome and Its Role in Cardiovascular Diseases," *Current Opinion in Cardiology* 32, no. 6 (2017): 761–766.

8. M. Carlström, J. O. Lundberg, and E. Weitzberg, "Mechanisms Underlying Blood Pressure Reduction by Dietary Inorganic Nitrate," *Acta Physiologica* (Apr. 25, 2018): e13080; C. D. Koch et al., "Enterosalivary Nitrate Metabolism and the Microbiome: Intersection of Microbial Metabolism, Nitric Oxide, and Diet in Cardiac and Pulmonary Vascular Health," *Free Radical Biology and Medicine* 105 (2017): 48–67.

9. C. Bogiatzi et al., "Metabolic Products of the Intestinal Microbiome and Extremes of Atherosclerosis," *Atherosclerosis* 273 (2018): 91–97.

10. M. F. Sun and Y. Q. Shen, "Dysbiosis of Gut Microbiota and Microbial Metabolites in Parkinson's Disease," *Ageing Research Reviews* 45 (2018): 53–61; Z. Q. Zhuang et al., "Gut Microbiome Is Altered in Patients with Alzheimer's Disease," *Journal of Alzheimer's Disease* 63, no. 4 (2018):1337–1346.

11. Z. Chen et al., "Comparative Metaproteomics Analysis Shows Altered Fecal Microbiota Signatures in Patients with Major Depressive Disorder," *NeuroReport* 29, no. 5 (2018): 417–425; T. T. Nguyen et al., "Overview and Systematic Review of Studies of Microbiome in Schizophrenia and Bipolar Disorder," *Journal of Psychiatric Research* 99 (2018): 50–61.

12. M. A. Ghebre et al., "Biological Exacerbation Clusters Demonstrate Asthma and COPD Overlap with Distinct Mediator and Microbiome Profiles," *Journal of Allergy and Clinical Immunology* 141 (2018): 2027–2036.

13. A. Lerner, R. Aminov, and T. Matthias, "Dysbiosis May Trigger Autoimmune Diseases via Inappropriate Post-Translational Modification of Host Proteins," *Frontiers in Microbiology* 7 (2016): 84.

14. M. Lee et al., "Large-Scale Targeted Metagenomics Analysis of Bacterial Ecological Changes in 88 Kimchi Samples during Fermentation," *Food Microbiology* 66 (2017): 173–183.

15. M. L. Marco et al., "Health Benefits of Fermented Foods: Microbiota and Beyond," *Current Opinion in Biotechnology* 44 (2017): 94–102.

16. V. Plengvidhya, F. Breidt Jr., Z. Lu, and H. P. Fleming, "DNA Fingerprinting of Lactic Acid Bacteria in Sauerkraut Fermentations," *Applied and Environmental Microbiology* 73, no. 23 (2007): 7697–7702.

17. Becky Plotner, "Sauerkraut Test Divulges Shocking Probiotic Count," Nourishing Plot, June 21, 2014, https://www.nourishingplot.com/2014/06/21/sauerkraut-test-divulges-shocking-probiotic-count; M. L. Marco et al., "Health Benefits of Fermented Foods: Microbiota and Beyond," *Current Opinion in Biotechnology* 44 (2017): 94–102.

18. C. Raak, T. Ostermann, K. Boehm, and F. Molsberger, "Regular Consumption of Sauerkraut and Its Effect on Human Health: A Bibliometric Analysis," *Global Advances in Health and Medicine* 3, no. 6 (2014): 12–18.

19. A. F. Athiyyah et al., "Lactobacillus Plantarum IS-10506 Activates Intestinal Stem Cells in a Rodent Model," *Beneficial Microbes* (May 4, 2018): 1–6.

20. M. Tolonen et al., "Plant-Derived Biomolecules in Fermented Cabbage," *Journal of Agricultural and Food Chemistry* 50, no. 23 (2002): 6798–803.

21. American Chemical Society, "Sauerkraut Contains Anticancer Compound," EurekAlert, Oct. 17, 2002, https://www.eurekalert.org/pub_releases/2002-10/acs-sca101702.php.

22. E. J. Park et al., "Bacterial Community Analysis during Fermentation of Ten Representative Kinds of Kimchi with Barcoded Pyrosequencing," *Food Microbiology* 30, no. 1 (2012): 197–204.

23. Y. J. Oh et al., "*Lentibacillus kimchii* sp. Nov., an Extremely Halophilic Bacterium Isolated from Kimchi, a Korean Fermented Vegetable," *Antonie Van Leeuwenhoek* 109, no. 6 (2016): 869–876.

24. H. J. Kim, J. S. Noh, and Y. O. Song, "Beneficial Effects of Kimchi, a Korean Fermented Vegetable Food, on Pathophysiological Factors Related to Atherosclerosis," *Journal of Medicinal Food* 21, no. 2 (2018): 127–135.

25. S.-H. Kwak, Y.-M. Cho, G.-M. Noh, and A.-S. Om, "Cancer Preventive Potential of Kimchi Lactic Acid Bacteria (*Weissella cibaria, Lactobacillus plantarum*)," *Journal of Cancer Prevention* 19, no. 4 (2014): 253–258.

26. M. K. Kwak et al., "Cyclic Dipeptides from Lactic Acid Bacteria Inhibit Proliferation of the Influenza A Virus," *Journal of Microbiology* 51, no. 6 (2013): 836–843.

27. S. Y. An et al., "Beneficial Effects of Fresh and Fermented Kimchi in Prediabetic Individuals," *Annals of Nutrition and Metabolism* 63, no. 1–2 (2013): 111–119.

28. E. K. Kim et al., "Fermented Kimchi Reduces Body Weight and Improves Metabolic Parameters in Overweight and Obese Patients," *Nutrition Research* 31, no. 6 (2011): 436–443.

29. Z. Wang and Y. Shao, "Effects of Microbial Diversity on Nitrite Concentration in Pao Cai, a Naturally Fermented Cabbage Product from China," *Food Microbiology* 72 (2018): 185–192.

30. Z. Wang and Y. Shao, "Effects of Microbial Diversity on Nitrite Concentration in Pao Cai, a Naturally Fermented Cabbage Product from China," *Food Microbiology* 72 (2018): 185–192.

31. E. Gala et al., "Diversity of Lactic Acid Bacteria Population in Ripened Parmigiano Reggiano Cheese," *International Journal of Food Microbiology* 125, no. 3 (2008): 347–351.

32. X. He et al., "*Lactobacillus rhamnosus* GG Supernatant Enhance Neonatal Resistance to Systemic *Escherichia coli* K1 Infection by Accelerating Development of Intestinal Defense," *Scientific Reports* 7 (2017): 43305.

33. X. Li et al., "Effects of *Lactobacillus casei* CCFM419 on Insulin Resistance and Gut Microbiota in Type 2 Diabetic Mice," *Beneficial Microbes* 8, no. 3 (2017): 421–432.

34. A. Tiptiri-Kourpeti et al., "*Lactobacillus casei* Exerts Anti-Proliferative Effects Accompanied by Apoptotic Cell Death and Up-Regulation of TRAIL in Colon Carcinoma Cells," *PLOS One* 11, no. 2 (2016): e0147960.

35. G. Karimi et al., "The Anti-Obesity Effects of *Lactobacillus casei* Strain Shirota versus Orlistat on High Fat Diet-Induced Obese Rats," *Food and Nutrition Research* 59 (2015): 29273.

36. R. F. Slykerman et al., "Effect of *Lactobacillus rhamnosus* HN001 in Pregnancy on Postpartum Symptoms of Depression and Anxiety: A Randomised Double-Blind Placebo-Controlled Trial," *EBioMedicine* 24 (2017): 159–165.

37. K. Van Hoorde, M. Heyndrickx, P. Vandamme, and G. Huys, "Influence of Pasteurization, Brining Conditions, and Production Environment on the Microbiota of Artisan Gouda-Type Cheeses," *Food Microbiology* 27, no. 3 (2010): 425–433.

38. U.S. Food and Drug Administration, "Code of Federal Regulations, Title 21," Apr. 2018, https://www.accessdata.fda.gov/scripts/cdrh/cfdocs/cfcfr/CFRSearch.cfm?fr=1240.61.

39. O. Firmesse et al., "Consumption of Camembert Cheese Stimulates Commensal Enterococci in Healthy Human Intestinal Microbiota," *FEMS Microbiology Letters* 276, no. 2 (2007): 189–192.

40. M. Fisberg and R. Machado, "History of Yogurt and Current Patterns of Consumption," *Nutrition Reviews* 73, suppl. 1 (2015): 4–7.

41. D. J. Lisko, G. P. Johnston, and C. G. Johnston, "Effects of Dietary Yogurt on the Healthy Human Gastrointestinal (GI) Microbiome," *Microorganisms* 5, no. 1 (2017).

42. Y. Suzuki et al., "Association between Yogurt Consumption and Intestinal Microbiota in Healthy Young Adults Differs by Host Gender," *Frontiers in Microbiology* 8 (2017): 847.

43. A. Creus-Cuadros et al., "Associations between Both Lignan and Yogurt Consumption and Cardiovascular Risk Parameters in an Elderly Population: Observations from a Cross-Sectional Approach in the PREDIMED Study," *Journal of the Academy of Nutrition and Dietetics* 117, no. 4 (2017): 609–622.e1.

44. J. Peterson et al., "Dietary Lignans: Physiology and Potential for Cardiovascular Disease Risk Reduction," *Nutrition Reviews* 68, no. 10 (2010): 571–603.

45. Ben Guarino, "Scientists Have Discovered the Earliest Evidence of Bread, and It's Much Older than We Expected," Science Alert, July 17, 2018, https://www.sciencealert.com/researchers-have-found-crumbs-of-evidence-from-the-world-s-first-bread.

46. Q. Mu, V. J. Tavella, and X. M. Luo, "Role of *Lactobacillus reuteri* in Human Health and Diseases," *Frontiers in Microbiology* 9, no. 757 (2018); J. R. Lakritz et al., "Beneficial Bacteria Stimulate Host Immune Cells to Counteract Dietary and Genetic Predisposition to Mammary Cancer in Mice," *International Journal of Cancer* 135, no. 3 (2014): 529–540.

47. B. J. Varian et al., "Microbial Lysate Upregulates Host Oxytocin," *Brain, Behavior, and Immunity* 61 (2017): 36–49.

48. J. Zheng, X. Zhao, X. B. Lin, and M. Gänzle, "Comparative Genomics *Lactobacillus reuteri* from Sourdough Reveals Adaptation of an Intestinalsymbiont to Food Fermentations," *Scientific Reports* 5 (2015): 18234.

49. B. J. Varian et al., "Microbial Lysate Upregulates Host Oxytocin," *Brain Behavior and Immunity* 61 (2017): 36–49.

50. C. Menni et al., "Gut Microbiome Diversity and High Fibre Intake Are Related to Lower Long-Term Weight Gain," *International Journal of Obesity* 41, no. 7 (2017): 1099–1105.

51. C. M. Schlebusch et al., "Southern African Ancient Genomes Estimate Modern Human Divergence to 350,000 to 260,000 Years Ago," *Science* 358, no. 6363 (2017): 652–655.

52. R. K. Singh et al., "Influence of Diet on the Gut Microbiome and Implications for Human Health," *Journal of Translational Medicine* 15, no. 1 (2017): 73.

53. C. De Filippo et al., "Impact of Diet in Shaping Gut Microbiota Revealed by a Comparative Study in Children from Europe and Rural Africa," *Proceedings of the National Academy of Sciences USA* 107, no. 33 (2010): 14691–14696.

54. F. Ounnas et al., "Whole Rye Consumption Improves Blood and Liver omega-3 Fatty Acid Profile and Gut Microbiota Composition in Rats," *PLOS One* 11, no. 2 (2016): e0148118.

55. Y. K. Lee et al., "Kiwifruit (*Actinidia deliciosa*) Changes Intestinal Microbial Profile," *Microbial Ecology in Health and Disease* 23 (2012).

56. D. J. Morrison and T. Preston, "Formation of Short Chain Fatty Acids by the Gut Microbiota and Their Impact on Human Metabolism," *Gut Microbes* 7, no. 3 (2016): 189–200.

57. L. Kellingray et al., "Consumption of a Diet Rich in Brassica Vegetables Is Associated with a Reduced Abundance of Sulphate-Reducing Bacteria: A Randomised Crossover Study," *Molecular Nutrition and Food Research* 61, no. 9 (2017).

58. J. Loubinoux et al., "Sulfate-Reducing Bacteria in Human Feces and Their Association with Inflammatory Bowel Diseases," *FEMS Microbiology Ecology* 40, no. 2 (2002): 107–112.

59. X. Li, J. Guo, K. Ji, and P. Zhang, "Bamboo Shoot Fiber Prevents Obesity in Mice by Modulating the Gut Microbiota," *Scientific Reports* 6 (2016): 32953.

60. B. Routy et al., "Gut Microbiome Influences Efficacy of PD-1-Based Immunotherapy against Epithelial Tumors," *Science* 359, no. 6371 (2018): 91–97.

61. A. K. Pandey and V. Ojha, "Precooking Processing of Bamboo Shoots for Removal of Anti-Nutrients," *Journal of Food Science and Technology* 51, no. 1 (2014): 43–50.

62. "The Precise Reason for the Health Benefits of Dark Chocolate: Mystery Solved," American Chemical Society, Mar. 18, 2014, https://www.acs.org/content/acs/en/press room/newsreleases/2014/march/the-precise-reason-for-the-health-benefits-of-dark -chocolate-mystery-solved.html; D. J. Morrison and T. Preston, "Formation of Short Chain Fatty Acids by the Gut Microbiota and Their Impact on Human Metabolism," *Gut Microbes* 7, no. 3 (2016): 189–200.

63. F. P. Martin et al., "Metabolic Effects of Dark Chocolate Consumption on Energy, Gut Microbiota, and Stress-Related Metabolism in Free-Living Subjects," *Journal of Proteome Research* 8, no. 12 (2009): 5568–5579.

64. R. Vanholder, R. De Smet, and G. Lesaffer, "p-Cresol: A Toxin Revealing Many Neglected but Relevant Aspects of Uraemic Toxicity," *Nephrology Dialysis Transplantation* 14, no. 12 (1999): 2813–2815; T. Pallister et al., "Hippurate as a Metabolomic Marker of Gut Microbiome Diversity: Modulation by Diet and Relationship to Metabolic Syndrome," *Scientific Reports* 7, no. 1 (2017): 13670.

65. X. Tzounis et al., "Prebiotic Evaluation of Cocoa-Derived Flavanols in Healthy Humans by Using a Randomized, Controlled, Double-Blind, Crossover Intervention Study," *American Journal of Clinical Nutrition* 93, no. 1 (2011): 62–72.

66. C. Bamberger et al., "A Walnut-Enriched Diet Affects Gut Microbiome in Healthy Caucasian Subjects: A Randomized, Controlled Trial," *Nutrients* 10, no. 2 (2018).

67. H. D. Holscher et al., "Walnut Consumption Alters the Gastrointestinal Microbiota, Microbially Derived Secondary BileAcids, and Health Markers in Healthy Adults: A Randomized Controlled Trial," *Journal of Nutrition* 148, no. 6 (2018): 861–867.

68. J. M. Monk et al., "Navy and Black Bean Supplementation Primes the Colonic Mucosal Microenvironment to Improve Gut Health," *Journal of Nutritional Biochemistry* 49 (2017): 89–100.

69. W. Rossouw and L. Korsten, "Cultivable Microbiome of Fresh White Button Mushrooms," *Letters in Applied Microbiology* 64, no. 2 (2017): 164–170.

70. J. Varshney et al., "White Button Mushrooms Increase Microbial Diversity and Accelerate the Resolution of *Citrobacter rodentium* Infection in Mice," *Journal of Nutrition* 143, no. 4 (2013): 526–532.

71. X. Xu, J. Yang, Z. Ning, and X. Zhang, "Lentinula Edodes-Derived Polysaccharide Rejuvenates Mice in Terms of Immune Responses and Gut Microbiota," *Food and Function* 6, no. 8 (2015): 2653–2663.

72. E. Biagi et al., "Through Ageing, and Beyond: Gut Microbiota and Inflammatory Status in Seniors and Centenarians," *PLOS One* 5, no. 5 (2010): e10667.

73. Y. Ren et al., "Polysaccharide of *Hericium erinaceus* Attenuates Colitis in C57BL/6 Mice via Regulation of Oxidative Stress, Inflammation-Related Signaling Pathways, and Modulating the Composition of the Gut Microbiota," *Journal of Nutritional Biochemistry* 57 (2018): 67–76.

74. M. Schneeberger et al., "*Akkermansia muciniphila* Inversely Correlates with the Onset of Inflammation, Altered Adiposetissue Metabolism, and Metabolic Disorders during Obesity in Mice," *Scientific Reports* 5 (2015): 16643; B. Routy et al., "Gut Microbiome Influences Efficacy of PD-1-Based Immunotherapy against Epithelial Tumors," *Science* 359, no. 6371 (2018): 91–97.

75. S. M. Henning et al., "*Pomegranate ellagitannins* Stimulate the Growth of *Akkermansia muciniphila* In Vivo," *Anaerobe* 43 (2017): 56–60.

76. Z. Li et al., "Pomegranate Extract Induces Ellagitannin Metabolite Formation and Changes Stool Microbiota in Healthy Volunteers," *Food and Function* 6, no. 8 (2015): 2487–2495.

77. F. F. Anhê et al., "A Polyphenol-Rich Cranberry Extract Protects from Diet-induced Obesity, Insulin Resistance, and Intestinal Inflammation in Association with Increased *Akkermansia* spp. Population in the Gut Microbiota of Mice," *Gut* 64, no. 6 (2015): 872–883.

78. J. B. Blumberg et al., "Cranberries and Their Bioactive Constituents in Human Health," *Advances in Nutrition* 4, no. 6 (2013): 618–632.

79. F. F. Anhê et al., "Triggering *Akkermansia* with Dietary Polyphenols: A New Weapon to Combat the Metabolic Syndrome?" *Gut Microbes* 7, no. 2 (2016): 146–153.

80. Z. Zhang et al., "Chlorogenic Acid Ameliorates Experimental Colitis by Promoting Growth of Akkermansia in Mice," *Nutrients* 9, no. 7 (2017).

81. J. F. Garcia-Mazcorro et al., "Effect of Dark Sweet Cherry Powder Consumption on the Gut Microbiota, Short-Chain Fatty Acids, and Biomarkers of Gut Health in Obese

db/db Mice," *PeerJ* 6 (2018): e4195; S. Y. Kang, N. P. Seeram, M. G. Nair, and L. D. Bourquin, "Tart Cherry Anthocyanins Inhibit Tumor Development in Apc(Min) Mice and Reduce Proliferation of Human Colon Cancer Cells," *Cancer Letters* 194, no. 1 (2003): 13–19.

82. M. Larrosa et al., "Effect of a Low Dose of Dietary Resveratrol on Colon Microbiota, Inflammation, and Tissue Damage in a DSS-Induced Colitis Rat Model," *Journal of Agricultural and Food Chemistry* 57, no. 6 (2009): 2211–2220.

83. A. Jiménez-Girón et al., "Towards the Fecal Metabolome Derived from Moderate Red Wine Intake," *Metabolites* 4, no. 4 (2014): 1101–1118.

84. S. Al-Lahham et al., "Propionic Acid Affects Immune Status and Metabolism in Adipose Tissue from Overweight Subjects," *European Journal of Clinical Investigation* 42, no. 4 (2012): 357–364.

85. A. Cuervo et al., "Red Wine Consumption Is Associated with Fecal Microbiota and Malondialdehyde in a Human Population," *Journal of the American College of Nutrition* 34, no. 2 (2015): 135–141.

86. E. Barroso et al., "Phylogenetic Profile of Gut Microbiota in Healthy Adults after Moderate Intake of Red Wine," *Molecular Nutrition and Food Research* 61, no. 3 (2017); L. J. Marnett, "Chemistry and Biology of DNA Damage by Malondialdehyde," *IARC Scientific Publications* 150 (1999): 17–27.

87. H. Sun et al., "The Modulatory Effect of Polyphenols from Green Tea, Oolong Tea, and Black Tea on Human Intestinal Microbiota In Vitro," *Journal of Food Science and Technology* 55, no. 1 (2018): 399–407.

88. S. Wang et al., "Dietary Teasaponin Ameliorates Alteration of Gut Microbiota and Cognitive Decline in Diet-Induced Obese Mice," *Scientific Reports* 7, no. 1 (2017): 12203.

89. Christen Brownlee, "The Skinny on Sweeteners: How Do They Work?" *ChemMatters*, Oct. 2011, https://www.acs.org/content/dam/acsorg/education/resources/highschool/chemmatters/archive/chemmatters-oct2011-sweeteners-brownlee.pdf.

90. J. Suez et al., "Artificial Sweeteners Induce Glucose Intolerance by Altering the Gut Microbiota," *Nature* 514, no. 7521 (2014): 181–186.

91. J. Suez et al., "Non-Caloric Artificial Sweeteners and the Microbiome: Findings and Challenges," *Gut Microbes* 6, no. 2 (2015): 149–155.

92. A. Rodriguez-Palacios et al., "The Artificial Sweetener Splenda Promotes Gut Proteobacteria, Dysbiosis, and Myeloperoxidase Reactivity in Crohn's Disease-Like Ileitis," *Inflammatory Bowel Diseases* 24, no. 5 (2018): 1005–1020.

Chapter 9: Direct Your Genetic Fate

1. "Dietary Supplements Market Size Worth $278.02 Billion by 2024," Grand View Research, Feb. 2018, https://www.grandviewresearch.com/press-release/global-dietary-supplements-market.

2. S. J. Padayatty et al., "Vitamin C as an Antioxidant: Evaluation of Its Role in Disease Prevention," *Journal of the American College of Nutrition* 22, no. 1 (2003): 18–35.

3. Y. T. Szeto, T. L. To, S. C. Pak, and W. Kalle, "A Study of DNA Protective Effect of Orange Juice Supplementation," *Applied Physiology, Nutrition, and Metabolism* 38, no. 5 (2013): 533–536.

4. S. Bashir et al., "Oxidative DNA Damage and Cellular Sensitivity to Oxidative Stress in Human Autoimmune Diseases," *Annals of the Rheumatic Diseases* 52, no. 9 (1993):

659–666.; A. Szaflarska-Poplawska et al., "Oxidatively Damaged DNA/Oxidative Stress in Children with Celiac Disease," *Cancer Epidemiology, Biomarkers, and Prevention* 19, no. 8 (2010): 1960–1965; C. Pereira et al., "DNA Damage and Oxidative DNA Damage in Inflammatory Bowel Disease," *Journal of Crohn's and Colitis* 10, no. 11 (2016): 1316–1323.

5. A. Hoffmann, V. Sportelli, M. Ziller, and D. Spengler, "Epigenomics of Major Depressive Disorders and Schizophrenia: Early Life Decides," *International Journal of Molecular Sciences* 18, no. 8 (2017): 1711; E. Markkanen, U. Meyer, and G. L. Dianov, "DNA Damage and Repair in Schizophrenia and Autism: Implications for Cancer Comorbidity and Beyond," *International Journal of Molecular Sciences* 17, no. 6 (2016); L. Yu et al., "Association of Brain DNA Methylation in *SORL1*, *ABCA7*, *HLA-DRB5*, *SLC24A4*, and *BIN1* with Pathological Diagnosis of Alzheimer Disease," *JAMA Neurology* 72, no. 1 (2015): 15–24; E. Masliah, W. Dumaop, D. Galasko, and P. Desplats, "Distinctive Patterns of DNA Methylation Associated with Parkinson Disease: Identification of Concordant Epigenetic Changes in Brain and Peripheral Blood Leukocytes," *Epigenetics* 8, no. 10 (2013): 1030–1038; K. Saavedra et al., "Epigenetic Modifications of Major Depressive Disorder," *International Journal of Molecular Sciences* 17, no. 8 (2016): 1279; D. Simmons, "Epigenetic Influences and Disease," *Nature Education* 1, no. 1 (2008).

6. T. Weisel et al., "An Anthocyanin/Polyphenolic-Rich Fruit Juice Reduces Oxidative DNA Damage and Increases Glutathione Level in Healthy Probands," *Biotechnology Journal* 1, no. 4 (2006): 388–397.

7. Y. S. Park et al., "Bioactive Compounds and the Antioxidant Capacity in New Kiwi Fruit Cultivars," *Food Chemistry* 165 (2014): 354–361.

8. A. R. Collins, V. Harrington, J. Drew, and R. Melvin, "Nutritional Modulation of DNA Repair in a Human Intervention Study," *Carcinogenesis* 24, no. 3 (2003): 511–515.

9. S. B. Astley, R. M. Elliott, D. B. Archer, and S. Southon, "Evidence That Dietary Supplementation with Carotenoids and Carotenoid-Rich Foods Modulates the DNA Damage: Repair Balance in Human Lymphocytes," *British Journal of Nutrition* 91, no. 1 (2004): 63–72.

10. Z. Li et al., "Profiling of Phenolic Compounds and Antioxidant Activity of 12 Cruciferous Vegetables," *Molecules* 23, no. 5 (2018).

11. P. Riso et al., "DNA Damage and Repair Activity after Broccoli Intake in Young Healthy Smokers," *Mutagenesis* 25, no. 6 (2010): 595–602.

12. A. Gajowik and M. M. Dobrzyńska, "The Evaluation of Protective Effect of Lycopene against Genotoxic Influence of X-Irradiation in Human Blood Lymphocytes," *Radiation and Environmental Biophysics* 56, no. 4 (2017): 413–422.

13. J. K. Y. Hooi et al., "Global Prevalence of *Helicobacter pylori* Infection: Systematic Review and Meta-Analysis," *Gastroenterology* 153, no. 2 (2017): 420–429.

14. S. H. Jang, J. W. Lim, T. Morio, and H. Kim, "Lycopene Inhibits *Helicobacter pylori*–Induced ATM/ATR-Dependent DNA Damage Response in Gastric Epithelial AGS Cells," *Free Radical Biology and Medicine* 52, no. 3 (2012): 607–615.

15. C. Sakai et al., "Fish Oil Omega-3 Polyunsaturated Fatty Acids Attenuate Oxidative Stress-Induced DNA Damage in Vascular Endothelial Cells," *PLOS One* 12, no. 11 (2017): e0187934.

16. Q. Meng et al., "Systems Nutrigenomics Reveals Brain Gene Networks Linking Metabolic and Brain Disorders," *EBioMedicine* 7 (2016): 157–166.

17. M. Song et al., "Marine ω-3 Polyunsaturated Fatty Acids and Risk of Colorectal Cancer according to Microsatellite Instability," *Journal of the National Cancer Institute* 107, no. 4 (2015).

18. S. A. Messina and R. Dawson Jr., "Attenuation of Oxidative Damage to DNA by Taurine and Taurine Analogs," *Advances in Experimental Medicine and Biology* 483 (2000): 355–367; L. Gaté et al., "Impact of Dietary Supplement of *Crassostrea gigas* Extract (JCOE) on Glutathione Levels and Glutathione S-Transferase Activity in Rat Tissues," *In Vivo* 12, no. 3 (1998): 299–303.

19. H. Tapiero et al., "The Antioxidant Effects of *Crassostrea gigas* Extract (JCOE) in Human Volunteers," *In Vivo* 12, no. 3 (1998): 305–309.

20. S. Ghosh, J. K. Sinha, and M. Raghunath, "Epigenomic Maintenance through Dietary Intervention Can Facilitate DNA Repair Process to Slow Down the Progress of Premature Aging," *IUBMB Life* 68, no. 9 (2016): 717–721.

21. M. Z. Fang et al., "Reversal of Hypermethylation and Reactivation of p16INK4a, RARbeta, and MGMT Genes by Genistein and Other Isoflavones from Soy," *Clinical Cancer Research* 11, no. 19, pt. 1 (2005): 7033–7041.

22. W. Qin et al., "Soy Isoflavones Have an Antiestrogenic Effect and Alter Mammary Promoter Hypermethylation in Healthy Premenopausal Women," *Nutrition and Cancer* 61, no. 2 (2009): 238–244.

23. J. J. Pappas et al., "Allelic Methylation Bias of the RARB2 Tumor Suppressor Gene Promoter in Cancer," *Genes, Chromosomes, and Cancer* 47, no. 11 (2008): 978–993.

24. "CCND2 Cyclin D2 [*Homo sapiens* (human)]," National Center for Biotechnology Information, https://www.ncbi.nlm.nih.gov/gene/894.

25. I. Locke et al., "Gene Promoter Hypermethylation in Ductal Lavage Fluid from Healthy BRCA Gene Mutation Carriers and Mutation-Negative Controls," *Breast Cancer Research* 9, no. 1 (2007): R20.

26. M. Traka et al., "Transcriptome Analysis of Human Colon Caco-2 Cells Exposed to Sulforaphane," *Journal of Nutrition* 135, no. 8 (2005): 1865–1872.

27. S. Ropero and M. Esteller, "The Role of Histone Deacetylases (HDACs) in Human Cancer," *Molecular Oncology* 1, no. 1 (2007): 19–25; E. Ho, J. D. Clarke, and R. H. Dashwood, "Dietary Sulforaphane, a Histone Deacetylase Inhibitor for Cancer Prevention," *Journal of Nutrition* 139, no. 12 (2009): 2393–2396.

28. W. J. Lee and B. T. Zhu, "Inhibition of DNA Methylation by Caffeic Acid and Chlorogenic Acid, Two Common Catechol-Containing Coffee Polyphenols," *Carcinogenesis* 27, no. 2 (2006): 269–277.

29. M. Fang, D. Chen, and C. S. Yang, "Dietary Polyphenols May Affect DNA Methylation," *Journal of Nutrition* 137, no. 1 suppl. (2007): 223S–228S.

30. "GSTP1 Gene (Protein Coding)," GeneCards Human Gene Database, https://www.genecards.org/cgi-bin/carddisp.pl?gene=GSTP1.

31. Z. Liu et al., "Curcumin Is a Potent DNA Hypomethylation Agent," *Bioorganic and Medicinal Chemistry Letters* 19, no. 3 (2009): 706–709; Y. Guo et al., "Curcumin Inhibits Anchorage-Independent Growth of HT29 Human Colon Cancer Cells by Targeting Epigenetic Restoration of the Tumor Suppressor Gene DLEC1," *Biochemical Pharmacology* 94, no. 2 (2015): 69–78.

32. J. Hu et al., "Curcumin Modulates Covalent Histone Modification and TIMP1 Gene Activation to Protect against Vascular Injury in a Hypertension Rat Model," *Experimental and Therapeutic Medicine* 14, no. 6 (2017): 5896–5902.

33. S. K. Kang, S. H. Cha, and H. G. Jeon, "Curcumin-Induced Histone Hypoacetylation Enhances Caspase-3-Dependent Glioma Cell Death and Neurogenesis of Neural Progenitor Cells," *Stem Cells and Development* 15, no. 2 (2006): 165–174.

34. J. Paluszczak, V. Krajka-Kuźniak, and W. Baer-Dubowska, "The Effect of Dietary Polyphenols on the Epigenetic Regulation of Gene Expression in MCF7 Breast Cancer Cells," *Toxicology Letters* 192, no. 2 (2010): 119–125.

35. M. J. Gunter et al., "Coffee Drinking and Mortality in 10 European Countries: A Multinational Cohort Study," *Annals of Internal Medicine* 167, no. 4 (2017): 236–247.

36. G. H. Romano et al., "Environmental Stresses Disrupt Telomere Length Homeostasis," *PLOS Genetics* 9, no. 9 (2013): e1003721.

37. L. A. Tucker, "Caffeine Consumption and Telomere Length in Men and Women of the National Health and Nutrition Examination Survey (NHANES)," *Nutrition and Metabolism* 14 (2017): 10.

38. J. J. Liu, M. Crous-Bou, E. Giovannucci, and I. De Vivo, "Coffee Consumption Is Positively Associated with Longer Leukocyte Telomere Length in the Nurses' Health Study," *Journal of Nutrition* 146, no. 7 (2016): 1373–1378.

39. R. Chan et al., "Chinese Tea Consumption Is Associated with Longer Telomere Length in Elderly Chinese Men," *British Journal of Nutrition* 103, no. 1 (2010): 107–113.

40. M. Guasch-Ferré et al., "Frequency of Nut Consumption and Mortality Risk in the PREDIMED Nutrition Intervention Trial," *BMC Medicine* 11 (2013): 164; T. T. Hshieh, A. B. Petrone, J. M. Gaziano, and L. Djoussé, "Nut Consumption and Risk of Mortality in the Physicians' Health Study," *American Journal of Clinical Nutrition* 101, no. 2 (2015): 407–412.

41. L. A. Tucker, "Consumption of Nuts and Seeds and Telomere Length in 5,582 Men and Women of the National Health and Nutrition Examination Survey (NHANES)," *Journal of Nutrtion, Health, and Aging* 21, no. 3 (2017): 233–240.

42. M. Crous-Bou et al., "Mediterranean Diet and Telomere Length in Nurses' Health Study: Population Based Cohort Study," *BMJ* 349 (2014): g6674.

43. T. von Zglinicki, "Role of Oxidative Stress in Telomere Length Regulation and Replicative Senescence," *Annals of the New York Academy of Sciences* 908 (2000): 99–110.

44. Y. Gong et al., "Higher Adherence to the 'Vegetable-Rich' Dietary Pattern Is Related to Longer Telomere Length in Women," *Clinical Nutrition* 37, no. 4 (2018): 1232–1237.

45. D. Ornish et al., "Increased Telomerase Activity and Comprehensive Lifestyle Changes: A Pilot Study," *Lancet Oncology* 9, no. 11 (2008): 1048–1057.

46. J. Zhu, H. Wang, J. M. Bishop, and E. H. Blackburn, "Telomerase Extends the Lifespan of Virus-Transformed Human Cells without Net Telomere Lengthening," *Proceedings of the National Academy of Sciences USA* 96, no. 7 (1999): 3723–3728.

47. D. Ornish et al., "Effect of Comprehensive Lifestyle Changes on Telomerase Activity and Telomere Length in Men with Biopsy-Proven Low-Risk Prostate Cancer: 5-Year Follow-Up of a Descriptive Pilot Study," *Lancet Oncology* 14, no. 11 (2013): 1112–1120.

48. A. Perfilyev et al., "Impact of Polyunsaturated and Saturated Fat Overfeeding on the DNA-Methylation Pattern in Human Adipose Tissue: A Randomized Controlled Trial," *American Journal of Clinical Nutrition* 105, no. 4 (2017): 991–1000.

49. F. Rosqvist et al., "Overfeeding Polyunsaturated and Saturated Fat Causes Distinct Effects on Liver and Visceral Fat Accumulation in Humans," *Diabetes* 63 (2014): 2356–2368.

50. V. Shukla, C. Cuenin, N. Dubey, and Z. Herceg, "Loss of Histone Acetyltransferase Cofactor Transformation/Transcription Domain-Associated Protein Impairs Liver Regeneration after Toxic Injury," *Hepatology* 53, no. 3 (2011): 954–963.

51. J. A. Nettleton et al., "Dietary Patterns, Food Groups, and Telomere Length in the Multi-Ethnic Study of Atherosclerosis (MESA)," *American Journal of Clinical Nutrition* 88, no. 5 (2008): 1405–1412.

52. A. M. Fretts et al., "Processed Meat, but Not Unprocessed Red Meat, Is Inversely Associated with Leukocyte Telomere Length in the Strong Heart Family Study," *Journal of Nutrition* 146, no. 10 (2016): 2013–2018.

53. L. Shao, Q. H. Li, and Z. Tan, "L-Carnosine Reduces Telomere Damage and Shortening Rate in Cultured Normal Fibroblasts," *Biochemical and Biophysical Research Communications* 324, no. 2 (2004): 931–936.

54. J. Oellgaard et al., "Trimethylamine N-oxide (TMAO) as a New Potential Therapeutic Target for Insulin Resistance and Cancer," *Current Pharmaceutical Design* 23, no. 25 (2017): 3699–3712.

55. R. A. Koeth et al., "Intestinal Microbiota Metabolism of L-Carnitine, a Nutrient in Red Meat, Promotes Atherosclerosis," *Nature Medicine* 19, no. 5 (2013): 576–585.

56. C. W. Leung et al., "Soda and Cell Aging: Associations between Sugar-Sweetened Beverage Consumption and Leukocytetelomere Length in Healthy Adults from the National Health and Nutrition Examination Surveys," *American Journal of Public Health* 104, no. 12 (2014): 2425–2431.

57. M. Du et al., "Physical Activity, Sedentary Behavior, and Leukocyte Telomere Length in Women," *American Journal of Epidemiology* 175, no. 5 (2012): 414–422.

58. C. W. Leung et al., "Sugary Beverage and Food Consumption, and Leukocyte Telomere Length Maintenance in Pregnant Women," *European Journal of Clinical Nutrition* 70, no. 9 (2016): 1086–1088.

Chapter 10: Activate Your Immune Command Center

1. B. O. Rennard et al., "Chicken Soup Inhibits Neutrophil Chemotaxis In Vitro," *Chest* 118, no. 4 (2000): 1150–1157; M. A. Babizhayev and A. I. Deyev, "Management of the Virulent Influenza Virus Infection by Oral Formulation of Nonhydrolizedcarnosine and Isopeptide of Carnosine Attenuating Proinflammatory Cytokine-Induced Nitric Oxide Production," *American Journal of Therapeutics* 19, no. 1 (2012): e25–47.

2. Suzanne Wu, "Fasting Triggers Stem Cell Regeneration of Damaged, Old Immune System," USC News, June 5, 2014, https://news.usc.edu/63669/fasting-triggers-stem-cell-regeneration-of-damaged-old-immune-system.

3. L. C. Kidd et al., "Relationship between Human Papillomavirus and Penile Cancer— Implications for Prevention and Treatment," *Translational Andrology and Urology* 6, no. 5 (2017): 791–802; D. Song, H. Li, H. Li, and J. Dai, "Effect of Human Papillomavirus Infection on the Immune System and Its Role in the Course of Cervical

Cancer," *Oncology Letters* 10, no. 2 (2015): 600–606; L. Zhang et al., "Nonkeratinizing Squamous Cell Carcinoma In Situ of the Upper Aerodigestive Tract: An HPV-Related Entity," *Head and Neck Pathology* 11, no. 2 (2017): 152–161.

4. C. K. Hui and G. K. Lau, "Immune System and Hepatitis B Virus Infection," *Journal of Clinical Virology* 34, suppl. 1 (2005): S44–S48; C. Zhu et al., "Hepatitis B Virus Inhibits the Expression of Complement C3 and C4, *in vitro* and *in vivo*," *Oncology Letters* 15, no. 5 (2018): 7459–7463; Y. Liang et al., "Hepatitis C Virus NS4B Induces the Degradation of TRIF to Inhibit TLR3-Mediated Interferon Signaling Pathway," *PLOS Pathogens* 14, no. 5 (2018): e1007075.

5. P. Bandaru, H. Rajkumar, and G. Nappanveettil, "The Impact of Obesity on Immune Response to Infection and Vaccine: An Insight into Plausible Mechanisms," *Endocrinology and Metabolic Syndrome* 2 (2013): 113; J. J. Milner and M. A. Beck, "The Impact of Obesity on the Immune Response to Infection," *Proceedings of the Nutrition Society* 71, no. 2 (2012): 298–306.

6. H. J. Lee et al., "Immunogenetics of Autoimmune Thyroid Diseases: A Comprehensive Review," *Journal of Autoimmunity* 64 (2015): 82–90.

7. K. E. Lundin and C. Wijmenga, "Coeliac Disease and Autoimmune Disease—Genetic Overlap and Screening," *National Review of Gastroenterology and Hepatology* 12, no. 9 (2015): 507–515.

8. S. C. Jeong, S. R. Koyyalamudi, and G. Pang, "Dietary Intake of *Agaricus bisporus* White Button Mushroom Accelerates Salivary Immunoglobulin A Secretion in Healthy Volunteers," *Nutrition* 28, no. 5 (2012): 527–531.

9. K. I. Minato, L. C. Laan, A. Ohara, and I. van Die, "Pleurotus Citrinopileatus Polysaccharide Induces Activation of Human Dendritic Cells through Multiple Pathways," *International Immunopharmacology* 40 (2016): 156–163; H. Xu, S. Zou, X. Xu, and L. Zhang, "Anti-tumor Effect of β-Glucan from *Lentinus edodes* and the Underlying Mechanism," *Scientific Reports* 6 (2016): 28802; H. H. Chang et al., "Oral Administration of an Enoki Mushroom Protein FVE Activates Innate and Adaptive Immunity and Induces Anti-tumor Activity against Murine Hepatocellular Carcinoma," *International Immunopharmacology* 10, no. 2 (2010): 239–246; V. Vetcicka and J. Vetvickova, "Immune-Enhancing Effects of Maitake (*Grifola frondosa*) and Shiitake (*Lentinula edodes*) Extracts," *Annals of Translational Medicine* 2, no. 2 (2014): 14; D. Zhao et al., "Structural Characterization, Immune Regulation, and Antioxidant Activity of a New Heteropolysaccharide from *Cantharellus cibarius* Fr.," *International Journal of Molecular Medicine* 41, no. 5 (2018): 2744–2754.

10. M. P. Nantz et al., "Supplementation with Aged Garlic Extract Improves Both NK and γδ-T Cell Function and Reduces the Severity of Cold and Flu Symptoms: A Randomized, Double-Blind, Placebo-Controlled Nutrition Intervention," *Clinical Nutrition* 31, no. 3 (2012): 337–344.

11. H. Ishikawa et al., "Aged Garlic Extract Prevents a Decline of NK Cell Number and Activity in Patients with Advanced Cancer," *Journal of Nutrition* 136, no. 3, suppl. (2006): 816S–820S.

12. Y. L. Shih et al., "Sulforaphane Promotes Immune Responses in a WEHI-3-Induced Leukemia Mouse Model through Enhanced Phagocytosis of Macrophages and Natural Killer Cell Activities In Vivo," *Molecular Medicine Reports* 13, no. 5 (2016): 4023–4029; J. W. Fahey, Y. Zhang, and P. Talalay, "Broccoli Sprouts: An Exceptionally Rich Source

of Inducers of Enzymes That Protect against Chemical Carcinogens," *Proceedings of the National Academy of Sciences USA* 94, no. 19 (1997): 10367–10372.

13. L. Müller et al., "Effect of Broccoli Sprouts and Live Attenuated Influenza Virus on Peripheral Blood Natural Killer Cells: A Randomized, Double-Blind Study," *PLOS One* 11, no. 1 (2016): e0147742.

14. M. Rozati et al., "Cardio-Metabolic and Immunological Impacts of Extra Virgin Olive Oil Consumption in Overweight and Obese Older Adults: A Randomized Controlled Trial," *Nutrition and Metabolism* 12 (2015): 28.

15. Provided by Deoleo Company, in Cordoba, Spain.

16. A. Bonura et al., "Hydroxytyrosol Modulates Par j 1-Induced IL-10 Production by PBMCs in Healthy Subjects," *Immunobiology* 221, no. 12 (2016): 1374–1377.

17. C. Romero and M. Brenes, "Analysis of Total Contents of Hydroxytyrosol and Tyrosol in Olive Oils," *Journal of Agricultural and Food Chemistry* 60, no. 36 (2012): 9017–9022.

18. C. Ceci et al., "Ellagic Acid Inhibits Bladder Cancer Invasiveness and In Vivo Tumor Growth," *Nutrients* 8, no. 11 (2016).

19. S. Takahashi et al., "A Randomized Clinical Trial to Evaluate the Preventive Effect of Cranberry Juice (UR65) for Patients with Recurrent Urinary Tract Infection," *Journal of Infection and Chemotherapy* 19, no. 1 (2013): 112–117.

20. M. P. Nantz et al., "Consumption of Cranberry Polyphenols Enhances Human γδ-T Cell Proliferation and Reduces the Number of Symptoms Associated with Colds and Influenza: A Randomized, Placebo-Controlled Intervention Study," *Nutrition Journal* 12 (2013): 161.

21. Cranberry juice provided by Ocean Spray Cranberries.

22. Y. M. Yoo et al., "Pharmacological Advantages of Melatonin in Immunosenescence by Improving Activity of T Lymphocytes," *Journal of Biomedical Research* 30, no. 4 (2016): 314–321.

23. C. A. Rowe et al., "Regular Consumption of Concord Grape Juice Benefits Human Immunity," *Journal of Medicinal Food* 14, no. 1–2 (2011): 69–78.

24. A. R. Nair, N. Mariappan, A. J. Stull, and J. Francis, "Blueberry Supplementation Attenuates Oxidative Stress within Monocytes and Modulates Immune Cell Levels in Adults with Metabolic Syndrome: A Randomized, Double-Blind, Placebo-Controlled Trial," *Food and Function* 8, no. 11 (2017): 4118–4128.

25. Blueberry powder was made from two blueberry varietals, Rubel and Tifblue, and supplied by United States Highbush Blueberry Council.

26. L. S. McAnulty et al., "Effect of Blueberry Ingestion on Natural Killer Cell Counts, Oxidative Stress, and Inflammation prior to and after 2.5 h of Running," *Applied Physiology, Nutrition, and Metabolism* 36, no. 6 (2011): 976–984.

27. R. Yu, J. W. Park, T. Kurata, and K. L. Erickson, "Modulation of Select Immune Responses by Dietary Capsaicin," *International Journal for Vitamin and Nutrition Research* 68, no. 2 (1998): 114–119.

28. J. Beltran, A. K. Ghosh, and S. Basu, "Immunotherapy of Tumors with Neuroimmune Ligand Capsaicin," *Journal of Immunology* 178, no. 5 (2007): 3260–3264.

29. M. S. Gilardini Montani et al., "Capsaicin-Mediated Apoptosis of Human Bladder Cancer Cells Activates Dendritic Cells via CD91," *Nutrition* 31, no. 4 (2015): 578–581.

30. Y. K. Wang et al., "Oyster (*Crassostrea gigas*) Hydrolysates Produced on a Plant Scale Have Antitumor Activity and Immunostimulating Effects in BALB/c Mice," *Marine Drugs* 8, no. 2 (2010): 255–268.

31. J. Y. Cheng, L. T. Ng, C. L. Lin, and T. R. Jan, "Pacific Oyster-Derived Polysaccharides Enhance Antigen-Specific T Helper (Th)1 Immunity In Vitro and In Vivo," *Immunopharmacology and Immunotoxicology* 35, no. 2 (2013): 235–240.

32. K. Sakaguchi et al., "Augmentation of Cytolytic Activity in Murine Natural Killer Cells and Inhibition of Tumor Growth by the Ethanol Fraction of Oyster Extract," *Integrative Cancer Therapies* 17, no. 1 (2018): 31–40.

33. C. H. Cheng, H. Y. Wu, C. F. Wu, and T. R. Jan, "Pacific Oyster-Derived Polysaccharides Attenuate Allergen-Induced Intestinal Inflammation in a Murine Model of Food Allergy," *Journal of Food and Drug Analysis* 24, no. 1 (2016): 121–128.

34. J. Hendricks, C. Hoffman, D. W. Pascual, and M. E. Hardy, "18b-Glycyrrhetinic Acid Delivered Orally Induces Isolated Lymphoid Follicle Maturation at the Intestinal Mucosa and Attenuates Rotavirus Shedding," *PLOS One* 7, no. 11 (2012): e49491.

35. J. E. Tate, A. H. Burton, C. Boschi-Pinto, and U. D. Parashar, "World Health Organization–Coordinated Global Rotavirus Surveillance Network: Global, Regional, and National Estimates of Rotavirus Mortality in Children <5 Years of Age, 2000–2013," *Clinical Infectious Diseases* 62, suppl. 2 (2016): S96–S105.

36. H. R. Omar et al., "Licorice Abuse: Time to Send a Warning Message," *Therapeutic Advances in Endocrinology and Metabolism* 3, no. 4 (2012): 125–138.

37. X. Feng, L. Ding, and F. Qiu, "Potential Drug Interactions Associated with Glycyrrhizin and Glycyrrhetinic Acid," *Drug Metabolism Reviews* 47, no. 2 (2015): 229–238. https://www.ncbi.nlm.nih.gov/mesh/68019695.

38. P. A. Ayeka, Y. Bian, P. M. Githaiga, and Y. Zhao, "The Immunomodulatory Activity of Licorice Polysaccharides (*Glycyrrhiza uralensis* Fisch.) in CT 26 Tumor-Bearing Mice," *BMC Complementary and Alternative Medicine* 17 (2017): 536.

39. V. Andersen et al., "Diet and Risk of Inflammatory Bowel Disease," *Digestive and Liver Disease* 44, no. 3 (2012): 185–194.

40. P. Jantchou et al., "Animal Protein Intake and Risk of Inflammatory Bowel Disease: The E3N Prospective Study," *American Journal of Gastroenterology* 105, no. 10 (2010): 2195–2201.

41. A. Racine et al., "Dietary Patterns and Risk of Inflammatory Bowel Disease in Europe: Results from the EPIC Study," *Inflammatory Bowel Diseases* 22, no. 2 (2016): 345–354.

42. Y. Minami et al., "Diet and Systemic Lupus Erythematosus: A 4 Year Prospective Study of Japanese Patients," *Journal of Rheumatology* 30, no. 4 (2003): 747–754.

43. G. N. Y. van Gorkom et al., "Influence of Vitamin C on Lymphocytes: An Overview," *Antioxidants* 7, no. 3 (2018).

44. K. Oyarce, M. Campos-Mora, T. Gajardo-Carrasco, and K. Pino-Lagos, "Vitamin C Fosters the In Vivo Differentiation of Peripheral CD4+ Foxp3 T Cells into CD4+ Foxp3+Regulatory T Cells but Impairs Their Ability to Prolong Skin Allograft Survival," *Frontiers in Immunology* 9 (2018): 112; E. Nikolouli et al., "Alloantigen-Induced Regulatory T Cells Generated in Presence of Vitamin C Display Enhanced Stability of Foxp3 Expression and Promote Skin Allograft Acceptance," *Frontiers in Immunology* 8 (2017): 748.

45. D. Wu, J. Wang, M. Pae, and S. N. Meydani, "Green Tea EGCG, T Cells, and T Cell-Mediated Autoimmune Diseases," *Molecular Aspects of Medicine* 33, no. 1 (2012): 107–118.

46. D. Wu, J. Wang, M. Pae, and S. N. Meydani, "Green Tea EGCG, T Cells, and T Cell-Mediated Autoimmune Diseases," *Molecular Aspects of Medicine* 33, no. 1 (2012): 107–118.

47. D. Wu, "Green Tea EGCG, T-Cell Function, and T-Cell-Mediated Autoimmune Encephalomyelitis," *Journal of Investigative Medicine* 64, no. 8 (2016): 1213–1219.

48. K. Sayama et al., "Inhibitory Effects of Autoimmune Disease by Green Tea in MRL-Faslprcg/Faslprcg Mice," *In Vivo* 17, no. 6 (2003): 545–552.

49. Provided by Kisaku-en, Shizuoka, Japan.

50. P. Y. Tsai et al., "Epigallocatechiomega-3-Gallate Prevents Lupus Nephritis Development in Mice via Enhancing the Nrf2 Antioxidant Pathway and Inhibiting NLRP3 Inflammasome Activation," *Free Radical Biology and Medicine* 51, no. 3 (2011): 744–754.

51. H. R. Kim et al., "Green Tea Protects Rats against Autoimmune Arthritis by Modulating Disease-Related Immune Events," *Journal of Nutrition* 138, no. 11 (2008): 2111–2116; P. Hsu et al., "IL-10 Potentiates Differentiation of Human Induced Regulatory T Cells via STAT3 and Foxo1," Journal of Immunology 195, no. 8 (2015): 3665–3674.

52. Z. Shamekhi et al., "A Randomized, Double-Blind, Placebo-Controlled Clinical Trial Examining the Effects of Green Tea Extract on Systemic Lupus Erythematosus Disease Activity and Quality of Life," *Phytotherapy Research* 31, no. 7 (2017): 1063–1071.

53. R. N. Carmody et al., "Genetic Evidence of Human Adaptation to a Cooked Diet," *Genome Biology and Evolution* 8, no. 4 (2016): 1091–1103.

54. R. Peltonen et al., "Faecal Microbial Flora and Disease Activity in Rheumatoid Arthritis during a Vegan Diet," *British Journal of Rheumatology* 36, no. 1 (1997): 64–68.

55. M. Saresella et al., "Immunological and Clinical Effect of Diet Modulation of the Gut Microbiome in Multiple Sclerosis Patients: A Pilot Study," *Frontiers in Immunology* 8 (2017): 1391.

56. K. M. Danikowski, S. Jayaraman, and B. S. Prabhakar, "Regulatory T Cells in Multiple Sclerosis and Myasthenia Gravis," *Journal of Neuroinflammation* 14, no. 1 (2017): 117.

57. G. G. Konijeti et al., "Efficacy of the Autoimmune Protocol Diet for Inflammatory Bowel Disease," *Inflammatory Bowel Diseases* 23, no. 11 (2017): 2054–2060.

58. E. Scaioli et al., "Eicosapentaenoic Acid Reduces Fecal Levels of Calprotectin and Prevents Relapse in Patients with Ulcerative Colitis," *Clinical Gastroenterology and Hepatology* 16, no. 8 (2018): 1268–1275.

Chapter 11: The 5 × 5 × 5 Framework: Eating to Beat Disease

1. The clean plate campaign was started by U.S. president Woodrow Wilson in 1917 during a period of food shortage around World World I. It became designated as a "club" by U.S. president Harry S. Truman in 1947 to encourage food conservation by Americans to help Europeans recover from food shortages arising following World War II. It was never intended to encourage high caloric loads.

2. L. M. Redman et al., "Metabolic Slowing and Reduced Oxidative Damage with Sustained Caloric Restriction Support the Rate of Living and Oxidative Damage Theories of Aging," *Cell Metabolism* 27, no. 4 (2018): 805–815.e4.

Chapter 12: Rethinking the Kitchen

1. M. I. Greenburg and D. Vearrier, "Metal Fume Fever and Polymer Fume Fever," *Clinical Toxicology* 53, no. 4: 195–203.
2. E. Verzelloni, D. Tagliazucchi, and A. Conte, "From Balsamic to Healthy: Traditional Balsamic Vinegar Melanoidins Inhibit Lipid Peroxidation during Simulated Gastric Digestion of Meat," *Food and Chemical Toxicology* 48, no. 8–9 (2010): 2097–2102; R. Del Pino-García, M. L. González-SanJosé, M. D. Rivero-Pérez, and P. Muñiz, "Influence of the Degree of Roasting on the Antioxidant Capacity and Genoprotective Effect of Instant Coffee: Contribution of the Melanoidin Fraction," *Journal of Agricultural and Food Chemistry* 60, no. 42 (2012): 10530–10539.
3. N. H. Budak et al., "Effects of Apple Cider Vinegars Produced with Different Techniques on Blood Lipids in High-Cholesterol-Fed Rats," *Journal of Agricultural and Food Chemistry* 59, no. 12 (2011): 6638–6644.
4. D. Suresh and K. Srinivasan, "Tissue Distribution and Elimination of Capsaicin, Piperine, and Curcumin following Oral Intake in Rats," *Indian Journal of Medical Research* 131 (2010): 682–691.
5. "Food Storage: Dry Beans," Utah State University Extension, https://extension.usu.edu/foodstorage/howdoi/dry_beans.
6. "How Much Arsenic Is in Your Rice?" Consumer Reports, Nov. 18, 2014, https://www.consumerreports.org/cro/magazine/2015/01/how-much-arsenic-is-in-your-rice/index.htm.
7. M. J. Oh et al., "Immunomodulatory Effects of Polysaccharide Fraction Isolated from Fagopyrumesculentum on Innate Immune System," *Biochemical and Biophysical Research Communications* 496, no. 4 (2018): 1210–1216.
8. Erol Uman et al., "The Effect of Bean Origin and Temperature on Grinding Roasted Coffee," *Scientific Reports* 6 (2016): 24483.
9. A. J. Tonks et al., "A 5.8-kDa Component of Manuka Honey Stimulates Immune Cells via TLR4," *Journal of Leukocyte Biology* 82, no. 5 (2007): 1147–1155.
10. L. Li and N. P. Seeram, "Maple Syrup Phytochemicals Include Lignans, Coumarins, a Stilbene, and Other Previously Unreported Antioxidant Phenolic Compounds," *Journal of Agricultural and Food Chemistry* 58, no. 22 (2010): 11673–11679.
11. Y. Liu et al., "Isolation, Identification, and Biological Evaluation of Phenolic Compounds from a Traditional North American Confectionery, Maple Sugar," *Journal of Agricultural and Food Chemistry* 65, no. 21 (2017): 4289–4295.
12. Sherri A. Mason, Victoria Welch, and Joseph Neratko, "Synthetic Polymer Contamination in Bottled Water," report, Department of Geology and Environmental Sciences, Fredonia State University of New York, https://orbmedia.org/sites/default/files/FinalBottledWaterReport.pdf.
13. Creatine and creatinine are the precursors for carcinogenic heterocyclic amines in meat.
14. E. Persson et al., "Influence of Antioxidants in Virgin Olive Oil on the Formation of Heterocyclic Amines in Fried Beefburgers," *Food and Chemical Toxicology* 41, no. 11

(2003): 1587–1597; M. Gibis, "Effect of Oil Marinades with Garlic, Onion, and Lemon Juice on the Formation of Heterocyclic Aromatic Amines in Fried Beef Patties," *Journal of Agricultural and Food Chemistry* 55, no. 25 (2007): 10240–10247; P. V. Nerurkar, L. Le Marchand, and R. V. Cooney, "Effects of Marinating with Asian Marinades or Western Barbecue Sauce on PhIP and MeIQx Formation in Barbecued Beef," *Nutrition and Cancer* 34, no. 2 (1994): 147–152.

15. R. D. Semba, E. J. Nicklett, and L. Ferrucci, "Does Accumulation of Advanced Glycation End Products Contribute to the Aging Phenotype?" *Journal of Gerontology Series A: Biological Sciences and Medical Sciences* 65, no. 9 (2010): 963–975.

Chapter 13: Exceptional Foods

1. The flowers are health powerhouses, containing up to sixteen times more bioactive polyphenols than cabbage, parsley, or celery. The blossoms possess spinasterol, a bioactive that helps protect cells against DNA damage from chemicals called genotoxins. Spinasterol inhibits angiogenesis and has been shown to kill breast and ovarian cancer cells. These blossoms are also a source of immune-boosting vitamin C and the carotenoids that give the flowers their bright orange color. E. N. Aquino-Bolanos et al., "Physicochemical Parameters and Antioxidant Compounds in Edible Squash (*Cucurbita pepo*) Flowers Stored under Controlled Atmospheres," *Journal of Food Quality* 36 (2013): 302–308; I. M. Villaseñor, P. Lemon, A. Palileo, and J. B. Bremner, "Antigenotoxic Spinasterol from *Cucurbita maxima* Flowers," *Mutation Research* 360, no. 2 (1996): 89–93; N. K. Sedky et al., "The Molecular Basis of Cytotoxicity of α-Spinasterol from *Ganoderma resinaceum*: Induction of Apoptosis and Overexpression of p53 in Breast and Ovarian Cancer Cell Lines," *Journal of Cellular Biochemistry* 119, no. 5 (2017); G. N. Y. van Gorkom et al., "Influence of Vitamin C on Lymphocytes: An Overview," *Antioxidants* 7, no. 3 (2018).

2. Extracts from the persimmon's orange flesh prevent colon and prostate cancer cells from growing. S. B. Park et al., "Anticancer Activity of Calyx of *Diospyros kaki* Thunb. through Downregulation of Cyclin D1 via Inducing Proteasomal Degradation and Transcriptional Inhibition in Human Colorectal Cancer Cells," *BMC Complementary and Alternative Medicine* 17, no. 1 (2017): 445; Y. Ding et al, "Flavonoids from Persimmon (*Diospyros kaki* L.) Leaves Inhibit Proliferation and Induce Apoptosis in PC-3 Cells by Activation of Oxidative Stress and Mitochondrial Apoptosis," *Chemico-Biological Interactions* 275 (2017): 210–217.

3. Wasabi contains the many bioactives, including isothiocyanates, that kill breast cancer and liver cancer cells. S. Yano, S. Wu, K. Sakao, and D. X. Hou, "Wasabi 6-(methylsulfinyl)hexyl Isothiocyanate Induces Apoptosis in Human Colorectal Cancer Cells through p53-Independent Mitochondrial Dysfunction Pathway," *Biofactors* (May 14, 2018), doi: 10.1002/biof.1431; Y. Fuke et al., "Wasabi-Derived 6-(methylsulfinyl) Hexyl Isothiocyanate Induces Apoptosis in Human Breast Cancer by Possible Involvement of the NF-κB Pathways," *Nutrition and Cancer* 66, no. 5 (2014): 879–887; P. Z. Trio et al., "DNA Microarray Profiling Highlights Nrf2-Mediated Chemoprevention Targeted by Wasabi-Derived Isothiocyanates in HepG2 Cells," *Nutrition and Cancer* 69, no. 1 (2017): 105–116.

4. The bitter melon's potent bioactives like triterpenes, alkaloids, and peptides also serve the plant as natural insecticides. Extracts from its flesh were seen to kill colon and

breast cancer cells. It may protect against cardiovascular disease by lowering blood lipids, and even control the growth of fat cells. The juice of bitter melon can reduce inflammation by downshifting immune T cells. V. P. Dia and H. B. Krishnan, "BG-4, a Novel Anticancer Peptide from Bitter Gourd (*Momordica charantia*), Promotes Apoptosis in Human Colon Cancer Cells," *Scientific Reports* 6 (2016): 33532; J. R. Weng et al., "Cucurbitane Triterpenoid from *Momordica charantia* Induces Apoptosis and Autophagy in Breast Cancer Cells, in Part, through Peroxisome Proliferator-Activated Receptor γ Activation," *Evidence-Based Complementary and Alternative Medicine* (2013): 935675; M. B. Krawinkel et al., "Bitter Gourd Reduces Elevated Fasting Plasma Glucose Levels in an Intervention Study among Prediabetics in Tanzania," *Journal of Ethnopharmacology* 216 (2018): 1–7; M. Cortez-Navarrette et al., "*Momordica charantia* Administration Improves Insulin Secretion in Type 2 Diabetes Mellitus," *Journal of Medicinal Food* 21, no. 7 (2018); Q. Chen and E. T. Li, "Reduced Adiposity in Bitter Melon (*Momordica charantia*) Fed Rats Is Associated with Lower Tissue Triglyceride and Higher Plasma Catecholamines," *British Journal of Nutrition* 93, no. 5 (2005): 747–754; Mahwish et al., "Hypoglycemic and Hypolipidemic Effects of Different Parts and Formulations of Bitter Gourd (*Momordica charantia*)," *Lipids in Health and Disease* 16, no. 1 (2017): 211; D. G. Popovich, L. Li, and W. Zhang, "Bitter Melon (*Momordica charantia*) Triterpenoid Extract Reduces Preadipocyte Viability, Lipid Accumulation, and Adiponectin Expression in 3T3-L1 Cells," *Food and Chemical Toxicology* 48, no. 6 (2010): 1619–1626; R. Fachinan, A. Yessoufou, M. P. Nekoua, and K. Moutairou, "Effectiveness of Antihyperglycemic Effect of *Momordica charantia*: Implication of T-Cell Cytokines," *Evidence-Based Complementary and Alternative Medicine* (2017): 3707046.

5. Fiddleheads contain high levels of immune-boosting vitamin A and C antiangiogenic bioactives such as omega-3 fatty acids, beta-carotene, gallic acid, lutein, and zeaxanthin. At least seven species of fern fiddleheads are harvested for food and eaten in France, India, Indonesia, Japan, and Nepal, and in Native American cultures. Unless you're experienced, do not forage for these on your own, as many are highly toxic. Studies have shown that zeaxanthin protects against macular degeneration and also enhances the ability of stem cells to regenerate the liver. Gallic acid helps promote the growth of healthy *Lactobacillus* in the gut. J. M. DeLong et al., "The Unique Fatty Acid and Antioxidant Composition of Ostrich Fern (*Matteuccia struthiopteris*) Fiddleheads," *Canadian Journal of Plant Science* 91 (2011): 919–930; Y. Liu et al., "Precise Regulation of miR-210 Is Critical for the Cellular Homeostasis Maintenance and Transplantation Efficacy Enhancement of Mesenchymal Stem Cells in Acute Liver Failure Therapy," *Cell Transplantation* 26, no. 5 (2017): 805–820; R. Pacheco-Ordaz et al., "Effect of Phenolic Compounds on the Growth of Selected Probiotic and Pathogenic Bacteria," *Letters in Applied Microbiology* 66, no. 1 (2018): 25–31.

6. Anamdamide also activates the immune system of the intestines, helps balance immune homeostasis, and also kills endometrial cancer cells. G. Pacioni et al., "Truffles Contain Endocannabinoid Metabolic Enzymes and Anandamide," *Phytochemistry* 110 (2015): 104–110; N. Acharya et al., "Endocannabinoid System Acts as a Regulator of Immune Homeostasis in the Gut," *Proceedings of the National Academy of Sciences USA* 114, no. 19 (2017): 5005–5010; B. M. Fonseca, G. Correia-da-Silva, and N. A. Teixeira, "Cannabinoid-Induced Cell Death in Endometrial Cancer Cells: Involvement

of TRPV1 Receptors in Apoptosis," *Journal of Physiology and Biochemistry* 74, no. 2 (2018).

7. X. Jiang et al., "The Anti-Fatigue Activities of *Tuber melanosporum* in a Mouse Model," *Experimental and Therapeutic Medicine* 15, no. 3 (2018): 3066–3073.

8. A. Rosa et al., "Potential Anti-tumor Effects of *Mugil cephalus* Processed Roe Extracts on Colon Cancer Cells," *Food and Chemical Toxicology* 60 (2013): 471–478; A. Rosa et al., "Effect of Aqueous and Lipophilic Mullet (*Mugil cephalus*) Bottarga Extracts on the Growth and Lipid Profile of Intestinal Caco-2 Cells," *Journal of Agricultural and Food Chemistry* 59, no. 5 (2011): 1658–1666.

9. David Tanis, "For Extraordinary Flavor, Add a Few Drops of Squid Ink," *New York Times*, Apr. 1, 2016, https://www.nytimes.com/2016/04/06/dining/squid-ink-risotto .html.

10. Y. P. Gu et al., "Squid Ink Polysaccharide Prevents Autophagy and Oxidative Stress Affected by Cyclophosphamide in Leydig Cells of Mice: A Pilot Study," *Iranian Journal of Basic Medical Sciences* 20, no. 11 (2017): 1194–1199.

11. T. Zuo et al., "Dietary Squid Ink Polysaccharide Could Enhance SIgA Secretion in Chemotherapeutic Mice," *Food and Function* 5, no. 12 (2014): 3189–3196; X. Wang et al., "Sepia Ink Oligopeptide Induces Apoptosis of Lung Cancer Cells via Mitochondrial Pathway," *Cell Physiology and Biochemistry* 45, no. 5 (2018): 2095–2106; Q. Tang et al., "Dietary Squid Ink Polysaccharides Ameliorated the Intestinal Microflora Dysfunction in Mice Undergoing Chemotherapy," *Food and Function* 5, no. 10 (2014): 2529–2535; A. Zong et al., "Anti-metastatic and Anti-angiogenic Activities of Sulfated Polysaccharide of *Sepiella maindroni* Ink," *Carbohydrate Polymers* 91, no. 1 (2013): 403–409.

12. Z. L. Kong et al., "Immune Bioactivity in Shellfish toward Serum-Free Cultured Human Cell Lines," *Bioscience, Biotechnology, and Biochemistry* 61, no. 1 (1997): 24–28.

13. B. M. Popkin et al., "A New Proposed Guidance System for Beverage Consumption in the United States," *American Journal of Clinical Nutrition* 83, no. 3 (2006): 529–542.

14. D. X. Xiang, S. S. Wei, and W. Q. Li, "Anticancer Activity and Mechanism of Xanthohumol: A Prenylated Flavonoid From Hops (*Humulus lupulus* L.)," *Frontiers in Pharmacology* 9 (2018): 530; R. Costa et al., "Modulation of VEGF Signaling in a Mouse Model of Diabetes by Xanthohumol and 8-Prenylnaringenin: Unveiling the Angiogenic Paradox and Metabolism Interplay," *Molecular Nutrition and Food Research* 61, no. 4 (2017); C. Gallo, K. Dallaglio et al., "Hop Derived Flavonoid Xanthohumol Inhibits Endothelial Cell Functions via AMPK Activation," *Oncotarget* 7, no. 37 (2016): 59917–59931; J. S. Samuels, R. Shashidharamurthy, and S. Rayalam, "Novel Anti-Obesity Effects of Beer Hops Compound Xanthohumol: Role of AMPK Signaling Pathway," *Nutrition and Metabolism* 15 (2018): 42.

15. The study examined 107,998 people. S. Karami, S. E. Daugherty, and M. P. Purdue, "A Prospective Study of Alcohol Consumption and Renal Cell Carcinoma Risk," *International Journal of Cancer* 137, no. 1 (2015): 238–242.

16. The benefits of beer are not in its alcohol content, but in the compounds that give it such a unique taste. For instance, one compound in hops is antiangiogenic. And in a Spanish study, men who drank beer saw an increase in their circulating stem cells—even when they were drinking nonalcoholic beer. G. Chiva-Blanch et al., "The Nonalcoholic Fraction of Beer Increases Stromal Cell Derived Factor 1 and the Number

of Circulating Endothelial Progenitor Cells in High Cardiovascular Risk Subjects: A Randomized Clinical Trial," *Atherosclerosis* 233, no. 2 (2014): 518–524.

17. E. Patterson, S. C. Larsson, A. Wolk, and A. Åkesson, "Association between Dairy Food Consumption and Risk of Myocardial Infarction in Women Differs by Type of Dairy Food," 143, no. 1 (2013): 74–79.

18. K. Nimptsch, S. Rohrmann, R. Kaaks, and J. Linseisen, "Dietary Vitamin K Intake in Relation to Cancer Incidence and Mortality: Results from the Heidelberg Cohort of the European Prospective Investigation into Cancer and Nutrition (EPIC-Heidelberg)," *American Journal of Clinical Nutrition* 91, no. 5 (2010): 1348–1358; K. Nimptsch, S. Rohrmann, and J. Linseisen, "Dietary Intake of Vitamin K and Risk of Prostate Cancer in the Heidelberg Cohort of the European Prospective Investigation into Cancer and Nutrition (EPIC-Heidelberg)," *American Journal of Clinical Nutrition* 87, no. 4 (2008): 985–992.

19. L. Djoussé et al., "Chocolate Consumption Is Inversely Associated with Prevalent Coronary Heart Disease: The National Heart, Lung, and Blood Institute Family Heart Study," *Clinical Nutrition* 30, no. 2 (2011): 182–187; C. Matsumoto et al., "Chocolate Consumption and Risk of Diabetes Mellitus in the Physicians' Health Study," *American Journal of Clinical Nutrition* 101, no. 2 (2015): 362–367; K. M. Strat et al., "Mechanisms by Which Cocoa Flavanols Improve Metabolic Syndrome and Related Disorders," *Journal of Nutritional Biochemistry* 35 (2016): 1–21; A. Spadafranca, C. Martinez Conesa, S. Sirini, and G. Testolin, "Effect of Dark Chocolate on Plasma Epicatechin Levels, DNA Resistance to Oxidative Stress and Total Antioxidant Activity in Healthy Subjects," *British Journal of Nutrition* 103, no. 7 (2010): 1008–1014.

20. L. Dugo et al., "Effect of Cocoa Polyphenolic Extract on Macrophage Polarization from Proinflammatory M1 to Anti-Inflammatory M2 State," *Oxidative Medicine and Cellular Longevity* 2017 (2017): 6293740.

21. Multiple large population studies have shown a connection between eating spicy food and health. The study in China was the China Kadoorie Biobank, which involved 487,375 people across China showed that eating spicy food at least once per day was associated with a 14 percent decreased risk of death from any cause, including cancer, heart disease, stroke, diabetes, respiratory diseases, and infections. This association was also observed in a large North American study that examined the National Health and Nutritional Examination Survey III data involving 16,179 people. M. Chopan and B. Littenberg, "The Association of Hot Red Chili Pepper Consumption and Mortality: A Large Population-Based Cohort Study," *PLOS One* 12, no. 1 (2017): e0169876.

22. C. Kang et al., "Gut Microbiota Mediates the Protective Effects of Dietary Capsaicin against Chronic Low-Grade Inflammation and Associated Obesity Induced by High-Fat Diet," *MBio* 8, no. 3 (2017).

23. S. Kubow et al., "Effects of Simulated Human Gastrointestinal Digestion of Two Purple-Fleshed Potato Cultivars on Anthocyanin Composition and Cytotoxicity in Colonic Cancer and Non-Tumorigenic Cells," *Nutrients* 9, no. 9 (2017); V. Charepalli et al., "Anthocyanin-Containing Purple-Fleshed Potatoes Suppress Colon Tumorigenesis via Elimination of Colon Cancer Stem Cells," *Journal of Nutritional Biochemistry* 26, no. 12 (2015): 1641–1649; G. P. Madiwale et al., "Combined Effects of Storage and Processing on the Bioactive Compounds and Pro-Apoptotic Properties of Color-Fleshed Potatoes

in Human Colon Cancer Cells," *Journal of Agricultural and Food Chemistry* 60, no. 44 (2012): 11088–11096.

24. This was in the EPIC study, which examined nut intake in 478,040 people. M. Jenab et al., "Association of Nut and Seed Intake with Colorectal Cancer Risk in the European Prospective Investigation into Cancer and Nutrition," *Cancer Epidemiology, Biomarkers, and Prevention* 13, no. 10 (2004): 1595–1603.

25. Temidayo Fadelu et al., "Nut Consumption and Survival in Stage III Colon Cancer Patients: Results from CALGB 89803 (Alliance)," ACCO Meeting Library, June 3, 2017, https://meetinglibrary.asco.org/record/147476/abstract.

26. Chicory also has cancer-suppressing properties. P. H. Tsai et al., "Dietary Flavonoids Luteolin and Quercetin Suppressed Cancer Stem Cell Properties and Metastatic Potential of Isolated Prostate Cancer Cells," *Anticancer Research* 36, no. 12 (2016): 6367–6380.

27. P. Flores, E. Sánchez, J. Fenoll, and P. Hellín, "Genotypic Variability of Carotenoids in Traditional Tomato Cultivars," *Food Research International* 100, pt. 3 (2017): 510–516.

28. Papaya is a sweet tropical fruit originating from Asia. Its bright orange-colored flesh is due to carotenoids, lycopene, and beta-crytoxanthin that has antiangiogenic, antioxidant, and immunity-fostering activity. R. M. Schweiggert et al., "Carotenoids Are More Bioavailable from Papaya than from Tomato and Carrot in Humans: A Randomised Cross-Over Study," *British Journal of Nutrition* 111, no. 3 (2014): 490–498; S. Pandey, P. J. Cabot, P. N. Shaw, and A. K. Hewavitharana, "Anti-Inflammatory and Immunomodulatory Properties of *Carica papaya*," Journal of Immunotoxicology 13, no. 4 (2016): 590–602.

Chapter 15: Food Doses

1. "Lifetime Risk of Developing or Dying from Cancer," American Cancer Society, https://www.cancer.org/cancer/cancer-basics/lifetime-probability-of-developing-or-dying-from-cancer.html.

2. "Cancer Stat Facts: Cancer of Any Site," National Cancer Institute, https://seer.cancer.gov/statfacts/html/all.html.

3. "Lifetime Risk of Cancer," Cancer Research UK, http://www.cancerresearchuk.org/health-professional/cancer-statistics/risk/lifetime-risk.

4. J. X. Moore, N. Chaudhary, and T. Akinyemiju, "Metabolic Syndrome Prevalence by Race/Ethnicity and Sex in the United States, National Health and Nutrition Examination Survey, 1988–2012," *Preventing Chronic Disease* 14 (2017): 160287.

5. A. Azzarà et al., "Increased Level of DNA Damage in Some Organs of Obese Zucker Rats by γ-H2AX Analysis," *Environmental and Molecular Mutagenesis* 58, no. 7 (2017): 477–484.

6. D. S. Kim et al., "Attenuation of Rheumatoid Inflammation by Sodium Butyrate through Reciprocal Targeting of HDAC2 in Osteoclasts and HDAC8 in T Cells," *Frontiers in Immunology* 9 (2018): 1525.

7. Two powerful patient stories about how they overcome their autoimmune disease by a stem cell transplant were told at the (2016) Vatican conference Cellular Horizons. Their presentations can be seen here: https://www.youtube.com/watch?v=Iafkr-qRnm0.

8. "Neurodegenerative Diseases," National Institute of Environmental Health Sciences, https://www.niehs.nih.gov/research/supported/health/neurodegenerative/index.cfm.

9. "Age-Related Eye Disease Study—Results," National Eye Institute, https://nei.nih.gov/amd.

10. M. S. Zinkernagel et al., "Association of the Intestinal Microbiome with the Development of Neovascular Age-Related Macular Degeneration," *Scientific Reports* 7 (2017): 40826.

11. "US Approves First Cancer Drug to Use Patient's Own Cells—with $475,000 Price Tag," *Guardian* (US ed.), August 30, 2017, https://www.theguardian.com/us-news/2017/aug/30/cancer-drug-kymriah-leukemia-novartis.

12. Rachael Rettner, "Meet Your Interstitium, a Newfound 'Organ,'" Live Science, Mar. 27, 2018, https://www.livescience.com/62128-interstitium-organ.html; Fiona MacDonald, "It's Official: A Brand-New Human Organ Has Been Classified," Science Alert, Jan. 3, 2017, https://www.sciencealert.com/it-s-official-a-brand-new-human-organ-has-been-classified.

Appendix B: Assess Your Risks

1. G. A. Bello, G. G. Dumancas, and C. Gennings, "Development and Validation of a Clinical Risk-Assessment Tool Predictive of All-Cause Mortality," *Bioinformatics and Biology Insights* 9, suppl. 3 (2015): 1–10.

2. S. S. Khan et al., "Association of Body Mass Index with Lifetime Risk of Cardiovascular Disease and Compression of Morbidity," *JAMA Cardiology* 3, no. 4 (2018): 280–287.

3. "Children's BMI Formula," Centers for Disease Control and Prevention, https://www.cdc.gov/healthyweight/assessing/bmi/childrens_bmi/childrens_bmi_formula.html; "Calculating BMI Using the English System," Centers for Disease Control and Prevention, https://www.cdc.gov/nccdphp/dnpao/growthcharts/training/bmiage/page5_2.html.

4. "United States Cancer Statistics: Data Visualizations," Centers for Disease Control and Prevention, https://gis.cdc.gov/grasp/USCS/DataViz.html.

5. "Diagnosed Diabetes, Age-Adjusted Percentage, Adults with Diabetes—Total," Centers for Disease Control and Prevention, https://gis.cdc.gov/grasp/diabetes/DiabetesAtlas.html.

6. "Countries with the Highest Rates of Diabetes," World Atlas, https://www.worldatlas.com/articles/countries-with-the-highest-rates-of-diabetes.html.

7. "FDA Allows Marketing of First Direct-to-Consumer Tests That Provide Genetic Risk Information for Certain Conditions," U.S. Food and Drug Administration, Apr. 6, 2017, https://www.fda.gov/newsevents/newsroom/pressannouncements/ucm551185.htm.

8. Arthur L. Frank, "Taking an Exposure History," in *Environmental Medicine: Integrating a Missing Element into Medical Education*, ed. A. M. Pope and D. P. Rail (Washington, DC: National Academies Press, 1995), https://www.ncbi.nlm.nih.gov/books/NBK231990.

9. "Secondhand Smoke Is a Health Threat to Pets," Science Daily, Sept. 3, 2007, https://www.sciencedaily.com/releases/2007/08/070831123420.htm.

10. S. Manohar et al., "Associations of Rotational Shift Work and Night Shift Status with Hypertension: A Systematic Review and Meta-analysis," *Journal of Hypertension* 35, no. 10 (2017): 1929–1937; X. Yuan et al., "Night Shift Work Increases the Risks of Multiple Primary Cancers in Women: A Systematic Review and Meta-analysis of 61 Articles," Cancer Epidemiology, Biomarkers, and Prevention 27, no. 1 (2018): 25–40;

J. Shilts, G. Chen, and J. J. Hughey, "Evidence for Widespread Dysregulation of Circadian Clock Progression in Human Cancer," *PeerJ* 6 (2018):e4327.

11. H. Xie et al., "Chronic Stress Promotes Oral Cancer Growth and Angiogenesis with Increased Circulating Catecholamine and Glucocorticoid Levels in a Mouse Model," *Oral Oncology* 51, no. 11 (2015): 991–997; K. Aschbacher et al., "Circulating Angiogenic Cell Function Is Inhibited by Cortisol In Vitro and Associated with Psychological Stress and Cortisol In Vivo," *Psychoneuroendocrinology* 67 (2016): 216–223.

12. Walter Willet, *Eat, Drink, and Be Healthy: The Harvard Medical School Guide to Healthy Eating* (New York: Simon & Schuster, 2001).

Index

About the Author

Dr. William Li is a world-renowned physician, scientist, and author. Best known for leading the Angiogenesis Foundation, Dr. Li began a crusade in 1994 to bring "angiogenesis" from the research laboratory to the patient's bedside. His work ultimately led to thirty-two game-changing, FDA-approved therapeutics and devices and has impacted more than fifty million people worldwide. Today, Dr. Li's original vision to make angiogenesis part of mainstream medicine has been realized. In addition to its benefits to patients, angiogenesis is now even being taught in high school classes.

Dr. Li's pioneering approach to disease fighting revolves around finding "common denominators." Using this approach, he has brought new solutions to the war on cancer, the fight against blindness, and the specter of chronic wounds in people living with diabetes. He's even worked with veterinarians around the world to bring new treatments to save pets and endangered species.

A health futurist, Dr. Li is active in collaborating with top universities, leading companies, and scores of advocacy groups, governments, and institutions across five continents. He has forged collaborations with the National Institutes of Health, the World Health Organization, and the Food and Drug Administration. His accomplishments have been recognized by the Milken Institute and the Bill and Melinda Gates Foundation. The Vatican has twice invited Dr. Li to present his vision for the future of health, and his wildly popular TED Talk "Can We Eat to Starve

Cancer?" has garnered more than eleven million views. Bono, the lead singer of the band U2, writing in the *New York Times*, called Dr. Li one of the top ten people to watch for in the coming decade "with the potential to change the world."

Dr. Li is passionate about the future of health. He firmly believes that a better future can be achieved by using science to shatter the barriers of the past. He is an alliance builder and collaborates with like-minded leaders, innovators, and culture changers striving to make the world a better place.

Dr. Li has authored more than a hundred scientific publications in leading journals, such as *Science,* the *New England Journal of Medicine, The Lancet,* and more. He has served on the faculties at Harvard, Tufts, and Dartmouth. A guest expert on *The Dr. Oz Show,* CNN, and MSNBC, Dr. Li has also been featured in *USA Today, TIME,* the *Wall Street Journal,* the *Atlantic,* O magazine, and *Wine Spectator* and on NPR. Dr. Li is a graduate of Harvard and the University of Pittsburgh School of Medicine. He completed his medical residency at Massachusetts General Hospital.

When he's not writing or disease fighting, Dr. Li enjoys traveling, cooking, and listening to an eclectic music playlist.